Alchemy of the Soul

DR GARY CONE

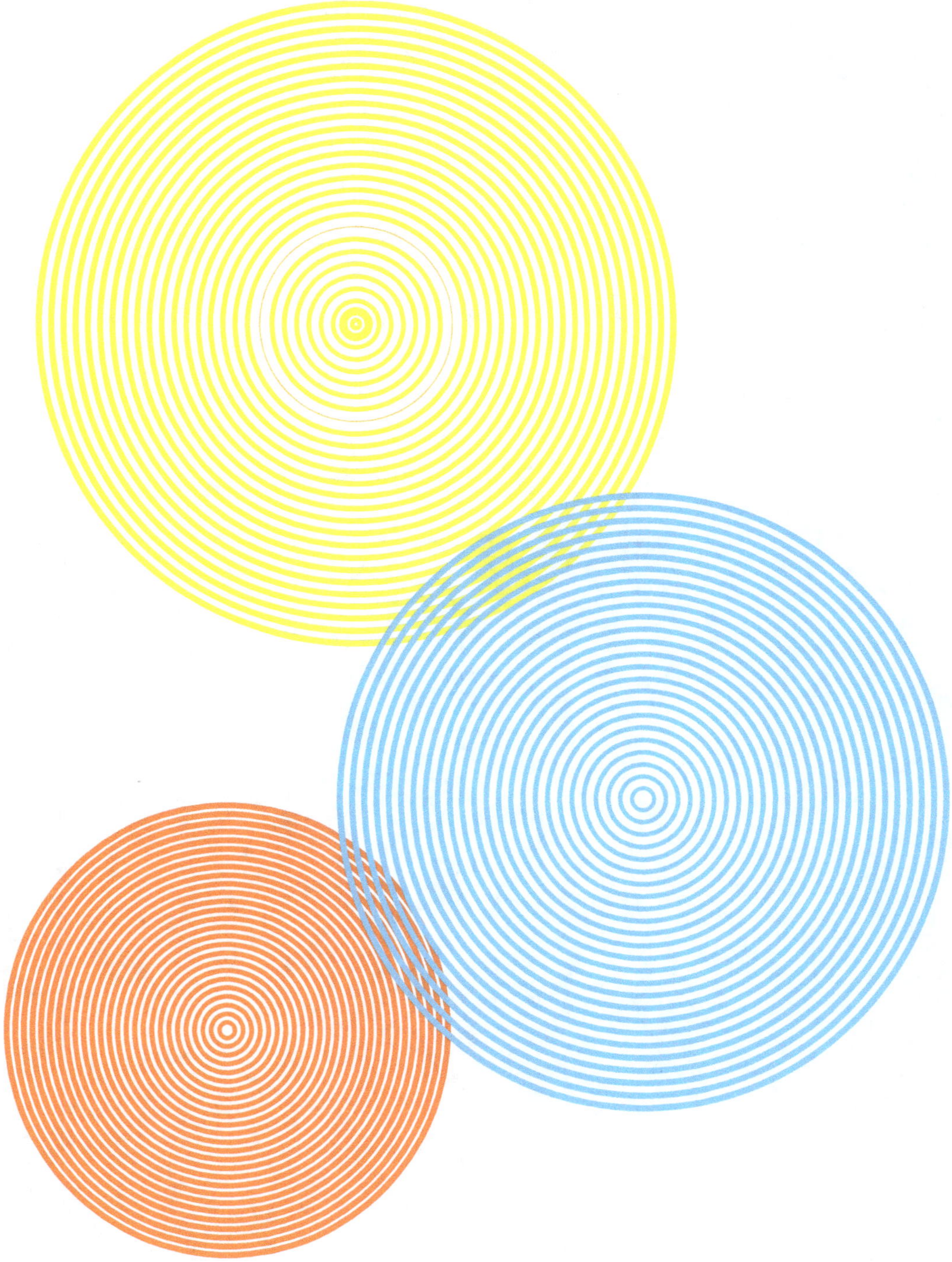

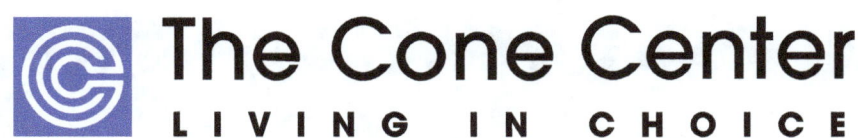
The Cone Center
LIVING IN CHOICE

ENERGY MATRIX CLEARING SYSTEM (EMCS)

A SACRED PRACTICE

An Energy Medicine/Energy Psychology process that transcends time and experience,

alchemically transforming the physical, mental, emotional, and spiritual bodies

GARY CONE

Ph.D., DCEP, L.A.D.C./MH, MAC

CONE CENTER—LIVING IN CHOICE

Revised 2025

Oklahoma City, Oklahoma

TABLE OF CONTENTS

ACKNOWLEDGEMENTS

Many people contributed to the research and production of this book, and I am grateful to every one of them. There is not enough space to recognize all those who have crossed my path and opened my eyes, so I name only a few.

Most of all, I am grateful to my loving partner, Allen Montandon. Your support, tolerance, and patience while I worked on this book have been beyond measure.

Next, I humbly thank my clients and students for their courage in exploring the depths of their beings. They have, indeed, been my greatest teachers.

To the great beyond, I send love and appreciation to my parents, Willard and Ruth Cone. They loved me, supported me, and cared for me in ways they never realized. Mom gave me her love of literature and discovery and pointed me toward life's front lines. Dad taught me determination. He believed that life's journey was always worth the troubles encountered along the way. I miss you, Mom and Dad. And to my sister, Karen, my greatest cheerleader and without whom I could not have made it through the darkest days of my life, words cannot express my gratitude.

I very much appreciate my children, Kendra and Steven. Kendra, for teaching me the value of letting go with love, and Steven, who taught me that without presence, love is not enough.

To all the countless mentors, teachers, and advisors who have inspired me along this course of energy work, I will name only a few: Caroline Myss, Norman Shealy, Colin Tipping, Tom Hyder, John Freedom, Gloria Arenson, Janet LeValley, Surrinder Kallar, Byron Gentry, and Eugene Whitworth, I thank all of you.

Additionally, a heartfelt "I am indebted to you" goes out to those who have shared their editing skills, love of this work, and precious time helping me compile this book.

I close with a "Thank you, Johnnie" to my spirit guide, who some fifty-odd years ago helped launch me onto this winding and fascinating road. I am forever grateful.

PREFACE

Some people seem to continuously 'show up' in your life. Dr. Cone, Gary, not only 'showed up' in my life but wholly and continuously shifted my perspectives about possibilities. Learning to Live in Choice became my mantra. In the words of Rumi, 'Your task is not to seek for love, but merely to seek and find all the barriers within yourself that you have built against it.' – Rumi

My favorite scientist of all time, Dr. Myron Tribus, best described Gary's work in this famous statement: "Knowledge without know-how is sterile." Gary's knowledgeable, loving presence and know-how make a difference in people's lives. Gary is a master!

As if in slow motion, I watched a friend's life soar despite an emotional disruption that would destroy most.

One of my friend's employees was not promoted as expected, and he committed suicide. My friend was emotionally devastated, blamed himself, quit his job, and got cancer.

He then met Gary Cone and lived under his care for the rest of his life.

My friend developed a proactive state of mind and followed the ECMS Model as a roadmap for a healthy existence. Emotionally, he had the COURAGE to imagine his life without the guilt he felt. He was WILLING to intentionally walk a new way that would not be destructive to his mind, body, and spirit for the rest of his life! Then, he discovered, with Gary's help, energy mechanisms that would help him begin to appreciate life again. He could put his life in NEUTRAL, like a car, and use this non-toxic space to address his FEELINGS.

He accepted that he owned some of the responsibility. He decided not to spend his life holding a reactive mindset about himself. He knew that a reactive life was short and painful. With reason, he forgave himself and began LOVING himself and others again.

My friend was LOVE. Each component of EMCS, identified by Dr. Cone, is designed to open the gates of our consciousness "above" and simultaneously reveal what is "below". This work illuminates the darkness "below" and floods it with the light of wisdom and truth "above". Thus, the Energy Matrix Clearing System effects a vibrational shift from "within" that naturally flows into "without" in an elegant flow of light, illuminating my friend's life from a whole new perspective.

He blossomed through Dr. Cone's work well into his 80s. He was always JOYFUL. Every cell in his body sang his wholeness. You could see the PEACE in his eyes, the trust, the alchemy of his soul. His shame, at every level, was cleared. His limiting beliefs, traumas, and other energy blockages that might distort his life energy were cleared. This was a man capable of ENLIGHTENMENT.

His path followed the Alchemy of the Soul. I wish for you to walk this new way with Dr. Gary Cone, as my friend did and as he coached me to do!

Kathy J Hagler, PhD

Author and Consultant

Art of Scars and ABC's of Murmuration

INTRODUCTION

For the sake of clarity regarding the evolution of the Energy Matrix Clearing System (EMCS), I share a few of the noteworthy experiences that continue to guide me on my journey toward enlightenment. A little indulgence as I tell my story.

As a result of my being president of my local FFA chapter, I was invited to participate in a "Good Neighbors Tour" that had been organized in 1961 by the FFA to visit Mexico. Our group consisted of local young people, medical doctors, optometrists, nurses, and various local political leaders. The mission of the FFA is to prepare its youth membership for leadership, personal growth, and career success through hands-on agricultural education, and the tour was organized in part to build better relationships between the people of Texas and Mexico by interacting with that country's dignitaries and citizens. We offered our friendship to the Mexican people, bringing doctors and optometrists for exams for the orphans and books for the libraries. I was fifteen years old and had never been out of Texas except for one short trip to Clovis, New Mexico. It still amazes me that my family made this remarkable opportunity possible for me. Summer was a busy season on the farm where I grew up, which meant my already busy family had to step up and do my work as well. My parents were also very protective, and in retrospect, it seems exceedingly out of character that they allowed this trip without their oversight. Today, I thank them, as this unique experience changed me forever and set me on a trajectory that I follow to this day.

A young Roman Catholic Mexican American boy named Juan Ramos was with us on the tour. During the tour, Juan and I became good friends. Juan, fluent in Spanish and already politically savvy, was familiar with many of the cities on our schedule. He ended up being a good friend and a valuable guide.

Juan loved dropping by the local cathedrals in the cities on our tour, and I, a complete novice concerning Catholicism, was so intrigued that I tagged along. It was during these impromptu visits that I first became aware of the unmistakable, palpable "energy" in those spaces. Some exuded disproportionate sadness and fear, while others generated sensations of joy and jubilation. My first experience with the scent of incense was in one of these cathedrals, where it permeated the air, enveloping me, flooding my senses, and mysteriously shrouding me as I viewed those beautiful, ornate, gold-encrusted inner sanctums. At every stop, Juan would find his way to the side altar to light a candle, praying for healing for the infirm and needy.

First, in San Louis Potosi and again in Mexico City, we joined small rallies of young people gathered in private groups. Not understanding their language, the reason for these meetings escaped me. I was young and inexperienced, and these mysterious secret gatherings both frightened and fascinated me.

On July third, near the American District of Zona Rosa in Mexico City, Juan and I joined yet another group, this one a private celebration for one of the authors of *The Ugly American*, a political novel about the failure of U.S. diplomacy in Southeast Asia that was published in 1958. Slowly, I began to realize these clandestine groups were peopled by profoundly angry, anti-American communists.

Years passed before I realized how much the covert danger associated with those groups stimulated me, causing me excessive anxiety and overwhelming my five young senses—but they also gave rise to a clarity previously unknown in the form of awakened intuition.

I share these remembrances purely to introduce events unfolding as we moved through the sacred sites at the Basilica of Guadalupe and at Teotihuacan, with its famous Pyramids of the Sun and the Moon, and at adjacent ruins outside Mexico City. At the Basilica, I witnessed men and women crawling on bare and bloody knees down the long *calzada* leading into the basilica as a way of giving thanks for prayers answered. I was both awed and confused by the sight.

Next on our tour was Teotihuacán. Long fascinated by the ancient Mayan and Aztecan cultures of Mexico, I had already learned of their subsequent disappearance from the planet somewhere around 900 CE.

Juan had already described the Pyramid of the Sun and Moon in breathtaking detail, but nothing could have prepared me for the experience of seeing it for the first time. As our taxi approached Teotihuacan and those ancient ruins first appeared on that warm sunny day, my heart soared with wonder, and my soul filled with strange and exciting sensations as I became one with the spiritual energy of this sacred place. Exiting the taxi, the pervasive smells of the ancient history contained within the walls of those ruins pierced my senses. As Juan and I walked toward the Pyramid of the Moon, which lay at one end of the long pathway known as the Avenue of the Dead, so many questions swirled in my mind: "Who were these people?" "How did they live?" "Where had they gone?"

Climbing the Pyramid of the Moon together, Juan and I could see the Pyramid of the Sun at the opposite end, anchoring the huge, open complex. Rushing to see this spectacular sight, my youthful legs, strengthened by farm work, deftly made the climb to the top of the pyramid. It did not disappoint. I stood in awe, gazing across the ruins to the horizon beyond, and felt the splendor of the ancient Mesoamerican civilization that had occupied it. During our descent toward the Pyramid of the Sun, I heard what sounded like singing and drumming in the distance. Intrigued, I decided to follow the sound, leaving Juan to climb the Pyramid of the Sun.

Strolling among the smaller pyramids and ruins, I arrived at an open space that appeared to be an ancient ball field. I read about the ritual importance of the Toltec ball games while at the Museum of Anthropology in Mexico City. I seated myself on what appeared to be the remains of ancient stone bleachers and closed my eyes, leaning toward the sun, letting the heat of the day surround me and enjoying the pleasure of a breeze cooling my sweat-drenched face.

Slowly, the singing and drumming faded. When I opened my eyes, I was shocked by what I saw on the field in front of me. There, a group of powerfully built young men with dark skin and flowing black hair dressed in colorful regalia were engaged in a competitive ball game accompanied by the rousing sounds of flutes, beating drums, and a cheering crowd. I was enraptured as one player made a grandstand play for what appeared to be an impossible opportunity for a winning score. Miraculously, he made the score, and the crowd cheered their approval. And then, just as suddenly as it had appeared, the scene dissolved.

I shook my head as if waking from sleep. It scared me to think that maybe this hadn't been a dream but, instead, a vision—something I'd never experienced before. The overwhelming realization of what would happen at the end of such a game frankly scared me. By making such a play and winning such a game, that beautiful, powerful young man would become a ritual sacrifice, his beating heart cut from his living body to demonstrate his people's devotion to their gods.

Sitting there and pondering what had occurred, I suddenly felt a presence behind me. I turned, expecting Juan, but instead found myself looking directly into a pair of kind eyes belonging to a brown-skinned old man. But his eyes were not the eyes of an old man. They were filled with light, and his aura was likewise radiant, a rainbow of electric colors. I sensed that he could read my mind because in response to my thinking, "How can you send out these beautiful colors? Can you teach me to do that?" he knowingly smiled and said, "The simplicity of your questions transports me back to a time when I asked my own teacher the same thing."

What happened next was inexplicable: our eyes locked, and with one swift movement, he opened his chest, reached inside, and quite literally pulled out his heart. I drew back in fear, but when I once again caught his eyes, I could see only gentleness and compassion emanating from the windows of his soul. I knew all would be well.

Next, I stared in amazement as he reached inside his chest, this time removing a radiant flame, which he then placed into the cavity that had somehow opened in my own chest. All fear had left me. Instead, I was filled with wonder at the extraordinary gift he had given me. To this day, I don't know if this was a lucid dream or a vision. But I do know that was my experience that day at Teotihuacan.

At that very moment at Teotihuacan, my soul—my very being—changed. The "I" of me became "one" with my physical body. The flame totally transformed my mind. I experienced my mind loving me, *being* me. Awestruck by the boundless quality of this uncontainable energy, the desire to share this love with every being, every animal, tree, flower, blade of grass, and rock—yes, every living thing—became a driving force. The magnitude of the love within the flame did not end even there. It kept traveling farther and farther out until it permeated the cosmos. I imagined this energy of love encompassing the sun, moon, and stars until we became one.

After this extraordinary spiritual experience in Mexico, I became fixated on religion, God, and all things mystical. I struggled with the feeling that God was calling me to the Baptist ministry. I was torn on the one hand to heed that call, but on the other, I recoiled at the thought. I did not want to disappoint Jesus, but I did not feel at peace with being a minister.

The following summer, my California cousins invited me to visit them, and again, I was amazed that my parents agreed to the trip. Before leaving, still struggling with my dilemma, I made a contract with God. I knew that my cousins lived in the vicinity of the famed Huntington Library, Art Museum, and Botanical Gardens in San Marino. I would ask them to take me there, and if I happened to see a painting of Jesus on the Cross, that would be my sign that God was calling me to his ministry.

Traveling alone, I took the train to my cousins' home in Anaheim, near Disneyland. I had no idea how far the Huntington Library was, exactly; I just knew I had to get there. Nelson, the husband of one of my cousins, graciously consented to the trip, and he and Lane, his son, drove me to Huntington early one Sunday morning. I was silently nervous about what I would see there, and as I scanned every room, making sure I saw every corner because I did not want to miss the painting of Jesus on the cross, I was relieved to find there was none. All thoughts of becoming a Baptist minister faded from my mind.

Eight years later, in London, the first stop on a European vacation with my wife, Cindy, I had my second experience with an alternate reality. Our hotel, the Charing Cross Hotel, was located near Trafalgar Square, home to Lord Nelson's column commemorating his defeat of the French Fleet at the Battle of Trafalgar on October 21, 1805. The day was bright and sunny; the sky was clear, unusual for

London in September. As I gazed upward toward the top of Lord Nelson's column, I heard the jingle of the trappings of horse-drawn carriages. I turned and was astonished at the scene before me. Everyone in the square, from liveried workers milling about on the sidewalks to young women hurrying along the cobbled streets, was dressed in nineteenth-century English attire.

What happened next was equally astonishing. As I dragged my eyes from the scene in the square, I locked upon the gaze of an old man standing across the street. It was none other than the old man from Teotihuacán. His eyes entranced me to the point that I could not move, and the thoughts emanating soundlessly from him reminded me of our previous meeting. "It is time for you to educate yourself with all things mystical," he said. Then, as quickly as the scene appeared, it disappeared. London was once again the London of the 1970s.

This would not be the last time the old man of Teotihuacán would appear to me as a guide along my journey of spiritual evolution. He would later come to me in a different form at a time when I felt all was lost. Eventually, he would pull me back from a precipice of self-annihilation into a world where all possibilities exist.

Still awe-filled from my London experience, I shifted my focus from tourist to metaphysical seeker as we visited the next two cities on our itinerary, Amsterdam and Paris. I wondered if my Mayan guide would present himself again, and as I strolled along the canals of Amsterdam, I looked for him in every face. I was disappointed not to see him there. When I reached Paris, the next and final stop on the trip, I knew without a doubt that I had been a resident there in a previous life. The Louvre—especially the Egyptian Room (holding prophecies of experiences yet to come)—sparked a past life memory of an Etruscan lifetime that felt so familiar that I was fascinated by the intense emotional response the sights elicited. Montmartre left me eerily aware of a dark period, full of foreboding that I had experienced in some past Parisian lifetime. I had a similar déjà vu moment while visiting the Palace of Versailles. I walked the gardens as if I knew what I would see next; it was familiar in a way that had nothing to do with the photos I'd seen or the books I had read. This intense, extrasensory knowledge was destined to become a theme in my life.

I explored the metaphysical world in earnest when I returned from Europe. I studied astrology, the Rosicrucian Order, and the work of Aleister Crowley of the Order of the Golden Dawn. I meditated by gazing into the flame of a candle to teach my mind to have a single focus. I sought the mystical and the mysterious anywhere I could find it. Eventually, however, the demands of "real" life began to erode my resolve. I shifted my focus from the metaphysical to the material. The pursuit of wealth became my religion.

During the next fifteen years, I bought into the desire for financial success and the "work hard, play hard" ethos that drives the pursuit of the "American Dream." My justification was that this was the only way I'd be able to enjoy my life—to travel widely and to acquire the trappings of success. Then, the house of cards that I'd built for myself tumbled down at the beginning of 1984, and I found myself at an all-time low. Knowing that I could not continue my life as it was, I experienced tremendous emotional despair. Yet, I also knew that the consequences of getting a divorce and leaving my family and my two young children were so overwhelmingly painful that I felt I could not handle it. I was caught between a rock and a hard place! To stay in the marriage would only delay the inevitable and cause further pain and suffering for us all. To leave would also be painful for us all. I chose to leave even with the knowledge I was not sure I had the mental, emotional or spiritual foundation to weather the storm.

I turned to drugs and alcohol. They become my daily companions. During one binge, I attempted to cut my wrists in a desperate cry for the help I was not able to give myself or ask anyone else to give me either. This crisis signaled the end of an era for me. I knew that life as it had been could no longer be. I no longer had the desire or the ability to continue living the lie that was my life. Financially and emotionally bankrupt, homeless, and without a car or job, depression became a constant in my life.

It took me three years after my initial crash to reach my bottom. Yet, within the darkness, I eventually realized that anger, resentment, bitterness, and revenge could not, and would not, restore my sanity. As had often happened in my life, when I found the courage to surrender, answers came. This time, surrender introduced me to a little book titled *The Superbeings* by John Randolph Price. In his preface, Price described a time in his life in which discontent propelled him to search for answers. Because I identified with his story, I continued reading, and the following statement caught my eye: "God wants man to be happy—that it is God's will for man to be successful, prosperous and totally fulfilled—and that nothing will be impossible to man once he learns to cooperate with his inner resources."[1] I wondered at that statement, for my conditioning had not conveyed that message; instead, I had learned to fear a god of wrath and condemnation. Finally, I realized that alcohol and drugs were neither my friends nor the answer to a life of despair. Alcoholics Anonymous and Al-Anon became my rock and fellow members of my family.

As I awoke from my long stupor, I also began seeking spiritual guidance. It came in an unusual manner. Since discovering the works of John Randolph Price, I have been meditating for several hours a day. I took long walks, and with each step affirmed peace, happiness, and prosperity for myself and others. Each night upon retiring, I spent time in meditation to quiet my mind, and I practiced being in the silence, listening. On most nights I just fell quietly asleep until morning woke me, but on one night in the spring of 1987, something quite different occurred. Awakened from a deep sleep by some foreign sound from elsewhere in the house, I bolted upright in bed. I glanced at the bedside clock—it was 2:07 a.m.

A little shaken but assured there was nothing amiss in the house, I lay back down and began meditating to get back to sleep. I noticed colors beginning to swirl behind my closed eyelids—blues, greens, and yellows, mixing and melting into each other like a swirling kaleidoscope. I watched the light show, fascinated by the display, until finally, the colors blended into one: purple. Entranced by the flow of the purple, I became calm and relaxed until I was aware of losing sense of my physical body, except for a slight numbing sensation. At the same time, I felt an incredible connection to the whole of the universe. There are no words to adequately describe the experience. It was similar to being hypnotized, my body asleep but my mind hyper alert. I was having so much fun in this altered state that I didn't want it to end. The more I let go of the physical, the more I experienced a world I did not know existed, and it filled me with awe.

I was so caught up in the "lightness of being" that it took me a moment to realize a voice was speaking, seemingly from somewhere in the room, although it seemed far away. Then I realized the voice was coming from my own mouth. The voice was saying, "I am Johnnie, and I have come to teach you." I was so startled that the purple light on which I had been focusing began to fade. The voice said, "Just stay with the purple light, keep your focus, and as long as you do, I will be with you. I will be with you as long as you need me." Johnnie's energy was palpable; it had a giddy quality about it, and yet I felt absolutely safe and secure in its presence.

I remembered another of Price's quotes: "The Cosmic Consciousness has always been within you, but you have been asleep to it. Now, you must awaken. You must feel the warmth of Love in your heart. You must sense the imprisoned Splendor of your True Nature."[2]

I thought, "Is that what is happening to me?" I loved how I felt in Johnnie's presence, and because I trusted him implicitly, I decided it did not matter. I knew I would follow his instructions to the letter. Soon, it dawned on me that Johnnie was the old man I had encountered during my visions at Teotihuacán and London.

Johnnie and I spent the next eight months in constant contact. I learned to tune out the mundane while listening to his instructions. Every night, we traveled together. He taught me to become a white dove so that I could fly with him to worlds unknown. My favorite destination was a beautiful purple pyramid in what I presumed to be ancient Egypt. We perched on top of the pyramid. From that vantage point, I could see the whole of Egypt laid out before us.

Johnnie instructed me to "become one" with specific entities: a scribe, a prince, a pharaoh, a slave, an animal, even God, so that I might learn important lessons from each one. I learned from the great Ra, the Egyptian god of the Sun, how all of life is possible because of the energy of the Sun. I understood that the Egyptians were not worshiping the Sun as a deity but instead recognized that without it, nothing could exist. Ra taught me his proper place in the cosmic order. Intuitively, I knew there was something else, some greater entity or source responsible for this order.

Johnnie intuited what I needed to break the chains of my Earthly conditioning. He knew I could not fully awaken until I knew *the truth*. He led me through the darkness into the light. I ran with wolves, flew with eagles, and crawled on my belly with snakes. He left no stone unturned until I could "fly" on my own. Then, abruptly, he left. Try as I might, I could not connect with him. I dedicated hours to focusing on the purple light. He did not come. I was angry, a signal that I was denying the grief arising from the feeling of abandonment and falling back into old patterns of helplessness and worthlessness. I could not imagine my days without contact with Johnnie. I did not want to return to my former state of apathy and depression—I just couldn't! I had come too far and learned too much to fall into that trap again.

Soon enough, I was able to concentrate and focus on what Johnnie had taught me. I began to practice metaphysical tools like automatic writing, clairaudience, and clairvoyance to keep myself on track. I noticed with some amusement that I received spiritual communication while in the shower. Sometimes the message was for me, and sometimes relatives or friends with whom I shared the message. With each experience, I became more comfortable with my connection to the unseen.

Years later, in 2010, I was presenting a workshop on the Mayan calendars. At the end of the presentation, an elegant woman (whom I later learned was a walk-in) said to me quietly but with great clarity, "The old man at Teotihuacán was your future self." Then she walked away, leaving me stunned by her declaration. I later wept at the knowledge of what I would become—no, I *had* become.

As I became more comfortable in my psychic shoes, I began to share with people the messages I received for them. Never sure how others would react, I realized I could trust the source of the messages and that I was only the channel through which Spirit chose to deliver those messages. This process became my life.

I began participating in psychic fairs, reading for those who were called to me. As time went on, I was approached by people who had family, friends, or lovers who had committed suicide. They intuitively knew I could contact the departed and lead them into the light and, therefore, peace. Even though I had not previously experienced this ability, I began to meditate on it, asking for guidance.

When guidance came, I was instructed to connect with the departed spirit by what I came to call *intuitive sensing* and, through that ability, lead them into the light. As I intuitively sensed the anguished energy of these spirits, I discovered them lost in a world of blackness, still connected in some sense to the material world but not able to communicate with it. They appeared to hang around loved ones left behind in the physical world, desperately trying to communicate their need for help but discovering only that they were not seen or heard.

It became my mission, then, in the darkness, to find a point of light and direct them toward it. When the spirits discerned my presence, they frantically attempted to hook into my energy. I found that if I allowed that, I could not help them, so I learned to focus the energy of love on them, which served to quiet and calm the entities. At that point, I telepathically told them to look for the light. I assured them that if they sought the light, they would find it. I was able to sense when they saw the light because their energy changed, grew and became lighter, and at that critical moment, I sent them the message to move toward the light. As they did, the light grew and illuminated the darkness, revealing other spirits waiting for them in the light, reaching out with love into the expanding light to brighten the way for the lost spirit. When the lost spirit moved into the light, I saw a huge flash of brilliant color, and at that moment, I knew my mission was complete.

I fondly remembered my lessons with Johnnie and attempted to contact him in the usual manner, but still to no avail. I began practicing automatic writing every day, and I noticed it took about three pages of writing before the "ego mind" gave up and a message from "the other side of the veil" came through. On one such occasion, I received a much longed-for message in my writing: "This is Johnnie. I haven't left you. It was time for you to 'fly' on your own. I taught you everything you need, and you have learned it well. I will always be with you. Always remember that I love *you*. You are me, and I am you. We are one for all eternity." As I read those words, the tears coursed down my cheeks and fell softly onto the yellow paper. The ink ran where they fell, the words fading, feathering, becoming illegible. It didn't matter. I had received what I needed.

The next step on my spiritual journey was working with an unseen spiritual group, which I called the Elohim. This work was different from the work I'd done with Johnnie. I went into a trance, and the Elohim took over my body, using my vocal cords with which to speak. People came for a reading from me in my Elohim state, seeking answers to their questions. Sometimes, I heard Elohim's answer; at other times, I was unaware of what they were saying unless the client consented to being audiotaped.

During a session with a client, I will call William, and I was not aware of either his query or Elohim's answer to it. After the session, William told me he appreciated the answer to his question and that, accordingly, he would not see me for a while. Six years later, I ran into him. He told me about his experience with the Elohim. He had asked them if certain illegal activities in which he had been involved would be found out. He said the Elohim told him, yes, he would, in fact, go to prison and that during his incarceration, he would become so despondent that he would contemplate suicide. But they said that they would be with him during this time and would keep him safe. They gave him a symbol on which to focus: a red rose. He was instructed to focus on this rose whenever he felt depressed or suicidal, and they would guide him through the darkness into the light. He shared his gratitude for the session and said he would have died in prison without that information. I was grateful to know that he was doing well and that the words of the Elohim had gotten him through a dark time in his life.

My life took yet another important turn in 1986 when a friend invited me to a Spiritualist Church one Sunday afternoon to hear Reverend Bobbie Roberts, a well-known local psychic and spiritualist. Rev. Roberts worked with spirit guides who assisted her with what she called Blindfold Billets. When the basket of billets was offered to me, I filled one out, writing my name at the top and three questions underneath. My first question was about my brother, Tommy, who made his transition into the spiritual world in 1968 at the age of twenty-five. The second asked, "What is my career path now?" My third concern was my grandmother, Mary Lee Owens Blackwell, who made her transition into spirit earlier that year.

Rev. Roberts took the billets in her hand and rubbed them on her head, her method of connecting with the energy of the writer. Her spiritual guides assisted her in connecting with souls on the "other side." After she made several connections, she said, "I want to come to Gary. Tommy is here and wants to give you a message."

I was stunned but found the voice to say, "Yes, Bobbie, this is Gary." She relayed the message that all was well with my brother and grandmother. Both told her to tell me they loved me and indicated they were watching over me from their spiritual vantage point. Then Rev. Roberts said, "I see you in a room working with people one-on-one, as if you were in a counseling setting."

With this affirmation of the direction I should take with my life, the following week, I enrolled at a local university to begin the studies that would lead me to a career in mental health counseling. As an undergraduate, I focused my studies on drug and alcohol counseling and received a Bachelor of Science degree.

While pursuing my undergraduate degree, I worked nights at a facility for the long-term, persistently mentally ill. The facility residents, who were diagnosed with schizophrenia and Alzheimer's disease, taught me about the world of mental illness.

There was Mary, an elderly woman who occasionally awakened from the effects of Alzheimer's to ask me where she was. In those moments, her normally cloudy and lifeless eyes glistened with awareness. She would ask if Bob, her son, had been to see her. When I assured her that he had, she would flash a smile only a mother's love can portray. Then, just as quickly, she would revert to a state of confusion and unawareness. I learned to treasure those moments of clarity, knowing I might be the only witness to share the brief, precious moments when she once again became aware of her identity and her life.

Hazel, another resident, had spent most of the past twenty years of her life homeless. She lived the "patterns of survival" she had learned on the street, i.e., hoarding food from the dining room. Hazel saved bread, meat, and fruit from her tray, took it to her room, and hid it under her bed. When anyone went into her room, Hazel raised holy hell for fear they would take her stash. She loathed taking her weekly bath, a major undertaking for her and the aides who bathed her. During her bath, the staff, myself included, would remove the spoiled food she hoarded under her bed. Because she wore her hair in dreadlocks, washing her hair was a full-blown battle. During the bath, she struggled with all her might against the aides as they put her in the shower, clothes and all. No one had the strength or ability to coerce Hazel into taking off her clothes or even changing them.

Then there was Cleve, who, depending on his mood, was sometimes known as Cleveta. He spent most of his days walking the halls and grounds. Cleve loathed wearing shoes and loved walking barefoot around a nearby lake. He had ongoing conversations with other "voices," some of which were kind, some of which were mean. When he heard the mean voices, he argued with them and told them to "shut up." Nonetheless, he was an intelligent man, and I found him to be a pleasant companion as he walked with me on my rounds. I worked for nine months at this facility, and my experiences there were invaluable, laying the foundation for my understanding of mental illness.

My next job was at a local mental health center, again working with the long-term, persistently mentally ill. By this time, I was pursuing my master's and certification in drug and alcohol counseling. One of the criteria for that certification included an internship in a drug and alcohol recovery facility. I found such an internship at a local hospital and completed it while working at the mental health center.

Once I received my certification as a drug and alcohol counselor, the alcohol and drug treatment facility hired me as an outpatient counselor. During the next two years, however, I realized that this was not going to be the focus of my career. I spent more time doing paperwork than I did working with clients. The job and internship did provide me with valuable experience working with addictions, dysfunctional families, and abuse and trauma issues, but traditional treatment approaches often failed, leading to continual patient relapse. The facilities were like revolving doors; patients would receive treatment, leave, relapse, and return for more treatment. Although I could not determine the factors missing in treatment, I suspected it was an unresolved shame. This hypothesis was my motivation for researching and exploring methods for identifying and addressing what I would come to call "cellular shame."

In 1991, a flyer came across my desk advertising individual treatment sessions using a technique called Transformational Kinesiology. I made an appointment with Rev. Tom Hyder, the practitioner. He used the muscle-based therapeutic modality known as kinesiology to gain access to the body's holographic information. (Holographic, as used here, means that each molecule of the body holds the information necessary to replicate the whole.) I was skeptical at first, but halfway into the process, I began to feel a kind of emotional release. At the end of my ninety-minute session, I was filled with a sense of freedom I had not experienced since childhood. As time passed, I noticed it became difficult for me to access the emotionally charged issues addressed in the session. I could still remember the traumatic childhood experiences but only as fact, without any emotion attached to them. It was very freeing.

I wanted to learn kinesiology, so I called Rev. Hyder to find out if he taught the technique. He did not. He said he learned it from a couple in Copenhagen. Unfortunately, they did not offer training in the United States, and traveling to Copenhagen was financially out of the question.

Nevertheless, I was certain this would be the direction of my study. A few weeks later, I discovered that One Brain certification classes would be held locally. One Brain also uses kinesiology to access information from the human energy system. After completing the two-day class, I spent the next four years studying the modality and became a certified practitioner and teacher. In addition to studying with

One Brain master practitioner Marjorie Bovard of Dallas, Texas, I trained with Daniel Whiteside and Gordon Stokes, creators of One Brain.

The One Brain system became a hallmark of my private counseling practice until 1998. During those years, I continued to learn and incorporate other energy-based psychology techniques like Thought Field Therapy and Emotional Freedom Technique into my counseling practice. Thought Field Therapy, developed by Roger Callahan, Ph.D., uses algorithms of grouped meridian points to treat specific issues such as phobias. His success using this technique has been astounding. Gary Craig, who studied with Dr. Callahan, expanded on what he learned and created the simpler but equally effective Emotional Freedom Technique (EFT).

In 1996, after reading *Anatomy of the Spirit* and other works by Caroline Myss, I decided to focus my studies on energy medicine. I also enrolled in the doctoral program focusing on energy medicine at Greenwich University in Hilo, Hawaii, directed by Caroline Myss and Dr. Norman Shealy. In 2001, I completed the program with honors.

It was during this period that I began to develop my own therapeutic methodology, the Energy Matrix Clearing System, a living system not limited by time or space. I am grateful for all clients throughout the years who have been open and courageous enough to stand up, hold out their arms, and trust in me and the process. I, in turn, trust that the client's energy system will lead the way. I am always amazed at the results.

I saw the process guide a client who, out of desperation to leave an abusive marriage, turned to the lucrative job of dancing in a men's club in order to save the funds to do so. She eventually became a child advocate attorney.

With another client, age recession took us into their time in the womb. The information we gleaned from this time indicated that the man she had long thought was her biological father clearly was not. She was so startled by the information that she did not return to counseling with me for two years. When she finally did make another appointment, she told me this story:

> During the summer, following my appointment with you, I went to a family reunion in my hometown. An elderly man, whom I recognized as a family friend, approached me and introduced himself as my biological father. I had forgotten what you told me in my session. The moment he introduced himself, it all came flooding back. I could not believe it. At least I had some forewarning. Had I not, I question my reaction in that situation. I am not sure whether to thank you or be angry with you because now I question everything about my life. That is why I came back. I am sure you can help me.

I have countless stories like this, but I will leave them for another book. *This* book is about the process.

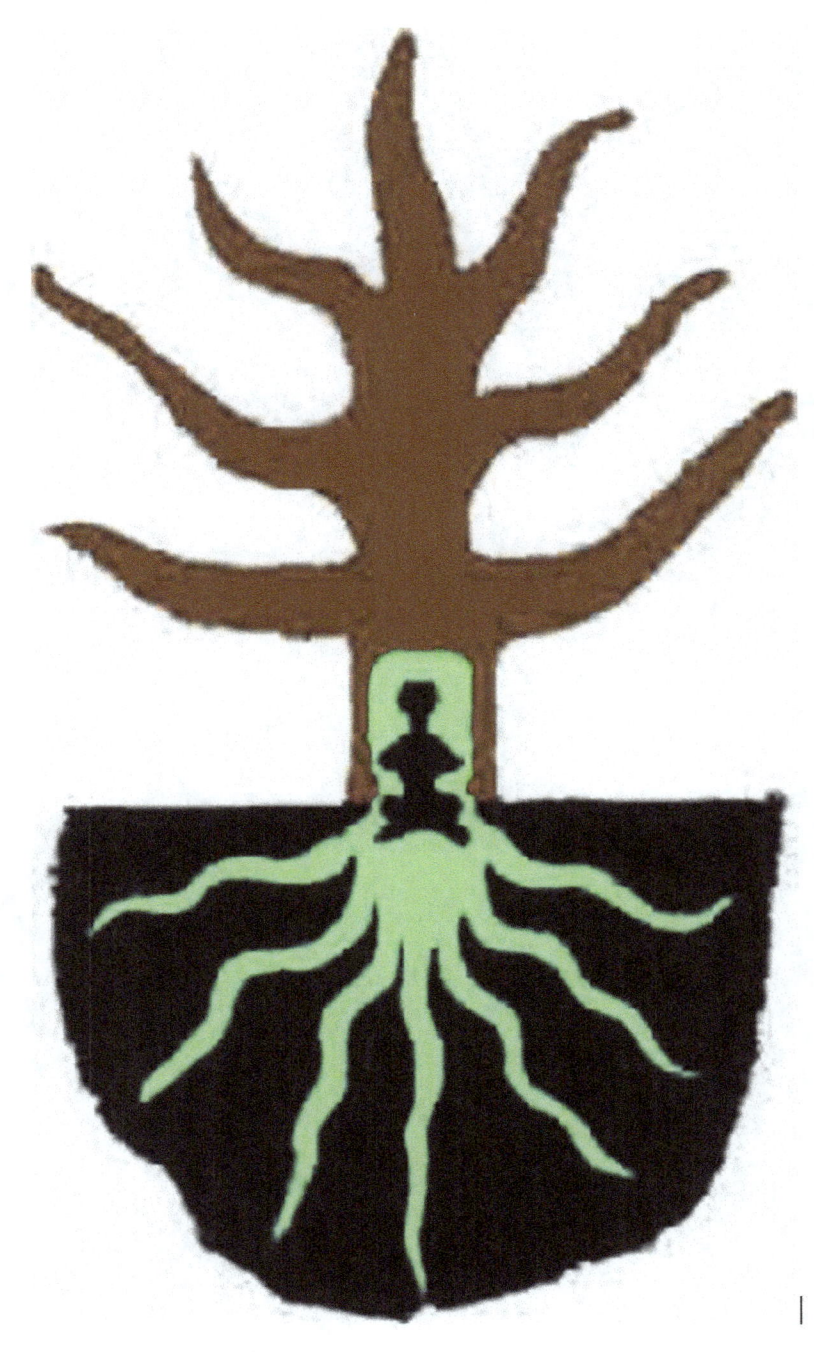

THE ESSENE TREE OF LIFE

CHAPTER ONE

THE ENERGY MATRIX CLEARING SYSTEM

AND

THE HOLOGRAPHIC HUMAN ENERGY SYSTEM

External nature moulds the shape of internal nature, and if nature vanishes, the inner nature is also lost; for the outer is the mother of the inner.

— PARACELSUS

The Energy Matrix Clearing System (EMCS) is based on the principle "as above, so below." This centuries-old premise, espoused by such great thinkers as the sixteenth-century Swiss physician Paracelsus and eighteenth-century German physician Samuel Hahnemann, has more recently been rediscovered as the "holographic principle" of Albert Einstein, David Bohm, William Tiller, and Donald Watson. This holographic paradigm is the foundation of EMCS.

EMCS uses a specialized form of kinesiology to search out blockages in the subtle force of energy that surrounds and interpenetrates the physical. The interruption of the flow of this vital force can negatively impact one's physical, mental, emotional, and spiritual health. EMCS uses energy medicines—gems, minerals, animal and flower essences, essential oils, creative imagery, light, color, and sound frequencies—to eradicate energy distortions or blockages.

EMCS views the human body as a holographic-halographic energy system and, therefore, is itself a form of energy medicine. When any part of this system is dysfunctional, the whole system suffers. The schematic or "matrix" of EMCS provides the medium for identifying and diffusing distortions. The Energy Matrix Clearing System identifies and removes patterns that limit, block, and prevent individual progress toward a happier and healthier life.

Self-insight is achieved following individual development of the spiritual core that is inherent in us all. Becoming aware of this spiritual core and its properties as an energy field allows alchemical conversion to take place through communication via electrical, chemical, and energetic interaction using the four levels of the holographic-halographic human energy field:

- The molecular world of the physical
- The psychic world of the atomical
- The spiritual world of the sub-atomical
- And the "being" world of the divine causal body

The spiritual process of EMCS also identifies and honors seven spiritual principles or levels of understanding. These seven spiritual principles are found in all spiritual traditions in one form or another. The following are the seven principles specific to the Hindu-Theosophical traditions:

Sthula Sarira, or Dense Physical Body—to Experience: This body is perceived through our five outer senses. It is a crystalized form and, in and of itself, lacks vitality as an entity clothed in dense chemical substances. It responds to lower-level vibrations. According to Bruce Fisher in volume one of his three-volume publication *Man, Grand Reflection of the Greater Cosmos: Studies in Occult Anatomy*, the dense physical body "is the medium through which Consciousness experiences and expresses *course physical blows.*"[3]

Linga Sarira, or Vital Body (etheric double)—to Sense: According to Fisher, the Vital Body serves two purposes:

> First, it is the medium through which the dense physical body is vitalized, maintained and propagated. Secondly, it functions as an intermediate for the transmission of psychic forces from the astral and mental bodies to the physical brain and nervous system.[4]

Prana, or preserving aspect of Life Force—to Live: This is best described as the integrating energy initiating the make-up of the physical, like molecules and cells.

Kama Rupa, or Desire Body (desires and emotions)—to feel: This is an "astral" body and is therefore less evolved than the physical. Originally a thought form, it is now a thought form clothed in desire or astral force-matter. It interpenetrates the etheric and physical and is in constant rapid motion, circulating in currents throughout the astral body. It has its own chakra system or force centers, and the main vortex is located near the liver. The astral functions as the human vehicle of feelings, emotions, and desires. It motivates us to action. Fisher relates that when we are asleep, the Higher Ego leaves the physical and vital bodies and functions in the astral body as its outer vehicle of consciousness. As a result, the physical body is rejuvenated. He suggests the astral body remains connected to the physical body through what he calls the "Silver Cord," which remains intact up to the moment we die."[5]

Lower Manas, or Mental Body (concrete mind)—to Think: As Theosophist A.E. Powell writes in *The Mental Body*:

> The mental body is thus the vehicle of the ego, of the real Thinker, who himself resides in the causal body. But, while the mental body is intended eventually to be the vehicle of consciousness on the lower mental plane, it also works on and through the astral and physical bodies in all manifestations that are usually called the "mind" in ordinary waking consciousness.[6]

Higher Manas, or Human Spirit—to Do: Fisher again explains in *Studies in Occult Anatomy*:

> The mind is a powerful creative force. Currently, it includes the mind sheath, astral and etheric head centers or chakras and the physical brain, and through this connection, we are learning to create with mineral substances. Which means we can consciously create

inanimate things like tables and chairs. The "highest level of the Region, the fourth and mid-level of the Thought World, is very important because it contains the *archetypal forces* involved in creative thought; is the *true location of the human mind*; is the focal point through which Spirit mirrors itself in Matter and contact Its vehicle of form in the Personality; and also the location of the *True "Memory of Nature"* or the "Akashic Records.*[7]

Buddhi (feminine), or Life Spirit—to Know: The Thought World is five-dimensional, the added dimension being one of the *consciousness of all possibilities at once* existing. This state, as can be seen, allows us the greatest possible wisdom because of the tremendously broad perspective that it provides while we are in it. So, too, does the *five-dimensional* consciousness of the mental state allow us to make more intelligent choices when we maintain a "clear head" in a difficult situation, as compared to the more limited four-dimensional consciousness of the emotional state, wherein only one possibility at a time can be perceived. [8]

Atman, or Divine Spirit: This is the individual soul, the essence that is eternal, unchanging, indistinguishable from the universe; to be.[9] Consciousness at the Atmic level (pure being) may be seven-dimensional because we realize possibilities beyond our total realm of Soul experience. In this ultimate oxalate state, we can create our own reality.[10]

The Energy Matrix Clearing System is a sacred process. Entering another person's biofield is entering into a sacred contract with them. This sacred contract calls for honor, respect, attunement, and integrity. Each of us is a divine being and, as such, is a role model for love, compassion, forgiveness, and enthusiasm.

The health of the whole self requires harmony at all levels of the holographic human energy system. Knowledge of this energy anatomy is the first priority of the EMCS process. EMCS includes energy medicine and vibrational medicine. Internalizing the truth that humans are more than physical beings is foundational to the understanding and practice of EMCS.

The following quotes from leaders in the field of holistic energy healing elucidate what is meant by energy and vibrational medicine:

Richard Gerber, MD: The Einsteinian paradigm, as applied to vibrational medicine, sees human beings as networks of complex energy fields that interface with physical and cellular systems. Vibrational medicine uses specialized forms of energy which positively affect those energetic systems that may be out of balance due to disease states. By rebalancing the energy fields that help to regulate cellular physiology, vibrational healers or "energicians" attempt to restore order from a higher level of human functioning.[11]

William Tiller, Ph.D.: Nature is a vast interpenetrating and interacting ensemble of substances at all ten dimensions of the universe. In addition, each individuation in every dimension is radiating and absorbing energy and information in a multiple variety of forms, such as sonic, EM, subtle, etc.; and over a wide variety of frequency ranges. Thus, these different spaces pulse with currents of different kinds of energy and information that flow back and forth between the different manifestations of substance. Sometimes the flow is gentle, and sometimes it is turbulent, but always, it is our environment. The ability of humans to sense and discriminate this information is essential for their survival and for their evolution.[12]

Julia Melges-Brenner (formerly Melges Jablonski): Recent technological developments have at last intellectually confirmed the ancient metaphysical knowledge that life is essentially energy and that life energy is observable in the auras emitted by all living organisms. Scientific research into the nature of this energy and the interactions between electromagnetic fields has produced results that mirror the observations and views of "sensitives" and healers. This research has provided evidence not only of the existence of the aura but also of the mechanisms behind and power of auric healing.[13]

Claude Swanson, Ph.D.: The "Life Force" is central to many forms of energy healing, such as Reiki and Qigong. It is the energy which flows in the acupuncture system of the body, and is basic to alternative medicine.[14]

The life-giving energy animating all things is known by a variety of names: chi or qi (Chinese), prana (Hindu), kundalini Ku (India) orgone, tachyon, vital life force, universal life force, and serpent fire. It is, in any case, energy that emanates from our Sun, and the Theosophists of the late nineteenth and early twentieth centuries divided it into three categories:

Fohat, or electricity. Some call this the primary force and relate it to the electromagnetic force of modern physics manifesting in the physical world as light, heat, and sound. Esoterically termed "the willpower or 'Father' Principle." The spiritual fire.

Prana, or vitality. In the West, we call this the vital life force. Hypothetically, it relates to gravitational and weak forces inherent in modern physics. Esoterically spoken of as the "Love-Wisdom Principle" or "Son-Daughter Principle." Its fundamental mode is mental fire.

Kundalini, or serpent fire.[15] This is known as the creative force. Esoterically known as actively creative intelligence or the Holy Spirit. It is the creator of form, the fire of matter.

These principles of energy-vibrational medicine will be discussed more fully in the following chapter as aspects of the holographic human energy anatomy.

Electromagnetic energy, found in practically all physical forces—electricity, magnetism, light, heat, sound, chemical affinity, and motion—is a necessary component of life. All these energies are convertible into one another. Many researchers speculate that kundalini is the universal life force, the creative and sustaining force of all life. Researchers such as William Tiller, Donald Watson, Claude Swanson, and Valerie Hunt have determined a certain balance of these forces is required to sustain life. All suggest the nervous system is a conductor for the absorption and processing of this energy. Further, they suggest that electromagnetic fields are the avenue or language through which the universal life force manifests and communicates. Kundalini is a force known only to a few. Masters of this art discuss it in yogic practices. Orthodox Western science does not mention its reality as a human force.

The Sanskrit word *prana* is a compound of *pra*, which means forth, and *an*, which means to breathe, move, and live. Thus, the closest English definition of prana means life breath, life energy, or to breathe forth. In Hindu thought, there is but one life, one consciousness. Prana also signifies the concept of the "Supreme Self," the energy of the one, and the "Life of the Logos," according to A.E. Powell.[16]

Powell states in *The Etheric Double,* "Too great an exuberance of it (Prana) in the nervous system may lead to disease and death, just as too little leads to exhaustion and ultimately death."[17] Therefore, the open, balanced flow of life force (prana) in the subtle energy bodies determines physical vitality, while blocked or disturbed balance or excessive prana results in disease and, ultimately, death. The Energy Matrix Clearing System provides a method that removes these imbalances in the holographic human energy system, leading to more vital physical, mental, emotional, and spiritual body expressions.

Allopathic medicine regards disease as an unexpected occurrence, appearing suddenly in healthy bodies. Because the science behind allopathic medicine is based upon the Newtonian view of man as a machine coupled with the Darwinist paradigm of evolution, the current Western medical model is one in which the doctor serves as a "mechanic" or "bio-technician" who repairs the damage. In the man-as-machine model, the "part" needing repair is the only consideration. "The whole" does not play a role in the allopathic treatment decision. Because of this view, conventional medicine is not meeting a host of challenges, including the exploding costs of crisis-oriented medical care and the rise of new diseases that do not respond to surgery or pharmaceutical intervention.

Alternative medicine may offer solutions to these crises. In an article by Barbara Starfield from the *Journal of American Medical Association,* vol. 284, she writes, "According to a recent study, U.S. medical care is falling behind European countries despite the belief by many in the United States that their health care is superior." She then lists the countries in order of their average ranking on certain healthcare indicators, with the first being the best: Japan, Sweden, Canada, France, Australia, Spain, Finland, the Netherlands, the United Kingdom, Denmark, Belgium, the United States, and Germany.[18] And Claude Swanson points out in *Life Force* that the American healthcare system is failing in part because of its escalating costs and resistance to innovation. "As a result," he continues, "More people are turning to alternative health care which uses the entire range of available remedies, including naturopathic and energetic approaches."[19]

The Energy Matrix Clearing System is an energy-based approach that includes the many systems making up the human holographic-halographic energy anatomy. This approach views these systems in categories or hierarchical components. First, there is the "outside" system: causal, mental, astral, etheric, and physical. Within these are interrelating systems, or "inside" and "outside" systems, recognized as the chakra and meridian systems. These systems communicate or transfer energy-information to the autonomic nervous system by way of the brain. The physical sciences tell us that the nervous system conducts electrical impulses that order the body's biological rhythms, such as heartbeat, breath, movement, and immune system functioning. Science has also established that all electric currents radiate an electromagnetic field. These facts are important in acknowledging the crucial role of energy-vibrational medicine in the healing arts.

Definitions of matter and consciousness are important in the holographic-halographic paradigm. The definition of matter is a waveform of the Essene Tree of Life's radiant energy transduced into the third dimension. This "matter" could be manifested or formed as the physical human body, a rock, a planet, or a galaxy. Regardless of its form, this matter is made up of different "waveforms" of "electromagnetic energy" at the third-dimensional level. It does not, however, exist in a vacuum; it exists within the larger "multidimensional" matrix system, which some call the "Grid of Consciousness." The word "halogram or halographic" is used by Carl Johan Calleman to differentiate the holographic model of David Bohm and Carl Pribram, in which the universe is a product of interference patterns of waveforms that provide for the universe an implicate order, i.e., a deeper underlying nature that unfolds into the explicate order that we normally perceive.[20] The halographic model Calleman presented included what he perceives as a missing link in the holographic model. This missing link is an understanding of the source of these waveforms and how they have generated an orderly universe. Mayan cosmology suggests that *Hunab Ku* ("the one god") imposes polarized fields on the universe, creating coherent organizations of life on different levels. Thus, a hierarchical organization of life manifests, and the boundaries and energies of the microcosms are ultimately defined by the macrocosms that could be called holonomic in alignment with the work of Arthur Koestler.[21] Calleman further states, "I prefer to talk about the universe as Halographic, since there is much data to indicate that the Holons are formed by Halos generated by spinning Trees of Life at different levels of the universe."[22]

Consciousness is the awareness of existence; thus arises the adage: "know thyself." Information is necessary for awareness; there are levels of awareness and, therefore, different levels of information for the many levels. In this current period of the evolution of consciousness, humans are evolving to "super-human" status or a divine state of being. Simply put, "a divine state of being" means we will have the ability to consciously co-create with the Source. Our divine nature has always been in existence, but our awareness of it has not. The next expression in the evolution of consciousness is to "be divine." Conscious awareness is one thing, *being* is another altogether. The purpose of the EMCS process is to provide greater awareness of our individual divine nature by clearing the beliefs and attachments that disconnect humanity from its divine nature and to offer tools to make divine expression possible.

It is common knowledge that the quality of our thoughts, feelings, and emotions indicates levels of consciousness. Consciousness is primary, meaning that consciousness activates the neurons of the brain to fire a certain pattern. Consciousness flows from the outside, which influences the quality of thoughts, feelings, and emotions that have a positive or negative impact not only on the system itself but on the surrounding environment, external as well as internal. Habitual survivalist thoughts eventually negatively impact the health of the cellular and energetic structure of the subtle energy of the holographic-halographic human energy system. The process of EMCS has proven to be an efficacious methodology for reestablishing the vital flow of life force, resulting in the overall vitality of the entire holographic human energy system.

As a result of famed Austrian psychoanalyst Wilhelm Reich's work and the work of his followers, there is clear recognition that the autonomic nervous system plays an integral part in the communication of the human energy system.[23] It has been determined that the autonomic nervous system is an interface between the physical body and emotional processes. Because of its close connection to the functions of internal organs, it serves as a messenger for emotional perception by way of the blood and plasma. The central nervous system's connection with areas of the cerebral cortex creates a connection with emotions[24].

The efficacy of the Energy Matrix Clearing System rests upon these scientific facts. To summarize, EMCS specifically focuses on removing blockages in the human holographic/halographic energy anatomy that involve the following:

- brain functions
- autonomic nervous system
- meridians

- chakras
- the etheric, astral, mental, and causal bodies
- and the guiding ray energy systems.

CHAPTER TWO

KINESIOLOGY

Kinesiology is a diagnostic tool used to access information from the human holographic energy anatomy. It is a key component in the EMCS process. American chiropractor George Goodheart introduced this new science, which he called Applied Kinesiology, in 1964. Since that time, the use of kinesiology has expanded into a wide range of therapeutic fields.

During the late 1970s, Australian physician and holistic practitioner John Diamond refined the science into a process he called Behavioral Kinesiology. He discovered that indicator muscles, i.e., the muscles being tested, would strengthen or weaken in the presence of negative emotional and intellectual stimuli. David Hawkins took Diamonds' work further through his discovery "that this kinesiology response reflects a capacity of the human organism to differentiate not only positive from negative stimuli, but also anabolic (life-enhancing) from catabolic (life-consuming) and, most dramatically, true from false."[25] Goodheart had already discovered that indicator muscles would do the same with physical stimuli. In other words, a negative response, such as "no," would cause the muscle indicator to go weak, and a positive one, such as "yes," would cause a strong muscle response. The Energy Matrix Clearing System uses yes and no questions to check for clear muscle response. A strong muscle response results when a yes question is asked, and a weak muscle response results when a no question is asked.

The Energy Matrix Clearing System grew out of my study of the One Brain system developed by Gordon Stokes and Daniel Whiteside. Research studies conducted by Stokes and Whiteside determining the accuracy of muscle testing have shown that muscle checking or "brain-testing" is accurate to the ninety-seventh percentile when "issues are accurately identified."[26]

We have already determined that the holographic human energy system has the capacity to hold information as well as respond to it. This means the system holds within it all the information about the person being tested. This explains the accuracy of kinesiology shown through the research of Stokes and Whiteside and the predictable, repeatable, and universal results that John Diamond demonstrated.

Physician and spiritual healer David Hawkins, intrigued by Diamond's work, began his own research using kinesiology to determine human levels of consciousness. He discovered kinesiological testing could accurately "calibrate human levels of consciousness so that an arbitrary logarithmic scale of whole numbers emerges, stratifying the relative power of levels of consciousness in all areas of human experience."[27] He further determined that the calibrated levels of human consciousness correlated with emotional and intellectual phenomena found in sociology, clinical psychology, and traditional spirituality.

The Kinesiology Federation defines kinesiology as " . . . literally the study of body movement." In their Thorsons Introductory Guide to Kinesiology, Maggie la Tourelle and Anthea Courtenay describe kinesiology as a "holistic approach" to balancing the interaction of movement and energy systems.[28] Kinesiology, according to the guide, can be used as a method to determine where blockages and/or imbalances are impairing physical, emotional, or energetic well-being. It follows that identifying blockages and bringing those blockages back to balance can lead to increased physical, mental, emotional, and spiritual health. That is what EMCS accomplishes.

The Mechanics of Muscle Testing

Muscle testing using the traditional kinesiology method has the testing subject stand erect, the right arm relaxed at the side of the body, the left arm out parallel to the floor, and the elbow straight. The person conducting the muscle checking places one hand on the opposite shoulder of the client for stability while placing light pressure using the pointer and middle fingers on the opposite hand just above the wrist of the arm being used for checking.

Specialized kinesiology departs from this traditional form by asking the client to hold both arms parallel to the floor simultaneously at about a thirty-degree angle. This provides a comfortable position for the subject, and since the body works in a cross pattern—the right brain hemisphere operating the left side of the body and vice versa—this checking procedure accesses both brain hemispheres. As Diamond proved, this method bypasses the belief system, providing accurate results because the belief system cannot interfere.

The "energician," in this case, applies only the lightest amount of pressure with the fingers just above the subject's wrists. It is only necessary to make contact with the subject's skin so that the energician can be aware of any movement of the arms. The pressure applied by the energician on the wrists should be no more than the weight of a nickel coin. A release of the arm indicated by a downward movement indicates a weak response—a no or indicator change. If the arms do not move, this is considered a strong indicator—a yes response or a blocked muscle circuit.

The range of movement of the anterior deltoid muscle is from the thirty-degree angle to just past the midline of the body. Educate your subject about this range of movement. Take their hands and move them through this range of motion before muscle checking. This will show them their "job" as a subject. The greatest extension of the anterior deltoid muscle is at the front thirty-degree position. The greatest contraction of the muscle is just past the midline of the body. Any greater extension or contraction results in other muscle involvement, which compromises accurate muscle checking.

Accurate Muscle Checking

To ensure accurate muscle checking, always ask checking questions in a way that achieves both an affirmative and negative response. It is possible to ask an entire series of yes questions, while receiving a hold strong response when the person is blocked or overwhelmed. To avoid this situation, either ask every question in a way that requires both a strong response and a weak one or stop along your checking process and verify a clear muscle circuit.

To begin, take a deep breath, avert your eyes to the left or right of the subject, and bring your consciousness to the palms of your hands as your fingers lightly touch the skin just above the wrist of the subject. Say, "Give me a yes," and wait for the response. The response will be no movement. After a moment, test by saying, "Give me a no," and wait for the response. The response will be a downward movement or "muscle release."

If you do not get a response, ask the subject to take a deep breath along with you and start again. Often, body circuits go into stress from dehydration, so make sure water is accessible for the client to drink if needed when muscle checking. Hydration is important for accurate muscle testing.

Terminology is also important in muscle checking. There are two methods of getting responses from the body through kinesiology. The first method is a "yes or no" question, as in *"Give me a yes"* and *"Give me a no."* The second method is to ask for indicator changes. For instance, *"Give me an indicator change for the priority number 1, 2, 3, [etc. . . .],"* until the arms release for the indicator change. *Do not* ask for an indicator change and then say, *"It is number 1, 2, 3, . . . ,"* because this is asking for a verbal response of "yes" or "no," not an indicator change. This causes fear and self-doubt to come on line, resulting in a "confused" answer. Be clear when asking questions or making statements while checking muscles; this will make checking easier and will result in increased muscle-checking assurance.

Accurate muscle checking requires both the subject and the "energician" to be "present in the moment." This means that both are relaxed, breathing and have both eyes open. Many people tend to close their eyes while being muscle-checked. Closing the eyes during muscle testing often triggers "past" issues, and as a result, the person may slip out of the present time, and fear may come on line, causing interference and making accurate muscle checking more challenging.

Identifying a clear muscle circuit involves getting an appropriate response given the question presented. For instance, when the "energician" asks, *"Give me a yes,"* the appropriate physical response is that the arms remain in a strong position. This position is the full extension of the anterior deltoid muscle or an approximate thirty-degree angle.

When the "energician" asks, *"What is a no?"* or *"Give me a no,"* the appropriate arm response is a slow muscle release in a downward motion. This happens because the proprioceptor located in the belly of the checked muscle (in this case, the anterior deltoid) communicates a negative response to the brain. The brain releases the muscle to use all its attention to respond to the negative situation at hand. When asked a negative question such as *"What is a no?"* the arms do not release; instead, they hold strong. This indicates a blocked, switched, or overloaded muscle circuit, now termed systemic energetic interference (SEI) by the Association of Comprehensive Energy Psychology.

The following describes the process through which energy psychology addresses three core psycho-energetic dimensions. Information from the Association for Comprehensive Energy Psychology (ACEP) states:

> One straightforward way to describe the key elements of the psycho-spiritual growth process is through the phrase, 'Ready, willing, able.' Energy-psychology methods address all three of these dimensions in new, elegant ways that, so far, appear to be more effective, rapid, and lasting than most previously available psychotherapeutic methods.[29]

The three core psycho-energetic dimensions, as described by the ACEP, are:

1. *Readiness*: established through removing any existing Systemic Energetic Interferences that prevent successful treatment of specific psychological issues. Gary Craig, of Emotional Freedom Technique (EFT) fame, says this core dimension is like setting up the pins at a bowling alley. Unless the pins are set correctly, the possibility of getting a strike diminishes; similarly, this treatment dimension concerns psycho-energetically preparing the human system to respond efficiently to treatment.

2. *Willingness*: established through removing any psycho-energetic objections to treatment with a specific issue. Many people say they want to lose weight or become wealthy but instead spend their time and energy in fear of achieving their goal. This treatment dimension is about securing psycho-energetic permission to succeed with treatment.

3. *Ability*: facilitated through "Resonance Recalibration," in which a person's energetic resonance with goal-interfering blockages (e.g., undigested life experiences, limiting beliefs, "baggage") is neutralized, and their resonance with a desired goal is amplified. Think of an image of someone whose resonance to any baggage that has kept her from her goal has completely faded, and in its place is a strong, unimpeded resonance that enhances her ability to manifest a goal.[30]

CHAPTER THREE

CHECKING FOR SYSTEMIC ENERGETIC INTERFERENCE (SEI)

Systemic Energetic Interferences (SEI) identified within EMCS include blocked, overloaded, and switched energetic circuitry. Many sources may cause interference within the holographic human energy system. Systemic Energetic Interferences may be the result of long-held negative beliefs that limit and restrict life expression and, therefore, interfere with the readiness to heal. Traumatic life experiences like trauma, physical, mental, emotional, and sexual abuse may also be a cause of SEI. These experiences may lead to a pattern of control or perfectionist behaviors that tend to overwhelm, deplete, or "blow out" the energetic system. An inability to set healthy emotional boundaries, nutritional or biochemical imbalances, food sensitivities, and toxicities like mold, pollen, household cleaning products, and air pollutants may also be causes of SEI.[31]

A blocked muscle circuit is indicated by a lack of movement no matter what question is asked; this is the result of extreme stress and fear. The stressor has virtually locked the muscle in place. The individual has "checked out" of present time to avoid, deny, or escape specific unacceptable emotions. Correction of a blocked circuit may be as simple as asking the person to take a deep breath followed by suggesting that she come back to the present time. Check again, asking a new question soliciting a "yes" response. Immediately rephrase the same question to produce a "no" response. Often, this will produce a clear muscle circuit, and you may continue with the defusion process. If that simple process does not clear the muscle circuit for accurate muscle checking, ask the client to join you in taking a drink of water and then lead the client in several rounds of cross-patterning by first crossing the right palm to the left knee and then crossing the left palm to the right knee. Next, switch to right hand to right knee and left hand to left knee, ipsilateral, for four or five rounds before returning to cross patterning. Always end on a cross pattern.

Overloaded Circuits

Overloaded circuits indicate sufficient fear held in the system causing it to "short circuit."[32] A reversal of polarity has occurred. A question designed to produce a yes answer will produce a no answer. This results in "switching" and can be verified by the polarity test. Muscle check one arm with the right hand, one polarity, and then with the left hand, another polarity. Notice what happens. Next, muscle check both arms at the same time in the usual manner, then recheck, crossing your hands. If there is an indicator change in any of these checks, an indication of belief system fears is on line. Correct this by assuring the subject that muscle checking is accurate and beneficial. Ask the client to breathe, assuring him that everything that needs to be accessed for defusion success will be.

Stokes and Whiteside identified an area in the left-brain hemisphere called the Common Integrative Area (CIA) that is located just above and behind the left ear[33]. Their research indicates the CIA houses and activates negative belief system information to facilitate survival. This area, identified as the CIA, is part of the limbic system of the brain. Researchers have also labeled it the survival, emotional, and reptilian brain, as well as the limbic system. This area interacts with what is known as the astral-emotional subtle energy body, which has made it possible for the human species to survive for hundreds of thousands of years. For this reason, it is valuable. Because it starts automatically, it is difficult for us to know when it is "running the show." This automatic survival response is holographic, meaning that the whole system is involved in the reactive response. It happens with such speed that we do not often notice that it is running the show. The primary purpose of the reactive response system is to determine the actions necessary to survive pain and fear, as well as the fear of future pain, according to Stokes and Whiteside. The limbic system does not have the capacity to think and "create new options." It can only react, and its reaction is based on the recorded actions that worked for survival. The system compares this stored data and chooses the path most likely to cause the least amount of pain. It does not have the option to choose a response based on peace, joy, love, or enlightenment because these can only be accessed by the neocortex or the reasoning brain, which the limbic bypasses in the survival reaction. The language of the survival brain is fear, self-doubt, anger, resentment, and separation. The survival brain has a limited ability to communicate with memory based on perceptions and emotions attached to a particular painful event.

We can, therefore, deduce that survival reactions are driven by negative emotion, the effect of blocked energy. This specifically happens in the meridian system. When the system heats up because of the blocked energy, the triple warmer meridian communicates the problem to the hypothalamus, which determines the extent of the problem and either sends the information to the neo-cortex or the amygdala. The actions necessary to resolve the problem with the least amount of pain are then set into motion.

EMCS Living in Choice Levels of Responsibility Chart

The EMCS Living in Choice Levels of Responsibility chart is central to the work of EMCS. On the left side of the chart (or the right if you are facing the chart), it demonstrates reactive beliefs and their corresponding thoughts, feelings, and emotions. On the right side of the chart, the thoughts, feelings, and emotions generated from a proactive state of mind are listed. The reactive side of the chart indicates the patterns of resistance to the pain. Diffusing the energy blockages that trigger these reactions resumes thinking and effective strategies for living life joyfully and spontaneously. Clients often make statements such as "I feel lighter" or "Wow, that was a crazy way to look at it, but it makes sense."

The EMCS Living in Choice Levels of Responsibility chart encourages self-responsibility. In this system, "energicians" are not in the business of making decisions for their clients. They are in the business of identifying information held within the holographic/halographic human energy system. They are trained in techniques that diffuse energy blockages, thus reinstating the flow of vital energy and returning the system to a state of health and wellness in the physical, emotional, mental, and spiritual realms.

ENERGY MATRIX CLEARING SYSTEMS

LEVELS OF RESPONSIBILITY

PRO-ACTIVE	RE-ACTIVE
COURAGE Affirming, empowered, feasible constructive, strong, active, positive, engaged, excited, imaginative, possible, feasible	**ANTAGONISM** Hides inadequacy, attached, annoyed, combative, indignant, bothered, counter-active, burdened, opposing
WILLING Intentional, optimistic, enthusiastic, prepared, courageous, adequate, creative, playful, invigorated, answerable, worthwhile, responsible	**PRIDE/INDIFFERENCE** Belligerent, demanding, scornful, pessimistic, immobilized, numb, unfeeling, stagnant, destructive, disconnected, rigid, detrimental
NEUTRAL Trust, satisfied, interested, fascinated, welcomed, needed, essential, tuned in, appreciated	**ANGER/RESENTMENT** Hides behind "You hurt me and that gives me the right to protect myself", confused, incensed, overwrought, wounded, hysterical, wrathful, fuming, furious, abused, unappreciated, rejected, numb, offended, hurt & used.
ACCEPTANCE Harmonious, forgiving, adaptable, worthy, open, amused, approachable, deserving, choosing to, owning	**DESIRE/HOSTILITY** Blaming, "Someone else is responsible for me not getting what I want.", Frustrated picked on, sarcastic, trapped, mean, deprived, withholding, vindictive
REASON Wise, understanding, bold, proud, daring, protected, selfless, thoughtful, motivated, considerate, understanding	**FEAR** Anxious, escape, "Something will be taken away from me." avoids, uncared for, trapped, disappointed, frightened, threatened, overlooked, unacceptable, unwelcome
LOVE Reverent, benign, revelatory, risking, trusting, caring, knowing, pleasurable, secure, respectful, giving, responsible	**GRIEF** Regretful, despondent, tragic, self-blaming, victim, depressed, unacceptable, morose, despondent, melancholy, defeated, deserted
JOY Serenity, whole, exuberant, fullfilled, energetic, complete, unencumbered	**SHAME** "I wont't survive", humiliation, cowardice, betrayed, disgraced, self-blaming, dishonored, bad (embarrassed), doubtful
PEACE Perfection, bliss, harmony, trust, thoughtfulness, nurturing, complete	**SEPARATION/GUILT** Self destructive, non-entity, "God does not love me, therefore, I am unlovable", lost, ruined, condemned, ineffectual, conquered
ENLIGHTENMENT Pure, sincere, ineffable, aware, respectful, appreciating, powerful	**APATHY** Waiting to succumb, resigned, hopeless, takes no responsibility for cause, uncared for, insignificant, powerlessness, distrustful & suspicious

EMOTION — FEELING — THOUGHT (left and right margins)

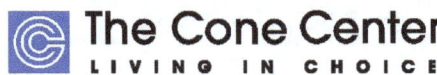

The Cone Center
LIVING IN CHOICE

CHAPTER FOUR

LEVEL OF CONSCIOUSNESS

Torkom Saraydarian writes in his book *The Ageless Wisdom*, "Advancement on the ladder of evolution is achieved by your consciousness, then growing toward it with your 'beingness.' 'Beingness' is transformed immediately when your consciousness moves ahead."[34]

Within the context of EMCS, identification of current levels of awareness is helpful in assessing the consciousness level driving a particular issue and individual personal choices. The Energy Matrix Clearing System uses the Living in Choice Levels of Responsibility chart and David Hawkins" 'Map of Consciousness" from his groundbreaking book *Power vs Force*. These powerful tools indicate the belief patterns that cause the energy blockages that eventually result in life-limiting expressions—physical, emotional, and spiritual dysfunction, or "dis-ease." A complete explanation of the chart and its use is in my book titled *The Power of Living In Choice*.

Energy Matrix Clearing System Format

The framework of EMCS consists of gathering information using kinesiology in order to address a specific identified issue. For instance, a client may present for treatment to resolve issues of depression, anger, relationship dysfunction, physical dis-ease, or financial lack. Muscle checking will assist the energician in determining the priority issue with which to work.

Discussing these issues with the client as limiting patterns rather than as problems is important because it begins to separate the person from the "problem." It also helps identify the habitual, self-effacing thoughts, feelings, and emotions causing the limitation. These habitual, self-effacing patterns are blocked or distorted energy-information pathways that result in lower frequency modulation. The presented issue, while obviously causing pain in the life of the individual, is only a symptom of a greater cause. It is this cause that the structural format of EMCS identifies and diffuses. Within the holographic perspective, discovery of the whole within the piece is possible. Client dialogue and muscle checking identify the exact language for defusion focus. After identifying the issue and specific language, muscle test for present time information indicated in the following EMCS Case Notes form.

Energy Matrix Clearing System

CASE NOTES SPECIFIC TO MATRIX I AND II

_____

NAME   DATE

_____

ISSUE

_____

NEE

_____

PEE

Subtle Energy Bodies: P E A M C   **Matrix System Effected I, II**

_____Level of Responsibility

_____Avoidance Behavior (15)

_____Specific Point (13)

_____Meridian (14)

_____Side of Body (R or L)

_____Polarity (Middle: +, Index: -, or Both: +, -)

_____Element (5)

_____Neurolymphatic point (use chart: go by muscle number)

_____Neurovascular point (use chart: go by muscle number)

Age of Cause _____ Age On Line _____

Correction:

SEB: P E A M C   **Matrix System Effected I, II**

_____Level of Responsibility

_____Finger

_____Specific point (13)

_____Meridian (14)

_____Side of Body (R or L)

_____Polarity

_____Element (5)

_____Neurolymphatic point (use chart: go by muscle number)

_____Neurovascular point (use chart: go by muscle number)

_____

HOMEWORK

_____

NOTES

_____

_____

_____

_____

_____

CHAPTER FIVE

EMCS PROTOCOL AND PROCEDURE

The protocol and procedure for EMCS are as follows:

Systems Energetic Interferences

1. Using muscle checking, identify root cause non-transient Systems Energetic Interferences and make notations on the EMCS Case Notes form of any of the patterns as indicated by muscle checking:

   - Core Negative Beliefs (chapter eleven)
   - Shadow Beliefs (Appendix IV)
   - Historical (past life carry-over)
   - Genetically inherited patterns

   Soul distortions, including:
   - Lost Will[35] (see Lost Will Casual Beliefs, chapter fourteen)
   - Divine Essence[36]
   - Soul Level Essence[37]
   - Dimensions[38]
   - Ancestrally inherited patterns

2. Continue muscle testing for blockages held in any of the subtle energy bodies: physical, etheric, astral, mental, or causal.

3. Identify the levels of responsibility on the issue from the EMCS Living in Choice Levels of Responsibility chart.

4. Muscle check for the negative emotional charge on the issue by first asking, "More than infinity?" Notice the response. If you receive a strong response, the Negative Emotional Energy (NEE) is as high as it can be because there isn't "more" than infinity. If you receive a weak or no response, make the statement, "Less than infinity." A strong response indicates the NEE is less than infinity.

5. Next, check for less than infinity by saying, "Give me an indicator change and then muscle check: 0 to 50, 50 to 100, 100 to 150 . . . " until you receive the indicator change. Note the NEE on the case notes sheet.

Repeat the process for Positive Emotional Energy (PEE) beginning with the statement:

"more than a thousand, less than a thousand." If the statement "more than a thousand" holds strong, continue in increments of 1000 until the indicator makes the change. Note the change on the case notes sheets. If the statement "less than a thousand," makes the indicator change begin at 0 to 50, as in the above example, until the indicator makes the change. Note the number on the case notes sheet in the designated place.

Negative Emotional Energy (NEE) represents the amount of resistance (doubt) or the amount of investment the client has in maintaining the survival pattern. The higher the number, the more identification the client has with the negative state. When infinity comes up as the ultimate amount of identification to resisting the negative state, it means there is nothing new to learn concerning the negative state. The negative state has become a "truth" or a "fact" that is believed to be unchangeable. In this case, the good news is the resistance is gone, and the pain of the "fact" is all that remains. It is much easier to deal with the pain because it is unacceptable, and willingness comes much easier. Resistance and denial are closely related and are strong adversaries.

Positive Emotional Energy (PEE), in its origin, represents the amount of willingness to release negative states or survival responses. The test is from 0 to 100. The lower the number, the less the willingness. The higher the number, the greater the willingness.

Several years ago, when testing clients for PEE, I began to get indicator changes greater than one hundred; most often, they were 1000. Curious, I began to seek an answer for this change while meditating. The revelation came that the change was due to consciousness evolving from the third dimension to the fourth dimension. The third dimension is the material world and represents the manifestations of the five senses. It is the dimension of linear space and time in which we humans live with other biological creatures, including the plant kingdom. The fourth dimension, according to Barbara Hand Clow,[39] operates in the third dimension as subtle frequencies. These frequencies are nonphysical realms expressed through archetypal thoughts, geometry, mythology, and the memory of humanity throughout all time. This dimensional shift was very important to the EMCS process because it allowed the energician and client to access, receive, and use the information for healing from this realm. Recently, muscle checking has turned up numbers greater than 1000, indicating another shift in the evolution of consciousness. The ramifications of this shift for EMCS are unclear; however, I can only speculate the shift will serve to elevate the efficacy of the process.

Miasms, Drainers, Entities, Curses

Miasms, drainers, entities, and curses are the next areas of interest in gathering information by way of muscle testing. All of these are past-time energies and patterns. According to psychiatrist Rudolph Ballentine, "The word 'miasm' dates to a time when diseases were attributed to the evil vapors that permeated a locale."[40] However, Samuel Hahnemann, the father of homeopathy, was able to see beyond the veil of superstition attributed to diseases to reveal the deeper foundation of consciousness feeding the recurrence of chronic disease. He was able to identify remedies to remove the miasmic pattern, thus freeing the sufferer from the disease.

Hahnemann identified three miasms: psora, sycosis, and syphilis. Psora's classical symptoms include skin disorders like rashes, scabies, psoriasis, and warts. Sycosis' symptoms affect the mucous membranes and include gonorrhea, genital warts, and discharges of phlegm and nasal mucus from the nose and throat. Classical symptoms of syphilis are ulceration and central nervous system erosion. Tuberculosis is the fourth miasm, and cancer is actually a combination of all the miasms. Miasms attach to the astral body partly because it has a chaotic nature and partly because it is the seat of fear-based survival programming, according to Byron Gentry, a wonderful friend and mentor, who wrote of entities, piggybacks, and demons in his powerful book *Miracles of the Mind*.[41]

Entities and drainers refer to both actual living beings and energetic beings that inhabit the holographic human energy system. They primarily feed off the negative energy of anger.[42] "Three of the most detrimental afflictions affecting my patients have to do with entities, piggybacks, and demons," Gentry writes in *Miracles of the Mind*, "As farfetched as it may sound, these unwelcome spirits are quite real and are able to produce some incredibly unpleasant conditions."[43]

These entities, he writes, are disembodied spirits of the deceased who, for some reason, have not moved to "the other side." He gives some reasons for this: mourners who refuse to let go; negative projections from the living, who still hold negative thought forms toward the deceased; and disembodied spirits who loved earthly life so much they don't want to leave.

In her book *Invisible Roots*, psychotherapist Barbara Stone writes that disembodied spirits or "earthbound spirits," as she terms them, appear to stay earthbound for some of the same reasons mentioned by Byron but adds they stay earthbound because of "having strong negative feelings at the moment of a traumatic death."[44] She also has determined in her work that some stay earthbound because they fear "retribution for misdeeds."[45]

"Piggybacks," according to Gentry, are another matter altogether. These disembodied spirits are not "transient in nature" and, therefore, join an individual at the moment of conception, fusing or "piggybacking" onto their living host. Gentry, who had a wonderful sense of humor, likened piggybacks to bad tenants—impossible to remove unless you got out the "big guns," which in his case were the Holy Spirit and His angels. Gentry collectively called the angels the White Brotherhood. He would call on them to escort piggybacks to the other side so that they could continue their soul paths.[46]

Curses and hexes are often associated with the voodoo practices of witch doctors. The energician's work is not, however, in any way related to "voodoo." The Energy Matrix Clearing System includes these types of energies as systemic energetic interferences that cause energy systems to be blocked or distorted, resulting in client dis-ease. Since thoughts are things that affect other things, curses and hexes can bind energy both to a person and to a location. The energician identifies curses, curse energy, or patterns that are related to long-held generational, past life, and ancestral survival patterns. The person, unconscious of these innate patterns, is not aware that the curse or hex is responsible for their diseased state. Canceling curse energy is the only way to resolve the pattern. A curse is similar to a miasm, except curses cover a wide range of "dis-ease": poverty mentality, entitlement, physical pain, racism, and negative life choices. When identified in an EMCS session, the energician determines through muscle checking whether the SEI must be cleared at the present time or age of cause. If the present time is identified as the point to clear the SEI, then the energician muscle checks to determine where the SEI (curse/hex) is attached to the energy system. This usually is one or more of the chakras. In EMCS, however, the energician must identify which level of the chakra system— etheric, astral, mental, or causal—the attachment is held. Once the attachment location or locations have been identified, the energician muscle checks to identify the method of clearing by way of the Energy Matrix Clearing System matrices, depending on the location of the SEI. The energician determines the order of clearing (if multiple chakras are involved) and follows normal EMCS protocol to clear. In honor of Gentry's calling in of the Holy Spirit and the White Brotherhood to assist in releasing piggybacks and entities, EMCS includes several lists of angels, archangels, and other archetypes, should those energies be identified as necessary for assistance in clearing any SEI.

Present Time Information

These next testing categories make up all present-time information for an EMCS session:

- FlorAlive Essences
- Pleiadian Glyphs if PEE is greater than 1000
- Animal Essences if PEE is less than 1000
- Avoidance Behavior
- Universal Fear
- Reflective Mirror
- Ten Elements
- Archetype
- Hexagram[47]
- Level of Consciousness
- Kabbalistic 72 Names of God[48]
- Matrix Systems

The explanation of these categories follows in succeeding chapters. They represent "placeholders" for the first half of the EMCS defusion process. Upon completion of present time data, present the information to the client, and then begin age recession.

Age Recession

Instruct the client to stand and hold their arms in the appropriate position to engage their anterior deltoid muscle.

Recheck to make sure you still have a clear muscle circuit, then begin testing to age of cause or the age that is best to correct.

Begin at the present age of the client by asking them to give you an indicator change to the age of cause. Descend in increments of five years until you receive an indicator change. An indicator change can mean this is the age of cause, which is the age that is best to correct. It can also mean an age online. Be sure to clarify by asking if this is or is not the age of cause.

A hold strong on "This is the age of cause" indicates a "yes" answer. If the answer is affirmative, continue to gather the information indicated on the EMCS case note sheet. Sometimes an age on line has made the indicator change. This being the case, adding this information into the circuitry (see instructions below) and diffusing it along with the age of cause information is an option.

Intentional use of energy is a powerful and effective method of energy medicine. Intention anchors information into the energetic memory or "circuits" to be retained for later use. When information comes up during a defusion process, other than the age of cause, loading that information into the system releases it at the age of cause.

There are several methods for "loading a circuit." The easiest to use is as follows:

- Say, "I am putting this age-information into the circuit to be corrected at the age of cause."

- Simultaneously, the energician "flicks" their thumbs on the skin of each wrist of the testee; this indicates storage of the information for further use.
- Next, muscle checks again to affirm you have the information in the circuit by testing or saying, "I have the information loaded in the circuit with the intention of clearing it at the age of cause. Is there any reason I do not have permission to correct at the age of cause?"

The age of cause can be any age on the timeline of life, including in the womb and at conception. It can also refer to generations, ancestral ages, past lives, and soul levels. Be sensitive to a client's past life belief system; if the client does not believe in past lives, simply asking that question may cause a blockage, switching, or reversal of energy. If you suspect this is the case, you can circumvent the issue by using other terminology, such as "energy of spirit before conception."

Energy never dies. It can change form, but it does not die. This being the case, the person must have been in some form before conception. To be complete in the defusion process, this must be included in the intentional process.

Information gathered at the age of cause is a repeat of the information gathered in the present time; however, the answers will be different because they relate to a different time in the person's life. Once all the information is gathered, including the matrix systems indicating outages or blockages, make the corrections. Matrix systems and corrections are covered in later chapters.

Next, muscle-check for the data, discuss it with your client and make the necessary corrections. (Corrections are covered in the chapters on matrix systems.) Follow with muscle checking to verify that NEE is zero and PEE is at least 100. If so, determine by muscle checking the infusion symbol; most often, this is the element identified at the age of cause. Instruct the client to focus on the positive image of the elemental energy and anchor that image back to the present time.

When in the present time, check to ensure the client is in the present time by asking, "Are you right here, right now, 100 percent in the present time?"

- Look for a hold strong. If you get a weak response, ask, "Give me an indicator change for the appropriate method to move you to the present time."

Next, ask/muscle check:

- Take a deep breath
- Perform cross patterning
- Drink water
- Make another correction

Usually, taking a deep breath will suffice.

After making sure the client is in the present time, PEE is at least 100, and NEE is 0, muscle check for homework. Homework usually consists of continuing the infusion symbol for a specified number of days. Muscle check by stating: "Give me an indicator change for a number of days: 1, 2, 3 . . . " until you receive an indicator change.

Then ask, "How many times a day: 1, 2, 3 . . . ?"

Congratulations! You have just completed the defusion.

EMCS Matrix Systems

The EMCS matrix systems contain specific energetic clearing methods for specific blockages. They correspond to specific areas of the holographic human energy system, including the physical, which can become blocked because of held beliefs, trauma, generational patterns, painful life experiences, and even past life trauma carried forward into this lifetime. Identification of the blocked energy enables the energician to:

1. Know which energetic process will clear the blockage and
2. Give specific information regarding the long-held pattern(s) that eventually led to the current disease.

Each matrix covers a specific area of the holographic human energy system. There are thirteen matrix systems identified in EMCS. Each matrix has multiple subsystems depending on the area of the holographic human energy system covered by the specific matrix. In energy psychology/medicine, energy *is* the medicine, therefore, each matrix uses a specific form of energy medicine to correct a specific energy blockage. In Matrix I, the energy medicine is the energy of the holographic human energy system itself. In other matrix categories, energy medicine includes homeopathic remedies or vibrations from gem and mineral, animal, and flower essences. Essential oils and the vibration of color and sound are options available in the EMCS protocol.

CHAPTER SIX

MATRIX I AND MATRIX II

Matrix I

If Matrix I makes the indicator change during muscle checking to clear an energy blockage, muscle check for the specific correction "by the number."

Make the statement," Give me an indicator change by the number for the priority clearing method for this blockage, 1, 2, 3, etc."

Then follow the instructions given below for correction.

Matrix I clearing techniques include the following:

1. *Cross patterning:* Start by walking in place, placing the right hand on the left knee as it comes up, and switch the left hand to the right knee as it comes up. This is the cross pattern. Do five or more repetitions of the cross, then switch to ipsilateral hand movements: parallel touching of right hand to right knee and left hand to left knee. Always end on the cross patterning.

2. *Hydration:* Drink water to hydrate the system.

3. *Frontal occipital hold:* Place one hand on the forehead and the other just at the occipital bone on the back of the head while taking deep breaths. Hold until the sense of a shift is felt.

4. *Polarity navel hold:* Hold one hand on the navel while massaging with thumb and index and pointer fingers (neutral touch) the kidney 27 acupuncture point just below the collar bone, move with neutral touch to the upper and lower lip (thumb below and fingers above), and finally move the neutral touch hand to the tailbone-coccyx and massage. Switch hands and repeat the process.

5. *Breathing:* Both the client and energician take several deep breaths.

6. *Shine a light on the glabella.* The glabella, a fissure in the skull located in the center of the forehead, is designed to let white light enter the forebrain. Researchers have determined that white light is the only energy that activates the forebrain.

Matrix II: The Meridian System

Health is the natural state of the universe and, therefore, of humankind. The constant dynamic flow of the universe defines health. Any interruption in this natural energy flow causes disease. I agree with Torkom Saraydarian's assertion that "health is equilibrium." The law of balance dictates that if your thoughts are out of balance, so too is your body out of balance. Our unbalanced thoughts cannot unbalance the universe, but the universe does balance that which is out of balance, i.e., for every action, there is an equal and opposite reaction. So, in a very real sense, when you are suffering from the symptoms of a cold, your physical system is in the process of bringing into balance that which was out of balance. The human energy system is constantly interacting with energy information from the ocean of energy in which it "swims" in a constant. Elegant process of equilibrium with it. This living system can and often does become so out of balance that it appears to be "ill." Traditional Western medicine has focused on this extreme disequilibrium state as "cause," and because of this perception, western medicine has built a model for "health" that supports continued disequilibrium rather than the system's inherent ability to find a new balance. Contrary to the focus of Western medicine, energy psychology and energy medicine focuses on assisting the holographic human energy system's inherent ability to find a new balance, making possible the flow of "life force" from system to system and bringing balance in each system and between the systems. Balance equals health!

The focus of Matrix II is the meridian system, which has been the foundation of traditional Chinese medicine for thousands of years. The Chinese use the term qi or chi (che) to indicate the natural force of life that flows into and through the human energy system, providing the "food of life" that vitalizes the entire system. Chi makes life possible. When we say that we don't have any energy, it means that our system is out of balance in some areas of life.

Chi moves through the physical body by way of the meridian system. The ancient Chinese art of acupuncture attempts to return the flow of chi to a state of balance or vitality as it moves through the meridian system, thus, to the major organs of the physical body that it serves. However, chi is not limited to the meridian system; it flows through the chakra system and subtle energy bodies, which also play significant roles in maintaining the vitality of the human holographic energy system and, thus, the physical body. The energy that flows through the chakra system flows into the meridian system, and the energy that flows through the subtle energy bodies surrounding the physical is the same energy. Each of these systems uses the energy/information carried upon or within the chi, modulating and transducing it according to the need of each.

After the chakras and subtle energy bodies have filtered the chi according to their specific need, it is then distributed through the meridian system to the nervous system and each of the physical organs. Like acupuncture, energy psychology and energy medicine use technology that strives to activate communication by way of the autonomic nervous system, thus inducing the system to seek a more vital and balanced state.

The Energy Matrix Clearing System honors the fourteen life-force pathways identified in traditional Chinese medicine. Twelve of these are found within the physical body and carry the names of the major organs they vitalize. Two are located outside the body and are known as the central and the governing vessels. Each meridian contains a chi surface collection and transportation component. All meridians are either "excitatory" or "inhibitory," depending on the polarity of the chi energy they control. Positive ions excite, and negative ions inhibit. The organs also function in this dual process of excitation and inhibition. The insertion of needles at the correct acupuncture point can affect the organ associated with that meridian; in turn, they influence other body systems at more distant points from the meridian.

The Energy Matrix Clearing System does not use acupuncture to affect the flow of chi; rather, it uses vibrational medicines and technologies. Photonics (light beams in the infrared wavelength) is a modern technology known to stimulate acupuncture points. Understanding the meridian clock or circadian cycle is important in effecting the flow of chi through the meridians. The circadian cycle is a 24-hour rhythmic cycle of the flow of chi through the entire meridian system, and each meridian reaches a peak energetic point at a particular time of day. This is important in determining when treatment will have the greatest effect on balancing of the flow of energy.

A meridian clock chart, reproduced here, was created by Dr. Jeff Harris to reflect this energy flow. Although not indicated on the chart, keep in mind that noon is located at the top of the chart, and midnight is located at the bottom.

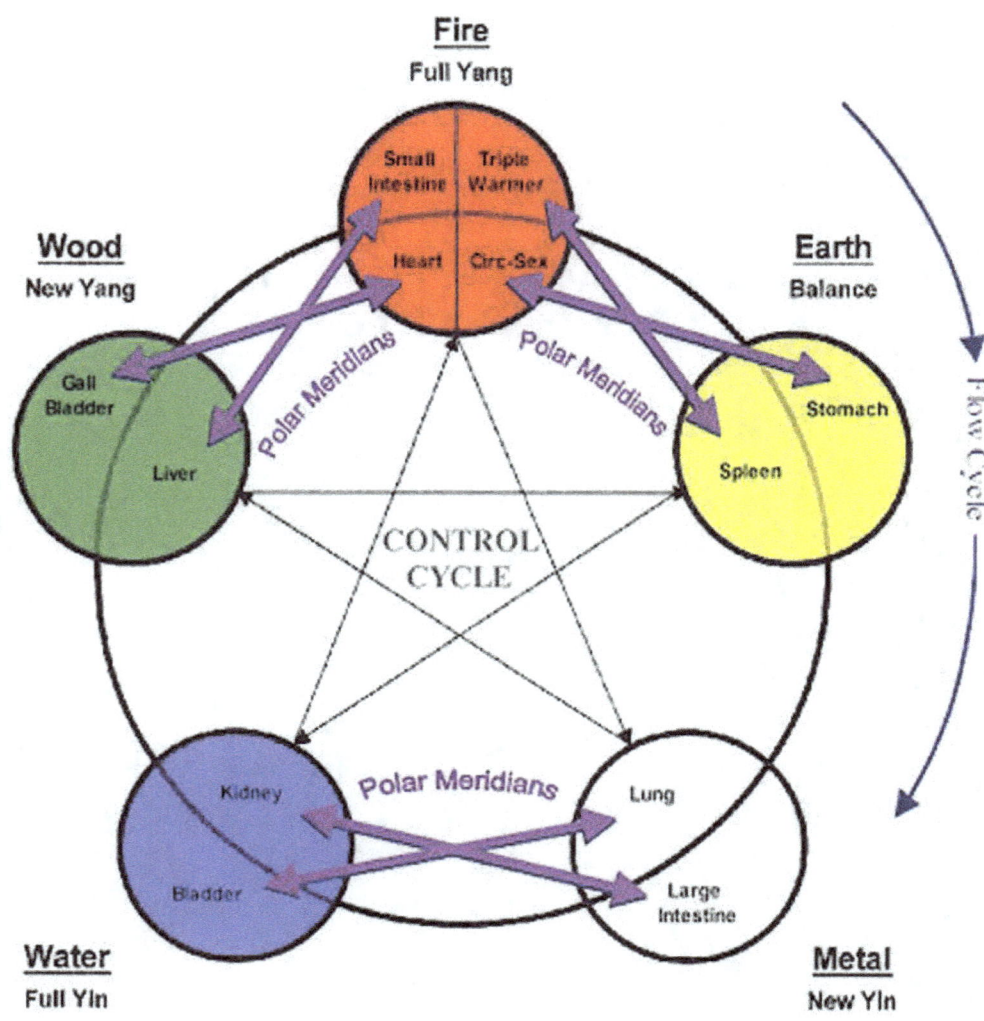

The Five-Element 24-Hour-Meridian Wheel

©2005, Jeff Harris, M.D

The theory of the Five Elements has its origins in ancient Chinese philosophy, in which all living things belong to one of five primary elements: wood, fire, earth, metal, and water. Whiteside and Stokes believe the five elements theory "has its roots in the concept of the eternal interplay of Yin and Yang."[49]

On the chart above, Dr. Harris places each polar meridian, which is twelve hours apart on the 24-hour cycle, in relationship to one of these five elements. Both meridians of a "polar pair" share certain characteristics with one another and, in other ways, are polar opposites. The polar meridians of the spleen and triple warmer are opposite one another on the 24-hour cycle. Both govern the immune system, and both are radiant circuits, yet they oppose one another in many of their actions. If the triple warmer meridian is overcharged, the spleen meridian is undercharged, and vice versa. Spleen meridian is at its maximum flow from 9 to 11 a.m.; the triple warmer is at its maximum from 9 to 11 p.m. They are like the shores on opposite sides of the ocean; when one is at high tide, the other is at low tide.

To understand a meridian that is involved in an energy medicine treatment, always be aware of its polar meridian, as well as the meridians involved in its control cycle (the inner arrows on the five-element diagram) and its flow cycle (the clockwise circle on the five-element diagram).[50]

You may find that it is easy to remember the polar meridians by visualizing their relationship on the five-element wheel. Note the following as well:

- A yin meridian is always twelve hours apart from a yang meridian.
- Metal and water meridians are polar meridians.
- Wood and fire meridians from the "left side" of fire are polar meridians.
- Earth and fire meridians from the "right side" of fire are polar meridians.

Chi, or vital energy, comes from the world around us: the air we breathe, the rays of the Sun, the foods we consume, and the energy or life force we inherited from our parents. The energetic process of gathering chi and distributing it throughout the system is automatic. However, each individual must be conscious of the choices they make that can positively or negatively affect this energy process, from the foods they eat to the quality of air in their immediate environment to inherited behavioral patterns. We are all capable of making choices that optimize the amount of life force available on a daily basis. Since life force animates and energizes every part of the holographic human energy system, its availability is necessary for health and well-being. Each energetic system must be open to the flow of chi, much like the flow of blood through the physical cardiovascular system of the human body.

The endocrine and nervous systems serve as pathways of interaction between the physical body and the subtle energy bodies that surround the physical. Dr. William Tiller, one of the world's leading scientists on the structure of matter, says, "We should think of the individual chakra-endocrine pairs as transducers of energy from the subtle levels to the physical level."[51]

The intercommunication between the acupuncture points and the nervous system explains the positive results of acupuncture with neurotic and psychotic patients. Dr. Richard Gerber suggests that addiction disorders, of all psychological disorders, are the most amenable to acupuncture therapy.[52] When working with hundreds of clients over the last twenty years, I have found that the Energy Matrix Clearing System supports Dr. Gerber's theory. Clients experience positive results with the EMCS protocol because it focuses on the whole human energy system and comprehensively addresses each client's goal to establish a more positive, life-affirming lifestyle.

Empirical data indicates that there are technologies that bring the meridian system into a state of natural balance, which is reflected in the physical organs as well as in psychological and spiritual states. Because of this empirical data and a growing body of anecdotal information supporting the data, it is not a difficult leap to ascertain that specific psychological states can be attributed to each meridian. Acupuncturists and holistic health practitioners associate the following emotional states or conditions with the corresponding meridian as follows:

Lung Meridian: Blockages in the lung meridian reflect a lack of trust in a supportive and nurturing universe, thus causing fear and anxiety. Change is a universal law, and the lung meridian represents this constant change through the inhalation and exhalation of breath. My work with clients who report anxiety, obsessions, and compulsions usually have lung meridian outages. Clients who show hypoactive lung meridians often indicate hypersensitivity and feelings of oppression, self-pity, and dejection. On the other hand, clients with a hyperactive lung meridian reflect issues of selfishness, greed, jealousy, and envy. Muscle testing has shown the EMCS Living in Choice Level of Responsibility position for these issues is most often Separation/Guilt (thought), Fear (feeling), and Pride/Indifference (emotion) as the reactive states of mind. This has proven to be the default survival reaction to most life experiences for these clients. The effect of this reaction is that they have very little joy in their lives. The EMCS protocol has proven to be effective in positively changing this default survival system to one in which the client is able to make proactive life choices, resulting in the return to more joyous states of mind and, therefore, a more fulfilling life.

Kidney Meridian: Traditionally, kidney meridian dysfunction suggests overwhelming fear issues accompanied by an inability to resolve them. A pronounced lack of trust in one's ability to handle life situations is often present. A special function of the kidney meridian is governing energy reserves that allow the system to adapt to life changes. A malfunctioning kidney meridian diminishes all life processes, including growth, the maintenance of a system's vitality, and the prevention of early aging. Hyperactive kidney meridian energy results in feelings of inadequacy, suspicion, paranoia, superiority, and arrogance. This condition is most often reflected on the Living in Choice Levels of Responsibility chart as Shame (thought), Desire/Hostility (feeling), and Antagonism (emotion). A hypoactive kidney meridian manifests in the development of phobias and feelings of fearfulness, inferiority, timidity, and panic. Chronic fear drains the reserve energy, which weakens the kidney meridian, which causes feelings of vulnerability, which in turn leaves the body susceptible to fears born of stress and fatigue. This condition most often reflects on the LCLR chart as Apathy (thought), Grief (feeling) and Anger/Resentment (emotion).

Distortions in the kidney meridian energy may also be a reflection of inherited family patterns or karmic patterns carried over from previous life experiences. It is important to keep these possibilities in mind when the kidney meridian makes the indicator change. A client of mine who reported chronic kidney pain shared that tests administered by their doctor did not indicate a physical reason for the pain, yet it persisted. While doing defusion work with this client, past life energy made the indicator change. Age recession took us to a previous life experience in which an unfaithful spouse murdered them with a sword plunged through the kidney on the right side of their body—exactly where the client's chronic pain manifested. After the defusion, the client reported having less pain in that area. At their next appointment, the client reported the pain was entirely gone. Continued monitoring of the kidneys over the next several months revealed no return of previous pain.

The lesson here is to keep an open mind to all possibilities for healing. What is important is that each person's holographic energy system is the authority, and your job as an "energician" is to follow its lead!

Bladder Meridian: The bladder meridian regulates the function of the bladder and moderates the entire energetic balance of the body. This meridian is the only one that has points relating to all the main organs. Located along the back of the body, the bladder meridian produces the information needed to protect oneself from perceived dangers. The muscles of the back are large and usually take the brunt of physical and emotional stress. The physical body expresses itself literally; therefore, back problems are indicative of issues from the past that linger but remain resolved, similar to "putting your problems behind you," or, as Scarlett O'Hara from *Gone with the Wind* would say, "I'll think about that tomorrow."

Bladder meridian dysfunction can result in not feeling safe in one's environment, a general sense of insecurity, and the fear of being hurt and left alone. The Living in Choice Levels of Responsibility chart positions for the bladder meridian most often are Separation/Guilt (thought), Fear (feeling), and Pride/Indifference (emotion).

Liver Meridian: The liver is the organ that metabolizes the foods we eat, breaking it down into the nutrients that fuel our bodies. One of the substances it uses to do this is bile, a bitter fluid stored in the gall bladder. While bile is necessary for digestion, if the liver secretes too much of it, it can disrupt this vital process, causing gastrointestinal upset. No wonder, then, that "bile" means bitterness of spirit and is the reason behind the age-old perception that the liver and anger are related. The overall well-being of the physical body is, therefore, dependent on the vitality of the liver. It is literally a life-supporting process (Chinese acupuncturists call it the "organismic intention to live") and, therefore, reflects issues of self-assertion, motivation, and responsibility.

A hypoactive liver manifests as issues of self-blame, guilt, lack of motivation, boredom, impotency, and depression. Clients who present with these issues generally show up on the Living in Choice Level of Responsibility chart position of Apathy (thought), Grief (feeling), and Anger/Resentment (emotion).

A hyperactive liver manifests in issues of irritability, resentment, hostility, and bitterness. Oriental practitioners, reflexologists, and iridologists know that many liver problems first appear in the eyes, thus, reflecting their connection with the nervous and digestive systems. Therefore, the eyes reflect the condition of the entire nervous system and every organ of the physical body. Clients presenting with issues reflective of a hyperactive liver meridian make the indicator change on the Living in Choice chart at the position of Shame (thought), Desire/Hostility (feeling), and Antagonism (emotion).

Heart Meridian: A balanced heart meridian expresses joy, happiness, self-confidence, and compassion. Joy is the result of wisdom rather than knowledge. Knowing ourselves is a prerequisite for joy. Compassion, understanding, empathy, and forgiveness are implied in the state of being called joy. Joy shows up when we operate from a place of self-worth and empowerment. Self-esteem is implicit in joy, and, of course, love is an expression of the heart. Balance in the heart meridian would muscle test at the Joy (thought), Acceptance (feeling), and Courage (emotion) position on the Pro-Active State of Mind side of the Living in Choice Levels of Responsibility chart.

A hypoactive heart meridian is recognizable for the emotional energy associated with it—sadness, discouragement, self-doubt, despair, emptiness, hopelessness, and depression. Experience indicates this would muscle test at the Apathy (thought), Grief (feeling), and Anger/Resentment (emotion) position on the chart. It would also be characterized by a lack of warmth and passion, resulting in an inability to reach out to others or ask for help when needed.

Symptoms of a hyperactive heart meridian are elation, restless gaiety, nervousness, anxiety, and hysteria, which have their foundation in the Levels of Responsibility chart indicating Separation/Guilt (thought), Fear (feeling), and Pride/Indifference (emotion).

Pericardium Meridian (Circulation Sex): Because the heart and pericardium meridians are linked, tension held in the breast and upper back areas mirrors the unconscious defense against heartfelt feelings. In the words of Eastern healing scholar Iona Marsaa Teeguarden (who is also a Jin Shin Do acupressurist), this might illustrate the struggle between the "desire for love and the fear of letting go to love."[53] It would not be remiss to regard the pericardium meridian as the protector of the heart. Chinese acupuncturists say the heart is the "emperor" of all the organs; therefore, it must be protected from "evil." It falls to the pericardium to bear that burden.

Emotional and behavioral symptoms of a hyperactive pericardium meridian include intellectualization and justification of feelings. A rigid need to control, perhaps, and suppress or oppress feelings of fear, anxiety, love, joy, and enthusiasm, to name a few. In my experience working with addicts and codependents, the pericardium is identified by muscle testing as needing to be balanced more often than any other meridian. The Living in Choice Level of Responsibility triggered when the pericardium is unbalanced is Separation/Guilt (thought), Fear (feeling), and Pride/Indifference (emotion). This position indicates the psychological survival technique of denial. The survival mind uses this technique to "protect" the individual from the fear that the feelings, thoughts, and emotions that are attached to the emotional and behavioral symptoms will result in extreme pain or even death. It is an acceptable response to an unacceptable situation. Hypoactive pericardium symptomatology includes poor emotional and physical boundaries and often registers on the Living in Choice Level of Responsibility chart as Apathy (thought), Grief (feeling), and Anger/Resentment (emotion).

Large Intestine: Naturopathic doctors say the large intestine is the "drainage ditch" of the physical body; this refers to its primary function, the elimination of toxic waste material. The large intestine or colon reabsorbs fluids in the body and serves to maintain the body's store of salt and water. If this system fails, salt and water, important bodily resources, can be quickly depleted, causing impaction of waste materials and an imbalance of electrolytes.

Perhaps the most common ailment related to the colon is "irritable bowel syndrome," which causes lower abdominal pain and constipation alternating with diarrhea. Psycho-neurobiologically, these symptoms can be triggered by anxiety caused by stress-related situations. Rigid "mindsets" manifest as rigid intestines. Hanging on to rigid belief systems concerning "right and wrong" and "good and bad" cause toxic waste to accumulate; this results in the reabsorption of these toxic materials. Defensive attitudes cause tension along the large intestine and manifest as defensive pride, which is defined by resistance to change and to incorporating new attitudes. Self-righteousness and perfectionistic expectations of self and others represent a rigid large intestine. Stubborn attitudes and fear of loss are also symptomatic of a rigid belief system and are reflected in a rigid large intestine. The Living in Choice

Levels of Responsibility position for this condition is Separation/Guilt (thought), Fear (feeling), and Pride/Indifference (emotion).

Small Intestine: An imbalance in the small intestine meridian often correlates with pain in the shoulders and arms. The small intestines assimilate the nutrition from the food we eat to nourish our bodies, but they also assimilate energy from our thoughts. Since our shoulders provide the support that enables us to carry the "weight" of our burdens, both physical and emotional, and our arms reach out and take in, one could, by putting these two together, formulate these questions: "What is the weight I am carrying that does not nurture me?" or "Whose burden am I carrying?"

The resulting stress may also cause digestive problems, diarrhea, or constipation. The small intestine is a yang organ, and by assimilating nutrients from food intake, it transports the waste products to the large intestine. Teeguarden describes its function this way:

> They have to do with processing food, so the body gets the nutrients and energy it needs, and they have to do with processing mental and emotional events so the psyche gets the information it needs. Tension at yang meridian points can be related to defensive attitudes, which inhibit the growthful processing of thoughts and feelings.[54]

It stands to reason that the small intestines have the job of sifting the pure from the impure, the truth from the lie. Many tend not to "put their houses in order," causing pileups of unsorted thoughts, feelings, and actions that eventually obstruct the pathways. After a while, they obstruct the assimilative function of the body/mind connection. This results in undernourished bodies, minds, and spirits.

Since there is a close relationship between the small intestine and heart meridians, an imbalance in the small intestine creates restricted shoulder muscles, which creates tension in the upper ribs, causing them to be restricted, move up, and inhibit lung function. Inhibition of lung capacity restricts the heart's openness. A closed heart signals a decreased capacity for love of self and the love of others. The heart cannot soar, and depression sets in. The LCLR position for a compromised small intestine meridian is Separation/Guilt (Thought), Fear (Feeling) and Pride/Indifference (Emotion).

Spleen/Pancreas: These linked meridians manifest emotional expressions such as empathy, sympathy, consideration, and recollection. The spiritual aspect expressed through a balanced spleen/pancreas meridian connection is "Oneness." Chi is delivered to the spleen chakra (third chakra) via the astral body, where it is then delivered throughout the physical system. This "oneness of spirit" or energy is expressed in the physical world as compassion, forgiveness, and empathy. The sheer joy of living is evident in the lives of those who possess a balanced spleen/pancreas meridian. Opposite thoughts, feelings, and emotions are present when the spleen/pancreas meridian is unbalanced. Blame, shame, inconsiderate behavior, narcissistic attitudes, and jealousy are expressions of an unbalanced spleen/pancreas meridian. An unbalanced condition may lead to any of the Living in Choice reactive states or a combination of all three levels.

Gall Bladder: Gall bladder meridian disturbances can cause tension that clamps down the back of the skull, knots up the neck, snarls the shoulders, constricts the chest, blocks diaphragms, and makes the hip joints rigid. Issues of control are the dominant psychological symptom related to a dysfunctional gall bladder meridian. Physical symptoms such as allergies and headaches result from chronic gall bladder control issues. The gall bladder meridian is responsible for the flow of energy to all the other meridians. Chinese acupuncturists compare the gall bladder meridian to an overworked army general. The overworked general shows stress in the shoulders, neck, jaw, stomach, and solar plexus. The feeling of having armor around the chest, stomach, or pelvic region may be symptomatic of gall bladder control issues. Gall bladder issues show up most often on the Living in Choice Levels of Responsibility chart as Shame (thought), Desire/Hostility (feeling), and Antagonism (emotion).

Triple Warmer Meridian: This is the only internal meridian that is not associated with the organs of the physical body. It functions as the regulator-coordinator of the other meridian activities and regulates the warmth of the body and mind. An imbalance manifests as an increased susceptibility to coldness or fever. The "three warmers" represent the three divisions of the body: chest, abdomen, and pelvis. The triple warmer meridian coordinates the processes of the respiratory, circulatory, digestive, and urogenital systems. This meridian oversees the transportation of fluids and energy throughout the physical system. A hypoactive triple warmer manifests in a lack of energy. Exhaustion and the depression it can cause make it difficult to handle stressful situations. This manifests as Apathy (thought), Grief (feeling), and Anger/Resentment (emotion) on the Living in Choice Levels of Responsibility chart. Hyperactivity of the triple warmer meridian manifests as Separation/Guilt, Fear, and Pride/Indifference (thought, feeling, emotion), respectively. Anxiety, hyperactivity, and restlessness typify hyperactivity in the triple warmer meridian.

Stomach Meridian: Issues of the stomach meridian range from eye to intestinal problems. As one of the largest meridians in the body, this meridian has forty-five identified acupuncture points. Some excess patterns associated with the stomach meridian include constant hunger, elevated blood pressure, knee problems, male genitourinary disorders, intestinal problems, ankle issues, and painful, swollen, or bleeding gums, to name just a few.

Since the stomach processes the food we eat, when problems appear there, ask the client to consider what is going on in their life that they can't "stomach." What have they "swallowed" that they can't, or won't, "chew"? Apathy, Grief, and Anger/Resentment are thought, feeling, and emotional positions on the Living in Choice Levels of Responsibility chart.

Governing Vessel: The governing meridian runs from the tailbone up the spine and over the head, ending at the upper lip at governing vessel 27 (GV27). The physical body is very literal; when physical issues occur at the back of the physical body, the issue is related to baggage from the past. "What are you hauling around on your back from the past?" might be the question to ask. To take a deeper look into the issue at hand, identify the vertebrae to which the GV point is adjacent. For example, GV14 corresponds with point 26, or alignment point, on the spine. According to Cyndi Dale, in her book *New Chakra Healing*, the purpose of the alignment point is to integrate all aspects of self, from material/spiritual to child/adult. Lack of integration in any aspect of the self will result in disharmony.[55]

Central Vessel: The central vessel runs from the pubic bone to just under the bottom lip. It suggests issues of the essential self. The midline of the physical body cellularly represents more clearly than any other area of the physical cells not colored by inherited information from mom or dad. Parental genetics come into play the further one travels to the right or the left of the midline. Remember, the left brain (father) governs the right side of the body, and the right brain (mother) governs the left side of the body.

The question to ask if the central vessel makes the indicator change might be, "How do I see myself?" or "What do I keep saying about myself?"

This listing of physical, emotional, and spiritual attributions to each meridian is not meant to be exhaustive. It is, however, meant to illustrate the role of the meridian systems in the holographic nature of the human energy system.

It is only reasonable to apply the epithet "as above, so below; so below, as above" to meridian system work—the emotional and physical manifestations are symptoms (below) of a greater cause within the hierarchy of subtle bodies (above). Researchers suggest the meridian system is not terminated at the skin. Rather, it extends beyond the skin into the etheric body and into a nadis and matrix system as a web, spinning itself throughout the energy bodies and perhaps out into the greater universe.

This holographic/halographic view of the meridian system affords the health practitioner the opportunity to view symptoms from a larger perspective. The health landscape begins to take on a holographic/halographic viewpoint that includes the whole person as a physical, mental, emotional, and spiritual being. This information can be used to develop a treatment plan that encompasses interventions addressing every level of dysfunction.

Corrections for Matrix II, Meridians follow in chapter seven.

CHAPTER SEVEN

THE PRINCIPLES OF WHOLENESS:

YIN AND YANG, SEVEN PRINCIPLES OF TRUTH,

TWELVE THEOREMS OF THE UNIFYING PRINCIPLES

Yin and Yang

The theory of yin and yang is the principle underlying oriental medicine. Yin and yang philosophy begins with the premise that all things in the universe exist in a continual state of flux. This dynamic flow consists of yin becoming yang and yang becoming yin. Yin and yang are not absolute but relative; all things exist in a state of complementary opposition. This opposition is the foundation of change. Without up, there would be no down. If there was no cold, there could be no hot. Natural universal resistance may be another way to address the idea of opposition. Inherent in every change is resistance. The seed is planted in the soil; the seed begins to sprout; the sprout must break through the resistance, or opposition, of the seed shell. If the little sprout makes its way through the opposition of the seed shell, it must make its way through the opposition resistance of the earth, and so on. This natural process strengthens the new idea, concept, plant, etc. so that it can be strong enough to grow and blossom.

When the universal flow is centripetal, yang is the dominant force. This contraction produces density, activity, heat, weight, and speed. An ice skater spinning is an example of yang energy. If movement is away from the center, the dominant force is yin. These dispersions of energy produce less density, less activity, lightness, and slower speed. At the extreme positions, yin and yang change into one another. We can witness this ebb and flow in the very process of life itself: the rise and fall of the lungs, the waxing and waning of the moon, the ebb and flow of the tides.

In his book *Oriental Diagnosis: What Your Face Reveals,* Michio Kushi lists the following truths based on the ancient philosophy of yin and yang. He credits George Oshawa, the founder of the macrobiotic diet, for first extracting these truths from that philosophy:[56]

1. All things are the differentiation of the One infinity
2. Everything changes
3. All antagonisms are complementary
4. There is nothing identical
5. Whatever has a front has a back
6. The bigger the front, the bigger the back
7. Whatever has a beginning has an end

These seven principles of truth can guide you through every experience life presents, including your interactions with others and how you see them. It is your ethical duty as an EMCS "energician" to "do no harm," as the Hippocratic Oath delineates for medical professionals, and you may find that these principles guide you to the cause and solution to a problem rather than finding yourself a part of the problem.

Kushi then goes on to list what he calls the Twelve Theorems of the Unifying *Principle:*[57]

1. One infinite source differentiates into yin and yang, which are the poles created when the infinite centrifugality arrives at the geometric point of bifurcation. Either it will transform itself into something entirely new, or it will destruct.

2. Yin and yang result continuously from this infinite centrifugality.

3. Yin is centrifugal and yang is centripetal. Yin and yang together produce energy and all phenomena.

4. Yin attracts yang. Yang attracts yin.

5. Yin repels yin. Yang repels yang.

6. The force of repulsion is proportional to the difference between the like components, and the force of attraction is proportional to the difference between the unlike components.

7. All phenomena are ephemeral, constantly changing their constitution of yin and yang components.

8. Everything involves polarity. Nothing is solely yin or solely yang.

9. There is nothing neutral. In every occurrence, either yin or yang is in excess.

10. Large yin attracts small yin. Large yang attracts small yang.

11. At their extremes, yin produces yang, and yang produces yin.

12. All physical forms and objects are yang at the center and yin at the surface.

The following is Kushi's chart discerning the differences between yin and yang as they occur in the physical realm:

	YIN	YANG
Motion	Expansion	Contraction
Category	Space	Time
Position	Outward	Inward
Direction	Ascent	Decent
Color	Purple, blue, green	Yellow, orange, red
Temperature	Cold	Hot
Weight	Light	Heavy
Catalyst	Water	Fire
Vibration	Short wave	Long wave
Atomic particle	Electron	Proton
Elements	K, O, P, C, A, N, etc.	H, AS, CI, NA, C, etc.
Biology	Vegetable	Animal
Sex	Female	Male
Nervous system	Orthosympathetic	Parasympathetic
Attitude	Gentle, negative	Active, positive
Activity	Psychological	Physical
Origin	Hot climate	Cold climate

58

Classification of the organs into yin and yang is based on the more solid and dense structure of yang—heart, liver, spleen, and kidneys. The more hollow organs—large intestine, small intestine, bladder, stomach, gall bladder—are classified as being yin.

The complementary-antagonistic relationships for the organs (TCM) are as follows:

Yin and Yang Classification of the Organs[59]

YANG	YIN
Lungs	Large intestine
Heart	Small intestine
Kidneys	Bladder

Spleen/pancreas	Stomach
Liver	Gall bladder

The complementary-antagonistic relationships for the organs, taken from the tenets of traditional Chinese medicine, are outlined here with the following chart as a guide (modified from Dr. Jeff Harris's by the TCM School):

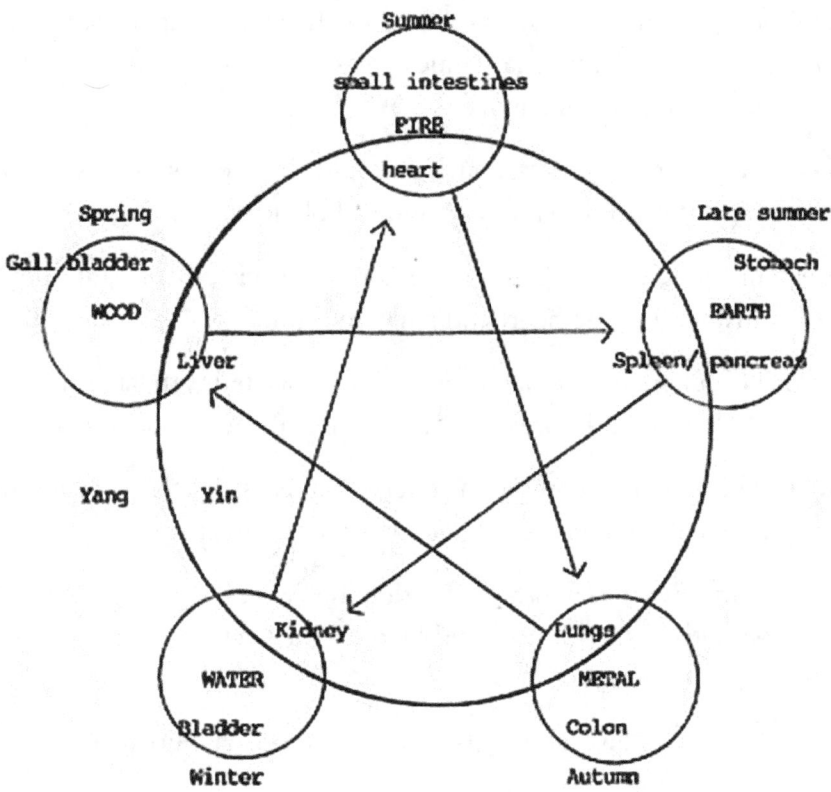

The Chinese 5-element System

In the diagram above, the outer arrows illustrate the process of energy flow. The heart strengthens the spleen-pancreas; the spleen-pancreas strengthens the lungs; the lungs strengthen the kidneys; the kidneys strengthen the liver; and the liver strengthens the heart. The interrelating processes of each organ draw strength from the preceding one and, thus, strengthen the one following. Therefore, strengthening a weak organ vitalizes the one following it.

The inner arrows in the illustration suggest the path of antagonism or destruction. Shown is the path of overactivity or too much yang energy. In other words, excessive yang kidneys result in a weak heart, or an excessively yang spleen makes weak kidneys; excessive yang lungs make a weak liver; an excessively yang liver results in a weak spleen. An excessively yang heart makes weak lungs.

The interaction suggested by the inner arrows does not reflect a circulating process. For example, if the lungs are excessive yang, they only affect the liver. The other organs are not affected as in the circulating aspect of the outer arrow indication. In reality, each element is associated with two organs because of the complementary-antagonist relationship between the meridians. Though not attributed to specific organs, a sixth meridian pair, known as the circulation-sex or pericardium (the heart protector) and triple warmer, make a total of twelve "organs" associated with meridians.

Additionally, there are two major meridians located outside the physical body, which are known as the Conception Vessel and the Governing Vessel. The Conception Vessel is located down the front or mid-line of the body, begins at the pubic bone, and ends just under the lower lip. The Governing Vessel begins at the tailbone, runs up the spine and over the head, and ends just under the nose.

The five natural elements that the Chinese associate with the meridian system, shown in the five smaller circles in the above diagram, are as follows:

1. *Wood*: This energy suggests birth and rebirth, like what one sees in the spring. It has a yang polarity and is related to the liver and gall bladder.

2. *Fire*: This energy promotes growth and is associated with summer. Its polarity is very yang and is attributed to the heart and small intestine.

3. *Earth*: This element is a maturing energy associated with late summer or early fall. Its polarity is more balanced and is associated with the spleen and pancreas.

4. *Metal*: This energy is completing energy and is associated with autumn. It is yin in nature and corresponds to the lungs and large intestine meridians.

5. Water: This energy is energetically identified as resting, very yin, and is associated with winter. It corresponds to the kidneys and bladder meridians.

The Five Elements and their Representations

Element	Wood	Fire	Earth	Metal	Water
Phase	New yang	Full yang	Yin/yang balance	New yin	Full yin
Color	Green	Red	Yellow	White	Black
Direction	East	South	Center (nadir/zenith)	West	North
Life Cycle	Infancy	Youth	Adulthood	Old age	Death
Energy Quality	Generative	Expansive	Stabilizing	Contracting	Conserving
Season	Spring	Summer	Between seasons	Autumn	Winter
Climate	Windy	Hot	Damp	Dry	Cold
Development	Sprouting	Blooming	Ripening harvest	Withering	Dormant
Smell	Rancid	Scorched	Fragrant	Putrid	Rotten
Flavor	Sour	Bitter	Sweet	Pungent	Salty

Mental Quality	Sensitivity	Creativity	Clarity	Intuition	Spontaneity
Negative Emotion	Anger	Hate	Anxiety	Grief	Fear
Positive Emotion	Patience	Joy	Empathy	Courage	Calmness
Body	Tendons	Pulse	Muscle	Skin	Bones
Aperture	Eyes	Tongue, throat	Lips, mouth	Nose	Ears
Bodily Fluids	Tears	Sweat	Saliva	Mucus	Urine
Primal Spirit	Green Dragon	Red pheasant	Yellow phoenix	White tiger	Black tortoise
Male Animal	Tiger	Horse	Dragon, dog	Monkey	Rat
Female Animal	Rabbit	Snake	Cow, sheep	Hen	Pig
Numbers	8, 3	2, 7	10, 5	4, 9	6, 1
I Ching	Wind	Fire	Earth, mountain	Heaven, lake	Water

The Five Elements and their Animal Representations

Lao Tzu, a sixth-century B.C. Taoist philosopher, developed a series of exercises created to assist in balancing the yin and yang flow of the five elements. He attributed these exercises symbolically to the movement of the following five animals (listed here with their corresponding elements).[60]

1. *Tiger (Wood)*: represents the energy of ambition, power, and physical effectiveness. This energy is goal-oriented and focused. The use of this energy is effective in balancing the liver and gall bladder meridians.

2. *Bear (Earth):* represents the energy of strength, courage, conceptualization, and decisiveness. It is grounding energy and benefits the spleen, pancreas, and stomach.

3. *Dragon (Fire)*: represents the energy of supreme wisdom, power, control, self-confidence, and social effectiveness. Utilization of this energy helps in overcoming depression, anger, hostility, powerlessness, and anxiety. The heart and small intestine can benefit from this energy.

4. *Monkey (Water)*: represents the energy of freedom, boundless energy, activity, and free will. Monkey energy supports and vitalizes the kidneys and bladder.

5. *Eagle (Metal)*: represents spirit, alertness, intelligence, overview, a complete awareness in the present time, attention to detail, and ease of movement. Eagle energy supports the lung and large intestine meridians.

These symbols become homework assignments in the EMCS process. Clients have found that practicing a short meditation focusing on the qualities of a specific animal, identified by muscle testing, has proven to be an effective tool for transcending self-defeating survival patterns.

Meridian Points

Think of the meridian system as a sophisticated communication system. The human body, through the meridian system, has the capacity to send and receive data from the world within and without. William Tiller describes it this way:

> The human body has this capacity in the autonomic nervous system (ANS) as a signal carrier via both the sympathetic and the parasympathetic branches, which influences secretions, smooth muscle response, blood vessel response, electrocardiograms, heart rate variability, respiration, etc. It also serves as an excellent waveguide by way of the myelin sheath surrounding each nerve axon to conduct a traveling wave to a multitude of "endpoints" just under the surface of the skin. . . . One set of antenna elements in this system [is] thought to be the acupuncture points (AP) of the body. Since these number in the thousands, they would provide an exquisitely rich array with capabilities exceeding the most advanced radar system today.[61]

Because the body/mind relationship represents the whole system and the mind defines everything concerning a system, each individual system is regulated by one of the organs, which also affects all other systems. This is known as the holographic perspective of the human energy system. If one of the systems is out of balance, the entire system is affected. I previously defined "chi" as the life-giving energy activating and maintaining all of life. I repeat this definition here to emphasize the point that while chi flows through every living cell and tissue of our bodies, there is also an external or surface (of the skin) circulation of chi linked by the meridians. When stimulated, key points found along each meridian stimulate energy flow and restore natural balance in the system. These key points have a number designation preceded by the abbreviation of the meridian, for example, K27, or the twenty-seventh point on the kidney meridian.

Meridian abbreviations may vary depending on the reference material used, but these are the most common:

K: Kidney	B: Bladder
T or TW: Triple Warmer	H: Heart
LV: Liver	LI: Large intestine
L: Lung	SI: Small intestine
GB: Gall Bladder	P: Pericardium or CS (circulation-sex)

Along each meridian, certain points have specific designated duties and are identified as follows:

SEDATION POINT: This point reduces the flow of chi from a meridian. When identified as being "out" through EMCS, it corresponds to Shame/Desire/Hostility/Antagonism on the Living in Choice Level of Responsibility chart.

DIVERGENT MERIDIANS: Yin energy literally piggybacks on its yang element partner in the neck to reach the head. If this energy connection does not take place, the yin energy remains in the torso and causes imbalanced meridian energy in the brain. The results may be lack of concentration, reading incomprehension, dullness of perception, pain, or allergies. (Refer to Appendix III for points to be tested.). When identified through EMCS as "out," it corresponds to Apathy/Grief/Anger/Resentment on the LCLR chart.

ASSOCIATED POINTS: Associated points correspond to Apathy/Grief/Anger/Resentment on the LCLR chart when "out." These points are found on the bladder meridian along the spinal column. They work together with the kidney meridian point 27 (K27) on the front of the body. K27 designates two points just below the clavicle (collarbone). To locate the points, place your fingers on the clavicle and move your fingers toward the center until you find the bumps that indicate the end of the bones on either side of the clavicle. Drop down about one inch below these bumps and out to the K27 points. Most people have a small indention at this location; your fingers will fall into it. Thousands of years ago, the Chinese determined that chronic imbalance of any organ would eventually negatively affect the bladder meridian. Psychologically speaking, the inability to eliminate feelings concerning the causal issue ultimately results in an imbalance in every meridian. The associated points lie on the midline of the body. When determined to be in an imbalanced state, it indicates emotional and psychological issues of lack of self-love.

TONIFICATION POINTS: Apathy/Grief/Anger/Resentment on the LCLR chart. When these points are made active, they allow chi to flow into the meridian on which the acupuncture point is determined.

MERIDIANS: Separation/Guilt/Pride/Indifference on the LCLR chart. Within the EMCS system, when meridians make an indicator change, use the following protocol to identify the correct activation point:

- Using the "yes/no" method, muscle test whether the Tsing point is the appropriate point to hold.
- If testing indicates the Tsing point is not the point to hold, use the body scan method or muscle test for the appropriate point on the identified meridian using the "indicator change" method by the number.
- Once the appropriate point has been identified, test for the side of the body where the point is to be held, right or left.
- Test the appropriate finger/polarity with which to hold the point. Hold the point with the appropriate finger for thirty seconds as the client intentionally focuses on moving their breath deeply into and through that point.

Right-Hand Finger Polarity
little finger - negative
ring finger - positive
middle finger - negative
index (pointer) finger - positive
thumb - neutral

Left-Hand Finger Polarity
little finger - positive
ring finger - negative
middle finger - positive
index (pointer) finger - negative
thumb - neutral

LOU POINT/JUNCTION POINT: This point represents either Pro-Active State of Mind or a Reactive State of Mind on the LCLR chart. This junction point forms connections between two connected meridians within an element, i.e., the kidney and bladder meridian of the water element or the lung and large intestine meridian of the metal element.

SOURCE POINT: A point of choice identified on the LCLR chart as Reactive or Pro-Active. Tradition indicates that these points have a direct relationship with or connection to the physical organ fed by the meridian.

ACCUMULATION POINT: Separation/Guilt/Fear/Pride/Indifference on the LCLR chart. This point is used when acute problems are present in the meridian energy field.

ALARM POINTS: Separation/Guilt/Fear/Pride/Indifference on the LCLR chart. These points indicate specific organ energy imbalances.

HORARY POINT: Shame/Desire/Hostility/Antagonism on the LCLR chart. This point corresponds to the element related to the specific meridian. Use the Five-Element chart to determine which element corresponds with a meridian. The oriental energy time cycle is also valuable when defusing horary points. Defusion during the time the energy is highest will be the most effective. If defusion during that time is not feasible, assign homework to be completed at the time of highest energy to augment the defusion process. It is unclear where this energy originates, but it seems to stem from geographical location. Jet lag, experienced when traveling long distances across several time zones, is evidence of this energy, and it can take the body several hours or even days to adjust to being in a new location.

ELEMENTS: Each meridian has specific points representing each of the Five Chinese Elements. In defusion work, once you have identified the meridian, check the chart of meridians to find the element point.

TSING POINT: Separation/Guilt/Fear/Pride/Indifference on the LCLR Chart. This point is found at the beginning or end points of the meridians. They are located on the fingers or the toes. Chinese medicine teaches that giving energy at these points protects the body from changes in climate, including the effects caused by the changes experienced when traveling between locations with extreme climate differences.

NEUROVASCULAR RECEPTORS: While not a part of the meridian point system, these receptors were identified as reflex points by chiropractor Terrence Bennett in the 1930s. Chiropractor George Goodheart, a pioneer in the use of kinesiology and former director of research at the International College of Applied Kinesiology, wrote extensively on the implications of Bennett's work.[62] Dr. Bennett associated these reflexes with the internal organs (Goodheart would go on to correlate the reflexes to specific muscles). Furthermore, Bennett said blockages in the neurovascular points prohibit the occurrence of normal lactic acid activity. The accumulation of lactic acid causes a blockage of its normal removal from the muscle by way of circulation or metabolic breakdown. Dr. Bennett's research focused on placing pressure on the neurovascular points, which proved to improve blood circulation to the muscle and related organs. (See Appendix III for Neurovascular Point Charts)

NEUROLYMPHATIC POINTS: Dr. Frank Chapman located these points, which are named for him.[63] The Chapman Reflex Points are located in the space between the ribs on the front and back of the body. He believed the stimulation of these points causes the afferent (bringing inward) and efferent (carrying away from) vessels that are draining these tissues to increase or decrease, and, as a result, the stimulation of the points permits the lymph flow to increase or decrease. Ten to fifteen seconds of gentle pressure on the Chapman Reflexes generally activate the points.

Meridian Energy Corrections

When the indicator changes on "meridians" as a correction during an EMCS defusion, first identify the specific point before identifying through muscle checking the priority meridian because the specific point determines the next step in the defusion process.

I. Muscle test for the specific energy point by the number:

1. Sedation	2. Divergent	3. Associate	4. Horary
5. Alarm	6. Notification	7. Meridians	8. Tsing
9. Lou	10. Source	11. Elements	12. Accumulation
13. Neuromuscular	14. Neurolymphatic	15. Conception Vessel	16. Governor Vessel

II. Identify the Avoidance Behavior through muscle testing.

III. Depending on the point identified by muscle checking, test for which side of the body—right or left—if appropriate, and then test for polarity. Test for appropriate polarity by placing first the middle finger on one arm and test with the other. If the indicator changes on the middle finger, then use that finger to hold the point. If the indicator does not make a change on the middle finger, then use the pointer finger to hold the acupuncture point. You are testing for body polarity with this procedure. Each finger represents an electrical polarity, either positive or negative, as I indicated earlier in this text. Remember, the thumb is neutral, just as using two fingers of opposite polarity is neutral. If you are holding the point with a finger representing the opposite polarity indicated for correction, it would serve to either further block the point or cause a short circuit. This is similar to the effect you would get by putting the negative polarity of a car battery booster cable on the positive pole. It would spark. Once you have identified the appropriate polarity, hold the specific point with the identified finger on the skin at the specific point. Identify the point position from the schedule of acupuncture points in Appendix I.

IV. If specific point number seven (meridians) makes the indicator change, identify the specific meridian by muscle testing. Once you identify the appropriate meridian, muscle test to determine if you will use the tsing point for correction or if there is a more appropriate point on the meridian. There may be more than one point to correct. Body scan or muscle test for the point on the meridian. The correction would consist of holding the frontal lobes with a neutral touch while holding the identified point with an appropriate polarity touch. If the position of the point makes it difficult for you to hold both the frontal eminences and the specific point, ask the client to hold the frontal eminences and you hold the point. If the client chooses to hold the point, retest for the polarity/finger they would need to use to touch the point themselves. It may be different.

V. If neurovascular or neurolymphatic points make the indicator change, muscle test for the appropriate meridian, look up the neurovascular or neurolymphatic points on that meridian, and apply pressure to those points using the appropriate polarity.

VI. If the conception vessel or governor vessel makes the indicator change, muscle test for the appropriate point or body scan for the appropriate body position to hold. Instruct the client to breathe deeply through the point while you hold the point with the appropriate polarity.

Energy Matrix Clearing System

CASE NOTES

DATE

ISSUE

LEVEL OF RESPONSIBILITY

NEE_____

PEE_____

FlorAlive_____

_____Pleiadian Glyph

_____Avoidance Behavior

_____Level of Consciousness

_____Universal Fear

_____Reflective Mirror

_____10 Elements

_____Archetype

_____Gene Key/Hexagram

_____Kabalistic 72 Names of God

NAME

CORE NEGATIVE BELIVE
Shadow Belief_____
Historial_____
Genetic, Lost Will, All Soul
LEVELS, ANCESTRAL, DIVINE SPIRIT, LEVELS, DIMENSIONS

SUBTLE ENERGY BODIES
__P   __E   __A   __M   __C
MIASM_____   DRAINER_____   ENTITY_____
CURSES_____   NEGATIVE ENERGETIC CORDS_____

MATRIX SYSTEM EFEECTED

_____Casual Age

_____Age on Line

_____NEE

_____Level of Responsibility

_____Avoidant Behavior

_____Universal Fear

_____Reflective Mirror

_____10 Elements

_____Archetype

Miasm_____   Drainer_____   Entity_____
SEB: __P   __E   __A   __M   __C

MATRIX SYSTEM EFFECTED

_____

_____

_____

_____

_____

_____

HOMEWORK:

_____

_____

_____

NOTES:

_____

_____

CHAPTER EIGHT

MATRIX III

THE LIMBIC AND ENDOCRINE SYSTEMS

Whether you say matter or body or essence, know that these also are energies of God and that materiality is the energy of matter, corporeality the energy of bodies and essentiality the energy of essence. And this is God, the All.

—CORPUS HERMETICUM XII

Holographic/halographic energy methods facilitate the re-integration of the appropriate flow of chi on all levels: physical, emotional, mental, and spiritual.[64] Chaos, when experienced as dis-ease, is often a bifurcation point or a steppingstone to a higher level of order. Each new level represents a higher expression of awareness/consciousness and may manifest on any level of the holographic/halographic system. The human energy system is dynamic; therefore, it must be constantly supplied with energy to maintain its vitality. When the human energy system is not aligned with the universal force of life, a dis-eased state is manifested.

The purpose and function of the Energy Matrix Clearing System is the realignment of each individual holographic energy system with the universal life force, the halographic resonance. The holographic and halographic realignment of the physical, etheric, emotional, mental, and causal bodies reinstates full access and alignment with the Universal One; this leads to balance and harmony in all aspects of life. The ability to tap into the primordial cosmic energy or halograph eventually allows the holographic human energy system to recalibrate to a vital balance, facilitating natural harmony within the whole system. Many people call this energy God; others call it chi, prana, orgone, life force, or, more recently, zero-point energy, a term taken from quantum mechanics. Labeling is an attempt to define a "thing." The "thing" itself is important, not the name or label it is given. Consciousness and "eternalness" can only occur when alignment with that primordial energy occurs, whatever "it" is called. The Energy Matrix Clearing System process is one method for reestablishing this connection.

The earlier chapters of this course set the stage for delving more deeply into the operating systems of the inner self. The venous arterial system, which includes the limbic and endocrine systems, is the "heart" of our physical, mental, and emotional selves. The interrelated functions of these systems make it possible for us to generate thoughts, feelings, and emotions and to express them into unique and individual actions, thereby choosing our futures.

The limbic system, also called the emotional, reptilian, or "old brain," records memory and initiates movement. It converts conscious reactions, memory, and instinctive desires into emotions. The endocrine system assists in spiritual development. It vibrates to the specific spiritual energies transmitted through the etheric chakras and acts as a battery, which powers separate and specific physical and psychic functions. The venous, arterial system synergizes and uses energy from the other two systems through the breath and blood; as a result, it vitalizes the holographic human energy system.

A concept known as the Domination System[65], to which all humans have become conditioned, has resulted in a mindset that has created levels of fear and self-doubt. This conditioning has resulted in the belief that we do not have the ability or even the right to a personal relationship with Source/God, etc., and therefore, we must rely on an authority outside ourselves as a go-between ourselves and Source/God. The consequence of having given up our power in this way has manifested in our slavery to negative energies—thought patterns manifesting in stagnant, destructive dis-ease. According to the Abraham-Hicks material, the conditioned habit is to focus on that which we don't want rather than focusing on what we do want, which results in actually attracting more of what we don't want.[66]

These systems operate from a central location—the physical body. The significance of this lies in the fact that these central cells more clearly access the essential self. The organs, glands, and systems along the spinal column, brain stem, and middle brain specifically communicate with the subtle body systems. These systems deliver energy/information from the "outside universe" to the "inside universe" and vice versa. This is in alignment with the Law of Correspondences (Hermetic Axiom), "As above, so below." This means that by increasing our knowledge of ourselves, the microcosm, we are better able to understand or infer knowledge of the worlds immediately above and below us, the macrocosm in which "we live and move and have our being." The study of our immediate world can be divided into two aspects: the objective, or personality, which consists of the gross physical, the etheric, emotional (astral), and the concrete mental (lower mind); and the subjective, or spiritual ego, which consist of three qualities known as will or pure being, wisdom or pure knowing, and active intelligence (abstract or higher mind) or pure doing. Knowledge of these systems facilitates the most effective way to use the technology inherent in humans to co-create a world experience in harmony with the evolving universe. The result of distortions or misuse of this primal creative energy over time manifests blockages/destructive patterns in any of these systems, which show up as life expression issues.

In a large sense, the physical body acts as a monitor for the expression of life force. The manifestation of disturbances, which are expressed physically, mentally, emotionally, or spiritually as malfunctions (fear, rage, resentment, and lack, i.e., the feeling that one doesn't have enough resources, love, time, money, etc.), illustrates the misuse of energy systems or their underdevelopment.

Holographically speaking, negative emotions represent distorted subtle energy patterns and destructive chemical reactions at the cellular level of the physical body, which eventually negatively affect physical organs and result in disease. Candace Pert, a research professor in the area of physiology and biophysics, says:

> For me, the key idea is that the emotions exist in the body as informational chemicals, the neuropeptides and receptors, and they also exist in another realm, the one we experience as feeling, inspiration, and love-beyond the physical. The emotions move back and forth, flowing freely between both places and, in that sense, they connect the physical and nonphysical. Perhaps this is the same thing that Eastern healers call the subtle energy, or prana—the circulation of emotional and spiritual information throughout the body mind.[67]

Researchers working over the past twenty or so years have proven the body–mind connection. This connection is complicated and involves every aspect of the human body's organs, nerve pathways, chemical/receptor processes, and brain. Pert says, "If we accept the idea that peptides and other informational substances are the biochemical of emotion, their distribution in the body's nerves has all kinds of significance . . . The body is the unconscious mind! Repressed traumas caused by overwhelming emotion can be stored in any body part and thereafter affect our ability to feel that part or even move it."[68]

Until recently, researchers believed that the emotional brain was limited to the amygdala, hippocampus, and hypothalamus. New technologies have now made it possible to identify areas of high concentration of neuropeptide receptors in the dorsal horn (backside of the spinal cord), which is where "all somatosensory information is processed."[69] More importantly, a high concentration of neuropeptide receptors can be found at any physical body site where information from any of the five senses is processed. Pert calls these sites "nodal points," and according to researchers, they are designed to process energy/information, prioritize it, and, in a sense, judge the quality of the energy/information as it influences neurophysiological changes. The processing of energy/information involves all sensory input (odor, touch, taste, sight, and sound); the quality and quantity of receptors, experiences, and current activities such as exercise, nutrition, and daily stresses, which color the efficiency of the filtering process. This translates into a dynamically changing momentary experience of life; even the joy of the moment is colored by fears from the past. Living in the moment, enjoying it for its own sake, is not as easy a task as it might seem at first. Making a decision is not as easy as just saying "No!" as former First Lady Nancy Reagan suggested in the 1980s campaign against drugs or the more recent campaign by the George W. Bush presidency, which advocated sexual abstinence as a method for combating teen pregnancy. The process of living is not that simple.

The Energy Matrix Clearing System protocol provides an avenue to cleanse the holographic human energy system of debilitating and distorted energy blockages, thus freeing the process of decision-making from past negative experiences and limiting belief systems. The EMCS process uses natural energies as a method of shifting and clearing the holographic human energy system. These energies include gem, mineral, and plant/flower essences; planets; sacred places; and computer-generated treatment programs, specifically the AOSCAN (developed by Solex, Inc.), which uses sound technology to assess the overuse and underuse of certain octaves in the human voice in order to determine emotional and health imbalances.

Since antiquity, essences of gems and minerals have been used for healing. Spiritual and healing facilities like tombs, burial grounds, and crystalline structures housed the spiritual customs and arts practiced by ancient and indigenous peoples from around the globe. Ancient records document these practices. The spiritual healer known as Melody speaks to this in her book *Love is in the Earth*:

> The consciousness of the planet is leading humanity to the rediscovery of an ancient and forgotten healing art in which the utilization of crystals is prominent. "Dis-ease" and disorder in one's life usually entails lessons, which will allow one to release the burdens of unconsciousness. Although one must ultimately heal oneself, the healing process may be facilitated by the catalytic presence of many things. To experience "dis-ease" is to

experience a total or partial disconnection from wholeness, a loss of awareness of the innate and universal source of perfection. The members of the mineralogical kingdom have been used for centuries to act as catalysts and to assist one in becoming reunited with that source. . . . The Universe is a constantly moving mass of energy waves, with equilibrium being defined as harmony and disequilibrium known as "dis-harmony" or "dis-ease." [70]

I introduce *Living in Choice gem and mineral essences* as used within the EMCS process as one method of producing harmony within the holographic human energy system.

My mission while researching my doctoral dissertation was to understand the connection between the chakra system and health. Intuitively, I felt the key to restoring health to the holographic human energy system was to understand how the chakra system communicated energy/information from the "outside" to the "inside," and that understanding would lead to an energetic method through which the subtle energy system could be manipulated from an unhealthy state to a healthy one.

Although I searched for answers, nothing came to me. Serendipitously, I was at this same time reading the book *Nine Faces of Christ: Quest for the True Initiate* by Eugene Whitworth. Dr. Whitworth's main character, Jeshuau Joseph-bar-Joseph, was being taught the secrets of Egypt by three wise men, who held that in Egyptian religion, man has nine bodies instead of the 7 bodies taught by most spiritual teachers.

This nine-body explanation interested me, and to clarify, I called Dr. Whitworth, who, fortunately, answered the phone. After rambling on about what I was trying to understand regarding the nine bodies and their relation to the chakra system, Dr. Whitworth finally exclaimed impatiently, "Gary! What you are looking for is not in the chakra system. Look to the subtle energy bodies." He suggested that I reread chapter 13, titled "Egypt, Mother of Religions," with the subtle energy bodies in mind.

I thanked him profusely for his patience and insight, reread chapter thirteen, and then shifted my focus from the chakra system to the subtle energy bodies surrounding the physical. My research journey then led me to the Theosophical Society's work compiled by A.E. Powell, but I did not find in these works methods for manipulation of the energy of these systems.

Seeking inspiration, I explored the subtle energy bodies in my daily meditations. After several weeks in quiet contemplation, I had a dream in which I was witness to the Big Bang. I saw an incredibly beautiful and powerful explosion in the blackness of the void, followed by gases flowing out from the central blast. Waves of brilliantly colored energy expanded out from its center, and a flow of molten lava followed the white-hot heat of the blast. The last vision of the dream was the cooling of this lava flow, resulting in a bank of colored stone around a molten core.

I woke that morning in awe of the dream, but it was not until later that day, as I was working with clients, that the lightbulb of awareness switched on in my brain. There was now no doubt in my mind that manipulation of the subtle energy bodies from a compromised vibration to a healthy vibration using the vibrational essence of gems and minerals was the answer. It just made sense to me. Research had revealed that ancient healers from many cultures used gemstones in their healing practices, but I had no clue how to create the essences. This became my next quest.

Fortunately, many great, wise and willing Native American shamans live in Oklahoma and understand the use of gemstones and minerals as healing tools. They were invaluable to my study. This was when I also first discovered Melody's wonderful book, which helped me identify the healing and spiritual qualities of gemstones. I then moved on to read both volumes of *Gem Elixirs and Vibrational Healing*, which were channeled through psychic researcher Kevin Ryerson (Ryerson was made famous by Shirley MacLaine in her book *Out on a Limb)*. These books became my major source for understanding how gem and mineral essences can affect healing in the holographic human energy system. This statement from volume one was particularly enlightening:

> In the final analysis, the body physical is healed through energy, energy upon the biomolecular level, not even upon the level of chemical reactions but more so upon molecular structures. Real healing extends from the biomolecular to the cellular level and eventually to the anatomical level, where it is wrought into harmony with other levels of the body physical. This is because the biochemical properties of the body physical in their final element are based upon vibration.[71]

I began witnessing in my own practice a shift in my clients' energy immediately following the ingestion of gem and mineral essences. Sometimes, they had a shocked look on their face, and then a smile would emerge, or they would comment that it felt like a ripple of energy had flashed through their body. I likened this to the ripples that occur on a lake when pebbles are thrown into a pond. When administered to a physical "vehicle," the stable molecular structure of the essences is transferred through the law of vibration permeating the physical body all the way to the molecular level, inspiring stability in the bimolecular level where there is a sympathetic resonance. This resonance entrains the energy fields to a harmonious synchronicity with the Universal One/Halograph. This quote from Gurudas was no less powerful:

> When the gem elixirs are ingested, they become an evolutionary force in the consciousness of the individual. This serves to affect not only the individual's ability to exercise free will in a positive way but becomes a progressive element that stimulates inspiration and eventual change. They are not the causal force, but they are the inspiration behind the causal force—the free will of the individual—to further develop the individual's consciousness.[72]

Research into the world of gem and mineral essences and their healing qualities culminated in the development of the Cone Center for Living in Choice gem and mineral essences. I used kinesiology to identify which single or combination of gem and mineral essences would be effective when paired with the EMCS process. I identified combinations of essences for the clearing and balancing of the chakra system on each of the four levels of the holographic human energy system—etheric, astral, mental and causal—plus 155 single essences that are used as specific treatments for each of the categories in thirteen matrix systems of the EMCS process. I developed fifteen combinations for specialized use and twelve combinations for use specifically when working with the Cranial Nerves in association with the twelve houses of the astrology chart. [73]

**EMCS© protocol for the administration of the
Cone Center for Living in Choice gem and mineral essences**[74]

Muscle testing indicated that all categories of Cone Center for Living in Choice gem and mineral essences should be included in testing the client to determine the best individual option for energetic treatment for the limbic system.

Instructions to help EMCS energicians identify and administer gem and mineral essences are as follows:

- Muscle test for the priority "by the number" until the indicator changes.
- Test for the number of drops.
- Test for the method of administration—on the tongue, under the tongue, or in water. On-the-tongue administration indicates energetic blockage through the fifth chakra—communication or intentional action. Under-the-tongue administration activates the cellular release of energetic blockages. In-water administration suggests elimination through internal processes.

EMCS Utilization of FlorAlive Flower Essences and Perelandra Rose and Garden Essences

The story of FlorAlive Essences, the work of chiropractor Brent W. Davis, is beautifully related in his book *The Floral Hand of God*. The magic and wonder of Machaelle Wright's Perelandra Essences is told in her many books but most poignantly in her magnum opus, *Pivot,* which is the story of her life. I have included both as clearing energies in the context of an EMCS session. I have found the clearing power inherent in both products to be the most efficacious. Time and experience in the use of Perelandra Rose and Garden essences have revealed them to be most powerful when karmic, ancestral, genetic, or past life carry-over information makes the indicator change.

Functions of the Limbic System

The human brain is composed of three sections or components, all of which have evolved over time. The oldest section, the bottom section, is called the archipallium, and it is also known as the "reptilian" or primitive brain. It is composed of the brainstem structures, which are the medulla, pons, cerebellum, mesencephalon (the oldest basal nuclei), globus pallidus, and olfactory bulbs. The famous neuroscientist Paul MacLean dubbed this part of the brain the "R-complex."[75] The paleopallium or intermediate brain (old mammalian) comprises the structures of the limbic system. The neopallium (new mammalian) brain comprises almost all of both brain hemispheres (neocortex), as well as some subcortical neuronal groups.

The primitive brain is responsible for self-preservation and manifests in aggressive and repetitive behaviors. Instinctive reactions and commands, which allow for some involuntary actions and the control of certain visceral functions (cardiac, pulmonary, intestinal, etc.), are indispensable to the preservation of life. In addition, recent research into previously undocumented details of evolutionary changes in our species indicates that the development of larger olfactory bulbs, a wider orbitofrontal cortex, and larger, forward-projecting temporal lobe poles likely contributed to the evolution of learning and social functions in early homo sapiens. Therefore, the development of the olfactory bulbs, a later development of the primitive brain, has made possible accurate analysis of olfactory stimuli, leading to honed interpretation of external/internal stimuli oriented by odors, such as approach, attack, flight, and mating.

The olfactory cortex, amygdala, and hippocampus are located on the medial surface of the temporal lobe; all are critical to normal human functioning. The olfactory tract's main target is the primary olfactory cortex. The operation of the olfactory system disobeys a principal sensor system in that it does not have to pass through the thalamus before reaching the cortex. This is because it is such an old and primitive structure and has only four cellular layers—mitral cell layer, internal granule cells, glomerular layer, and mitral cell axons—unlike the six layers of the neocortex. The general principle is that sensory information must pass through the thalamus to get to the cerebral cortex. In humans, the amygdala and the entorhinal cortex are the only limbic system structures that connect with the olfactory system. It is in the reptilian brain that the first ritual phenomenon began in the territorial habits of animals. According to the *Rand McNally Atlas of the Body and Mind*, "Recent evidence suggests that some odors are in fact recognized only subliminally—that is without our being consciously aware of their effect on our behavior."[76] This indicates the importance of the use of essential oils in the EMCS process, as well as explaining how smells are involved in traumatic events and need to be considered in the defusion process.

The nineteenth-century French anatomist and anthropologist Pierre Paul Broca discovered that the speech production center of the brain is located in a certain section of the frontal lobe, a region that has come to be called Broca's Area. He arrived at this discovery by studying the brains of aphasic patients (persons unable to talk), in particular, his first patient, Leborgne, who was a resident in the Bicêtre Hospital. Broca nicknamed this patient Tan, due to his inability to clearly speak any words other than "tan." Broca was also the first to notice the area containing several nuclei of gray matter (neurons) on the medial surface of the mammalian brain, which he named the limbic lobe. Broca's "Triune Brain" model demonstrates that the reptilian complex (R-complex) plays a major role in the formulation of hierarchical structures, rituals, territorial behavior, and aggression. This is the limbic *system*. It causes and modulates specific functions that allow for the determination between the agreeable and the disagreeable. Certain functions requiring a complexity of loving, joyful, protective, and empathetic feelings, such as caretaking of the young, originate in the limbic system. Likewise, opposite emotions, like anger, fear, and hate originate there as well.

Many theories have been postulated throughout the last seventy-five years regarding the process of stimulus/reaction in the brain. In 1929, Walter Cannon and Phillip Bardand put forth the Cannon-Bard theory[77], which states that when people face upsetting events, the nervous impulse travels straight to the thalamus. It is here that the message divides. One impulse goes to the cortex and originates subjective experiences like fear, sadness, and anger, while the other impulse goes to the hypothalamus to determine the peripheral neurovegetative changes (symptoms). This theory postulates that physiological reactions and emotional experiences happen simultaneously.[78] More recent research calls this theory into question, and as technological advances in the area of neuroscience develop a greater understanding of how the brain/body process happens, this process will become clearer. Tim Dalgleish, in a 2004 article for *Nature Reviews Neuroscience*, predicts these advances:

> A historical analysis of the development of affective neuroscience reveals that many more
> brain regions than initially supposed are involved in the processing of emotion and mood.

In many ways, this mirrors developments at the psychological level of explanation, where there is an increasing understanding of the pervasive influence of emotions on all forms of psychological processing. An impressive body of knowledge is accumulating about the roles of individual regions of the brain, such as the amygdala, in emotion processing. However, there is less consistency and little hard empirical data about the detailed interactions of these regions as part of a broader emotion system. A key challenge for the future is to address these issues.[79]

Perhaps it is instructive to look back at the work of early twentieth-century neuroanatomist James Papez, who believed the experience of emotion was determined by the cingulated cortex and, to a lesser degree, by other cortical areas. The expression of emotion was believed to be governed by the hypothalamus. The experience of emotion, determined by the gyrus cingulated, related to the hippocampus, which passed it on to the hypothalamus through a bundle of axons called the fornix. Papez[80] demonstrated in 1937 that emotion is not a function of any specific brain center. Emotion and its expression are interconnected through several nervous bundles: the hypothalamus (with its mammillary bodies), the anterior thalamic nucleus, the cingulated gyrus, and the hippocampus. This circuit, now called the Papez circuit, acting in a harmonic fashion, is responsible for the central functions of emotions, as well as for its symptoms.

Neuroscientist Paul MacLean accepted the bases of the Papez circuit and created the term limbic system, adding the orbitofrontal and medial-frontal cortices, parahippocampal gyrus, and other important subcortical groupings, like the amygdala, medial thalamic nucleus, septal area, prosencephalic basal nuclei, and some brainstem formations. None of these structures alone is responsible for any specific emotional state. They do, however, interconnect to enable emotion to happen. Some of the structures contribute more to certain types of emotion. We will take each of these in turn. I relied heavily on the work of Dr. Julio Rocha do Amaral and Dr. Jorge Martins de Oliveira for these descriptions of some of the main parts of the limbic system.

AMYGDALA: A small almond-shaped structure deep inside the antero-inferior region of the temporal lobe, which connects with the hippocampus, septal nuclei, the prefrontal area, and the medial dorsal nucleus of the thalamus. It serves to mediate and control major affective activities such as friendship, love, and affection, as well as the expression of mood and, mainly, fear, rage, and aggression. Being the center for the identification of danger, the amygdala is fundamental to self-preservation. When triggered, it leads to fear and anxiety, which in turn leads to "fight or flight." In order for the amygdala to get sensory input, it must be fairly highly processed, and to this end, the visual, auditory, and somatosensory cortices are the main input to the amygdala. The amygdala is the nucleus responsible for the lurch you feel in your stomach when you find yourself in a dark alley faced with a man in a ski mask holding a gun. The amygdala must be able to control the autonomic system to provoke such a response. Amygdala output is to the hypothalamus and brainstem autonomic centers.

HIPPOCAMPUS: Crucial to long-term memory. If both hippocampi are destroyed, nothing is retained in memory. An intact hippocampus allows for a complete comparison of situations and determination of the level of present threat with experience. This makes possible the best survival choice. The hippocampus is divided into five layers—dentate gyrus, subiculum, and entorhinal cortex (part of the parahippocampal gyrus), and specific areas called CA3 and CA1. There is essentially a one-way flow of information through the hippocampus entering the dentate gyrus by way of the gap between the subiculum and the dentate. This gap is called the perforant path because it perforates the space between the two. According to *News Medical*, an internet publication:

> The hippocampus contains high levels of glucocorticoid receptors, which make it more vulnerable to long-term stress than most other brain areas. Stress-related steroids affect the hippocampus in at least three ways: first, by reducing the excitability of some hippocampal neurons; second, by inhibiting the genesis of new neurons in the dentate gyrus; third, by causing atrophy of dendrites in pyramidal cells of the CA3 region.

> There is evidence that humans who have experienced severe, long-lasting traumatic stress (for example, Holocaust survivors) show atrophy of the hippocampus more than of other parts of the brain. These effects show up in post-traumatic stress disorder, and they may contribute to the hippocampal atrophy reported in schizophrenia and severe depression.

> Hippocampal atrophy is also frequently seen in Cushing's syndrome, a disorder caused by high levels of cortisol in the bloodstream. At least some of these effects appear to be reversible if the stress is discontinued. There is, however, evidence mainly derived from studies using rats that stress shortly after birth can affect hippocampal function in ways that persist throughout life.

FORNIX AND PARAHIPPOCAMPAL GYRUS: Stimulation of the medial dorsal and anterior nuclei of the thalamus are associated with changes in emotional reactivity. It is not the thalamus that regulates the emotional behavior but the connections of the nuclei with other limbic system structures. The medial dorsal nucleus makes connections with cortical zones of the prefrontal area and with the hypothalamus. The anterior nuclei connect with the mammillary bodies and through them, by way of the fornix, with the hippocampus and the cingulated gyrus, thus taking part in the Papez circuit.

HYPOTHALAMUS: With ample connections to other prosencephalic areas and the mesencephalic nucleus, lesions on or stimulation of the hypothalamic nuclei interfere with several vegetative functions and some of the so-called motivated behaviors, like thermal regulation, sexuality, competitiveness, hunger, and thirst. The hypothalamus is also believed to play a role in emotion. Pleasure and rage are associated with its lateral parts, while aversion, displeasure, and a tendency to uncontrollable and loud laughing are associated with its medial parts. Generally, the hypothalamus has more to do with the expression of emotions than with the genesis of the affective states. When physical symptoms of negative emotion appear, the threat they pose returns, by way of the hypothalamus, to the limbic center and finally to the prefrontal nuclei, increasing anxiety. This negative response mechanism can be so strong as to generate a situation of panic. There is a spatially oriented connection with the hypophysis or pituitary gland immediately beneath the hypothalamus. The pituitary is composed of two distinctive parts: the anterior pituitary (adenohypophysis), composed predominantly of cells that secrete protein hormones, and the posterior pituitary (neurohypophysis), which is not classified as a gland but an extension of the hypothalamic neurons.

CINGULATE GYRUS: Located between the cingulated sulcus and the corpus callosum on the medial side of the brain, it is known to coordinate smells and sights with pleasant memories of previous emotions. This region also participates in the emotional reaction to pain and the regulation of aggressive behavior.

BRAINSTEM: This is the region responsible for emotional reactions. The structures of the reticular formation and locus coeruleus, a concentrated mass of nor-epinephrine secreting neurons, are all part of the brainstem. These primitive structures remain active. Not only do they serve as alerting mechanisms that are vital for survival, but they also assist in the maintenance of the sleep–wake cycle.

VENTRAL TEGMENTAL AREA: Located in the mesencephalic part of the brain stem. Located here is a compact group of dopamine-secreting neurons whose axons end in the nucleus accumbens (mesolimbic dopaminergic pathway). The spontaneous firing or electrical stimulation of neurons belonging to that region produces pleasurable sensations, some of them similar to those felt during orgasm. Many people who, because of a genetic error, have a reduction of D2 (dopamine) receptors in the accumbens nucleus become, eventually, incapable of obtaining gratification from the common pleasures of life. As a result, they may turn to alcoholism, cocaine addiction, impulsive gambling and compulsion for sweet foods. Certain brainstem structures, like the nuclei of the cranial nerves, stimulated by impulses coming from the cortex and the striatum (a subcortical formation), are responsible for the physiognomic expressions of anger, joy, sadness, and tenderness.

SEPTUM: Lies anteriorly to the thalamus. This is the center for orgasm, and inside it, one finds four for women and one for men. This area, of course, is associated with different kinds of pleasant sensations, mainly those related to sexual experiences.

PREFRONTAL CORTEX: Comprises the entire non-motor anterior region of the frontal lobe. This area does not traditionally belong to the limbic circuit. Its intense bi-directional connections with thalamus, amygdala, and other subcortical structure account for the important role it plays in the genesis and, specifically, in the expression of effective states. The limbic system came into being long before the frontal lobe held its current dominant role. The neo-cortex, of which the frontal lobe is a part, is the domain of reason and the central processing area for all perceived sensations. It gives a fuller understanding of what is happening around us and how it affects us. The neocortex generates our thoughts, but it is the limbic system that provides feeling to those thoughts. Together, they create a richer harmony than either can provide alone.

My intention in presenting the anatomy and functions of the limbic system is not so much to impart anatomical knowledge as to illustrate how thoughts, feelings, and emotions are intricately and intensely interrelated. Like any system, knowledge of how it works provides for better maintenance and understanding of the system. The human system differs from mechanical systems in that each of the components of the human energy system is a living system within living systems.

David Bohm, in sharing his idea of the implicate order, clearly identifies and explains the concept of living systems within living systems when he says:

Every action starts from an intention in the implicate order. The imagination is already the creation of the form; it already has the intention and the germs of all the movements needed to carry it out. It affects the body and so on so that as creation takes place in that way from the subtler levels of the implicate order, it goes through them until it manifests in the explicate.[81]

Ancient cultures understood this idea and explained it using different words. Psychologist Edmond Bordeaux Szekely translated these words from the ancient Essene document *The Sevenfold Peace*, which is written in Aramaic:

Man, it was held, has three bodies that function in each of these departments: an acting body, a feeling body, and a thinking body. The thinking body's highest power is wisdom. The feeling body's highest power is love. The acting body's function is to translate the wisdom of the thinking body and the love of the feeling body into action in an individual's social and cultural worlds . . .[82]

Gregg Braden's work *Walking Between the Worlds*[83] synthesizes the Essene writings and traditions into a more modern language called compassion, which echoes Szekely's view that the Sevenfold Peace is the process through which we create peace and harmony in our individual lives and the greater society.

It is one thing to take for granted what seems to be an automatic process of thought, feeling, and emotion; it is quite another to have the wisdom and understanding that results in the knowledge to make the ultimate highest choice possible.

Functions of the Endocrine System

The endocrine system is made up of the following glands and organs:

Thyroid	Pineal Gland
Parathyroid	Thymus
Pituitary	Adrenal Glands
Hypothalamus	Ovaries
Heart	Testes
Kidneys	Stomach
Pancreas	Liver [84]

These glands and organs secrete chemical messengers called hormones. These chemical messengers relay signals through the blood to a target organ, which possesses an appropriate receptor in its cells. Hormones are classed into three groups—steroids, peptides, and amines. Steroids are lipids derived from cholesterol. Peptides are short chains of amino acids. Most hormones are peptides. Peptides are secreted from the pituitary, parathyroid, heart, stomach, liver, and kidneys. Amines are derived from the amino acid tyrosine and are secreted from the thyroid and the adrenal medulla.

The endocrine system uses cycles and negative feedback to regulate physiological functions. Negative feedback regulates the secretion of almost every hormone. Cycles of secretion maintain physiological and homeostatic control. These cycles can range from hours to months in duration. The endocrine system acts by releasing hormones that, in turn, trigger actions in specific target cells. Receptors on target cell membranes bind only to one type of hormone. More than fifty human hormones have been identified to date.

Endocrine system-related problems include:

- Overproduction of a hormone
- Underproduction of a hormone
- Nonfunctional receptors that cause target cells to become insensitive to hormones

The physiological effects of hormones depend largely on their concentration in blood and extracellular fluid. The concentration of hormone from the perspective of target cells is determined by the rate of hormone production, rate of hormone delivery, and rate of degradation and elimination. Control and regulation of this life cycle of a hormone is largely through feedback circuits. Feedback circuits are at the root of most control mechanisms in physiology and are particularly prominent in the endocrine system. Instances of positive feedback occur, but negative feedback is much more common.

Negative feedback is seen when the output of a pathway inhibits inputs to the pathway. The heating system in our homes is an example of a negative feedback system. The thermostat set at a specific temperature signals the furnace to kick on or off when the temperature either exceeds or is less than the set number. An example of negative feedback in the endocrine system is the regulation of concentrations of blood components such as glucose. When milk or sugar products are ingested, the following events will occur:

- Glucose from the ingested lactose or sucrose is absorbed in the intestine, and the level of glucose rises.
- Elevation of blood glucose concentration stimulates endocrine cells in the pancreas to release insulin.
- Insulin facilitates the entry of glucose into many cells of the body. As a result, blood glucose levels fall.
- When the level of blood glucose falls sufficiently, the stimulus for insulin release disappears, and insulin is no longer secreted.

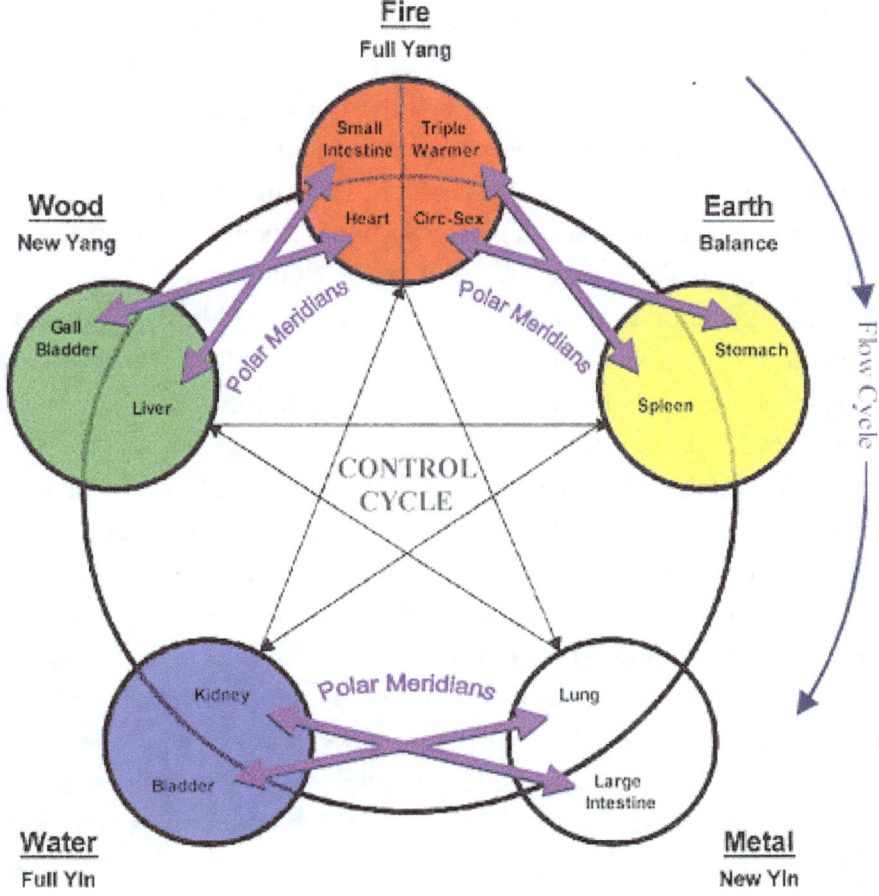

Fire
Full Yang

Wood
New Yang

Earth
Balance

Water
Full Yin

Metal
New Yin

Oriental Medicine is a system based on imbalance as the cause of disease, which corresponds to the pathologies sited for the production of hormone activity. In other words, malfunction is said to occur if there is too little hormone production. Revisiting the traditional Chinese Medicine perception of the five elements models from the previous chapter, we shall apply that model to the endocrine system.

The controlling cycle illustrated on that chart shows that the liver controls the spleen. If there is stagnation in the liver energy flow or chi, it will "over act" the spleen and interfere with its ability to transform and transport food. Using the generating cycle, the kidney supplies the liver with chi. According to the tenets of traditional Chinese medicine, the endocrine interaction occurs in the following way: The kidneys are the root of the yin of the body, and the liver stores the blood of the body. The spleen controls the kidneys; if the kidneys are in excess, they can insult the spleen. The heart supplies the spleen; if the heart is deficient, it cannot nourish the spleen. The lung is the son of the spleen, and if the lungs are deficient, they may drain too much energy from the spleen.

As the diagrams indicate, each individual organ has a direction in which the energy or chi flows. The liver chi goes in all directions to ensure that all organs send energy in the direction they were designed to send it. Thus, the liver can have a great influence on three major processes of the body—emotions, digestion, and the free flow of blood. Therefore, if there is distortion in the flow of liver chi, the mind cannot be at ease. Stagnant liver energy causes depression, sadness, oppression of the chest, or a lump in the throat. If liver chi is overactive, it causes restlessness, insomnia, dizziness, and vertigo. The liver assists in the smooth flow of stomach and spleen chi. If liver bile is not introduced properly, the liver will attack the stomach and spleen, resulting in nausea, vomiting, belching, reflux, chest pain, hypochondriac pain, and diarrhea. Because the blood cannot go where the chi does not flow, a stagnated liver causes blood to stagnate. Even though the heart and lungs are the promoters of blood circulation, stagnation of liver chi still causes stagnation of blood, resulting in the symptoms mentioned above.

Because the liver nourishes the body's tendons and sinews, allowing it to maintain its normal physiological functions, a deficient liver may deprive the tendons of nourishment and lead to weakness in the joints, tendons, and, ultimately, the limbs. A harmony of blood flow through the liver gives the eyes their brightness and shine. When liver blood is abundant, vision is clear and crisp. When it is deficient, vision is blurred, and the eyes are dry. This can lead to myopia.

From the perspective of traditional Chinese medicine, the lungs house the physical soul, and the liver houses the spiritual soul. It is the spiritual soul that gives the physical both life and purpose, without which a person would lose direction. When the liver blood is deficient, it cannot root the soul; thus, the person loses direction in life. Sensations of fear or floating, when experienced before sleep, indicate deficient liver blood. Even though the liver is not part of the endocrine system, it plays a major role in total health and well-being; it is intricately linked to the health and well-being of the endocrine system and, therefore, to the entire physical body.

Glands and Organs of the Endocrine System

PITUITARY GLAND: Also known as the hypophysis, the pituitary gland is located immediately beneath the hypothalamus. The pituitary gland is divided into two parts—the adenohypophysis and the neurohypophysis. Adenohypophysis (or anterior pituitary) is a classical gland that secretes protein hormones. The posterior pituitary is not a gland but an extension of the hypothalamus. It is composed largely of the axons of hypothalamic neurons. This system is a negative feedback system. Neurons in the hypothalamus secrete thyroid-releasing hormone (TRH), which stimulates cells in the anterior pituitary to secrete thyroid-stimulating hormone (TSH). Thyroid-stimulating hormone binds to receptors on epithelial cells in the thyroid gland, stimulating synthesis and secretion of thyroid hormones, which probably affect all body cells. When blood concentrations of thyroid hormones increase above a certain threshold, neurons secreting TRH in the hypothalamus are compromised; this stops the secretion of TRH.

The adenohypophysis or anterior pituitary mentioned in the preceding paragraph also produces and releases hormones called thyrotropin, adrenocorticotropin, luteinizing hormone, growth hormone, prolactin, melanocyte-stimulating hormone, endorphins, and enkephalins. The second part of the pituitary gland, the posterior pituitary or neurohypophysis, releases oxytocin and vasopressin. The pituitary/hypothalamus connection is essential in the maintenance of homeostatic levels of growth hormone.

Hypothalamus receptors monitor blood levels of thyroid hormones. The detection of low blood levels of TSH triggers the negative feedback process involving the anterior pituitary. The TSH promotes the production of thyroid hormones regulating metabolic rates and body temperatures. Gonadotropins, prolactin, and anterior pituitary secretions affect the gonads by stimulating gamete formation and the production of sex hormones. Gonadotropins include follicle-stimulating hormone(s) and luteinizing hormones.

The posterior pituitary stores and releases an antidiuretic hormone and oxytocin, which is produced by the hypothalamus, into the blood. The antidiuretic hormone controls water balance and blood pressure. Oxytocin stimulates uterine contractions during childbirth.

If the pituitary gland makes the indicator change in the EMCS defusion process, the emotional components or behavioral problems may manifest in feelings of self-distrust, loss of control of self or external situations, and lack of self-worth. They might cover these unwanted emotions with arrogance and use their "victim story" or "woundedness" as an excuse for self-determined failure.

THYROID AND PARATHYROID GLANDS: These are located in the neck close to the trachea. Thyroid hormones stimulate diverse metabolic activities in most tissues, leading to an increase in basal metabolic rate. One consequence of this activity is to increase body heat production, which seems to result, at least in part, from increased oxygen consumption and rates of ATP hydrolysis. By way of analogy, the action of thyroid hormones is akin to blowing on a smoldering fire.

A few examples of specific metabolic effects of thyroid hormones include:

- *Lipid metabolism*: Increased thyroid hormone levels stimulate fat mobilization, leading to increased concentrations of fatty acids in plasma. They also enhance the oxidation of fatty acids in many tissues. Finally, plasma concentrations of cholesterol and triglycerides are inversely correlated with thyroid hormone levels—one diagnostic indiction of hypothyroidism is increased blood cholesterol concentration.

- *Carbohydrate metabolism*: Thyroid hormones stimulate almost all aspects of carbohydrate metabolism, including enhancement of insulin-dependent entry of glucose into cells and increased gluconeogenesis and glycogenolysis to generate free glucose.

Thyroid hormones are derivatives of the amino acid tyrosine bound covalently to iodine. The two principal thyroid hormones are thyroxine and triiodothyronine. Physiologically, thyroid hormones affect all cells in the body. They have profound effects on the major physiologic processes of development, growth, and metabolism. Thyroid hormones stimulate almost all aspects of carbohydrate metabolism, including metabolism to enhance insulin-dependent and entry of glucose into cells.

Besides affecting development, growth, and metabolism, thyroid hormones increase heart rate, cardiac contractility, and out-put. These hormones promote vasodilatation, leading to enhanced blood flow to many organs. The central nervous system is affected by an increase or decrease in thyroid hormone concentration. This affects the mood or mental state of the individual. Too much concentration induces anxiety and nervousness, and too little causes mental sluggishness. The reproductive system is also affected by hypothyroidism; it is a common cause of infertility.

The emotional/behavioral response to a compromised thyroid may be best described as a feeling or experience interpreted as "no matter what I do, it is never my turn." Out of that comes a deep resentment and emotional unbalance based on past experience, which is perceived as one "never" getting what they want. Thyroid issues may also show up as life experiences that reflect deep resentment that they have never felt loved, respected, or supported in life.

THYMUS GLAND: The thymus gland is located just above the heart and below the thyroid and plays a critically important role in the body's response to disease invasion. Thus, it is crucial to a functioning immune system. One of its primary roles is to process white blood cells into T lymphocytes, which provide the following three defensive functions:

- Stimulate the production and growth of antibodies by other lymphocytes.
- Stimulate growth and action of the phagocytes, which surround and engulf invading viruses and microbes.
- Recognize and destroy foreign and abnormal tissue.

There is still much to learn about the operation of the thymus. Researchers currently agree that it is essential to the proper operation of the lymphatic system, and they agree its production of thymosin promotes the development of T-cells. The outer layer of the thymus is called the cortex; it contains lymphocytes with which it "seeds" the lymphatic organs and lymph nodes and diffuses lymphatic tissue with potential T lymphocytes. The T-cells attack the protein of certain tumor cells, foreign cells, and microorganisms.

The Energy Matrix Clearing System attributes a person's feelings of lack of fulfillment and difficult life circumstances to thymus gland problems. As a result, they may shirk responsibility for their actions as a form of self-defense. They are constantly plagued by the feeling that they will never have an opportunity to fully live life, and in extreme cases, may even believe that life is literally attacking them.

HEART: In traditional Chinese medicine, the heart is referred to as the "monarch" of the body. It is a magical and complicated place associated with love and joy as well as with the healing of sorrow and hurt. It is a place of compassion and unity.

Because the heart pumps the very "stuff of life" and regulates the flow of blood through the vessels that open into the tongue and face, Chinese medicine practitioners believe that the mind itself is housed in the heart. Dr. Bruce Fisher elaborates on this idea: "The blood absorbs those pictures of the outside world which the brain has formed within, transforms them into living constructive forces, and with them builds up the present human body."[85]

In a large sense, our present fascination with consciousness depends on the heart/mind connection. Without consciousness, human beings would just be animals surviving the elements. As Teeguarden suggests, "Following the 'path with heart' yields feelings of peace, love, and joy. There is a sense of inner harmony; all is well in the land of shen, and the sense of well-being pervades the whole self."[86]

Many books have been written about the heart from a purely anatomical perspective, as well as from a metaphysical/emotional/spiritual one. It is not my intention to add to the pile. The study of the human heart does, however, illicit in me the thought that the heart represents, in all ways, the ultimate processor of thought, feeling, and emotion. For all its mystery and function, it seems to hold within its "library" knowledge of our past, present, and future. I find especially fascinating a particular kind of cell known as purkinje, which generates electrical impulses in the gut, brain, and heart. In the heart, purkinje fibers comprise the muscle tissue that conducts electrical impulses into the ventricular cells. This tissue is comprised of very large cells modified to transmit electrical impulses, or action potentials, at a velocity many times greater than normal cardiac cells. Is it coincidental that 95 percent of the brain's volume is taken up with the abundantly multi-limbed branching of purkinje cells in the cerebellum and that each cell is capable of communication with some 30,000 other neurons? They are remarkable for their ability to integrate large amounts of information and learn by remodeling their dendrites.

The human brain has evolved over time to meet the need to solve problems within increasingly complex environments. Has the heart evolved as well? Have we, by virtue of evolution, become the "Children of Light" as the ancients predicted? In addition, is it our conscious awareness of the Unity of One, which our hearts represent, that makes this possible? Has the totality of our human physical system developed in such a way that we can now access information through our subtle energy fields, thus making it possible for us to move into a "new world" of peace and harmony with all things?

The Energy Matrix Clearing System considers that heart area problems arise from avoiding loving relationships in an effort to protect oneself from emotional injury, whether that be rejection or manipulation. In any case, love is regarded as a dangerous and even destructive force.

ADRENAL GLANDS: The adrenals produce three major classes of hormones, each assisting in processing stress arising from daily life. The two adrenal glands are located immediately anterior to the kidneys. Like the kidneys, the adrenal glands lie beneath the peritoneum. There are two distinct regions of the adrenals. The first is the inner medulla, which is a source of epinephrine and norepinephrine. The cell is the principal cell type of the medulla, which is also abundantly innervated by pregaglionic sympathetic fibers and is, in essence, an extension of the sympathetic nervous system. The other region, the outer cortex, secretes several classes of steroid hormones called glucocorticoids and mineralocorticoids, as well as sex hormones. The two sections of the adrenals, even though they are organized into one organ, are functionally different endocrine glands and have different embryological origins. The medulla derives from ectoderm, and the cortex develops from mesoderm.

The focus of the adrenal is to alert the system when "survival" is in question. The Energy Matrix Clearing System views adrenal problems from the perspective that the client is "running on empty." They have spent their life force in ways that did not return the investment. They may be suffering from overwork or are overloaded with responsibilities, resulting in anxiety, fear, and frustration to the point of exhaustion.

CELLS WITHIN THE ADRENAL MEDULLA: These cells synthesize and secrete norepinephrine and epinephrine. Following release into the blood, these hormones bind adrenergic receptors on target cells, where they induce essentially the same effects as direct sympathetic nervous stimulation, although their effect is longer lasting. Additionally, circulating hormones can cause effects in cells and tissues that are not directly innervated. The physiologic consequences of medullary catecholamine release are justifiably framed as responses that aid in dealing with stress. Major effects mediated by epinephrine and norepinephrine include the following:

- Increased rate and force of contraction of the heart muscle
- Constriction of blood vessels
- Dilation of bronchioles
- Stimulation of lipolysis in fat cells. Increased metabolic rate: consumption and heat production increase throughout the body in response to epinephrine
- Breakdown of glycogen in skeletal muscle, promoted by hormones, to provide glucose for energy production
- Dilation of pupils
- Inhibition of "nonessential" processes, such as gastrointestinal secretion and motor activity

Exercise, hypoglycemia, hemorrhage, and emotional distress are common stimuli for the secretion of adrenomedullary hormones. Removal of the adrenal glands results in death. Without mineralocorticoid activity, the concentration of potassium in extracellular fluid becomes dramatically elevated, urinary excretion of sodium rises to a high level, and the concentrations of sodium in extracellular fluid decrease significantly. The volume of extracellular fluid and blood plummets. The heart begins to function poorly causing cardiac output decline, resulting in shock. Mineralocorticoids maintain electrolyte balance, and glucocorticoids produce a long-term, slow response to stress by raising blood glucose levels through the breakdown of fats and proteins. Mineralocorticoids also suppress the immune response and inhibit the inflammatory response.

From an EMCS perspective, adrenal medulla issues relate to feelings of being overpowered by their own mind, causing feelings of not being able to control the thoughts it generates. In effect, they are "running on empty."

KIDNEYS: In *The Joy of Feeling,* Teeguarden suggests that the kidneys are associated with fear and the synergic feeling of resolution and willpower, along with certain physiological processes and characteristics, like the sense organ of the nose, bone marrow, and bodily fluids like urine. Traditional Chinese medicine refers to the bladder as the yang organ partner of the kidneys. Emotions and feeling associated with the kidneys are inadequacy, timidity, inferiority, panic, phobias, apprehension, and fear.[87]

The kidneys control water in the lower warmer, which helps them regulate water metabolism. Working hand in hand with the lungs, the kidneys receive the chi sent down into it from the lungs. If this interaction of chi does not occur, breathing issues can arise.

Marrow is associated with the kidneys; it is found in the bones, brain, and spinal cord. The chi of the kidney, or shen as it is referred to in TCM, is sometimes called the essence of the kidney; it produces the marrow. The marrow, in turn, makes the bones strong and fills the spinal cord and brain to activate intelligence and concentration. The brain is often called the "Sea of Marrow" for this reason. Everything involved in aging is governed by the kidneys. When the kidneys go weak, memory and quality of thought become poor (brain), the speed of the physical body's reactions are slowed (spine), teeth crack and fall out (bone), and bones become brittle. Other areas influenced by the health of the kidneys include the quality of hearing and the shine, health, and abundance of hair.

The Energy Matrix Clearing System perspectives related to kidney issues include:
1. Inability to cleanse the blood of waste products
2. Anxiety, worries, and fears around money
3. Lack of sense of well-being
4. An attitude of always saving for the future
5. Intense self-acceptance issues, self-doubt and shame
6. Fear of releasing negative emotions
7. Giving up - there is no hope

STOMACH: The main function of the stomach is digestive, i.e., to process the food we eat and turn it into energy that powers the body. Since every aspect of the human system relies on the stomach for nourishment, an imbalance in this organ's function quickly affects the whole system, impacting not only physical energy in the form of food but also mental, emotional, and spiritual energy. This translates into an increased susceptibility to stressors. From the holographic perspective, if we do not benefit from the food we take in, then how can we benefit from any kind of energy coming into us from the outside? One question might be, "What is it we can't stomach?" According to Teeguarden, "Traditional association of Stomach imbalance include[s] becoming antisocial, feeling restless, and being easily startled by the noise."[88]

The Energy Matrix Clearing System perspectives related to stomach issues include:

1. Digestive issues, including nausea
2. Dread and fear of the future
3. Difficulty "digesting" new ideas or life circumstances
4. Inability to see the lesson inherent in an experience
5. Denial, repression, and rationalization concerning a life experience
6. Inflexibility
7. Self-rejection leading to the deflection of nurturance and support

PANCREAS: This elongated organ is nestled next to the first part of the small intestine. Its gross anatomy and the structure of pancreatic exocrine tissue and ducts are associated with the digestive system. The endocrine portion of the pancreas takes the form of many small clusters of cells called the islets of Langerhans. They include three major cell types, each producing a different endocrine product. Alpha cells secrete the hormone glucagons (aka glycogens). Beta cells produce insulin, and delta cells secrete the hormone somatostatin. Islets are richly vascularized, allowing for the fact that even though they make up only 1 to 2 percent of the mass of the pancreas, they receive about 10 to 15 percent of the pancreatic blood flow. The islets are also innervated by parasympathetic and sympathetic neurons. Therefore, nervous signals clearly modulate the secretion of insulin and glucagons or glycogens.[89]

The Energy Matrix Clearing System perspectives related to pancreatic issues include:

1. Attitudes of sourness and bitterness about life
2. Difficulties integrating and expressing love
3. Inability to feel joy
4. Loss of creativity
5. Emotional excess, negative self-indulgence, and violence
6. Feeling that the world owes them a living

Traditional Chinese medicine places the spleen and pancreas together as partners in the flow of chi. Teeguarden says, "The Spleen-Pancreas is the official who distributes nourishment. When we absorb the fruits of the earth, they first go to the stomach. Then the powerful pancreatic juice is secreted (into the small intestine) and plays a leading role in digesting all kinds of food—starches, proteins and fats."[90] The pancreas is also called by some the "official of energy transport" throughout the body mind.

Emotional considerations are mental fatigue, codependency, lack, forgetfulness, anxiety, and obsessive-compulsive behaviors. Worry, over-thinking, and indifference are also issues related to the pancreas.

REPRODUCTIVE ORGANS*:* The human ability to procreate is the territory of the reproductive organs. This relative difference between men and women and the implications of sexual desire and expression have been a driving force throughout history. Nations have risen and fallen because of a leader's sexual alliances. Religions have relegated us to little more than animals because of our need—our innate drive to perpetuate the species. The reproductive organs represent our ability to create in all ways, not just offspring but also art, music, love, money, and relationships. They also color our sense of self-worth and value.

The Energy Matrix Clearing System perspectives related to reproductive organ issues include:

1. Feelings of being unwanted as a child
2. Feelings of being unacceptable the way they are
3. Difficulty in sharing love or being in a committed relationship
4. Sexual repression and repression of sexual identity
5. Frustrated in their ability to create
6. Traumatic sexual experiences include sexual exploitation or gender rejection

This discussion of the endocrine and limbic systems is perhaps most valuable for creating awareness of the human body as a vehicle—a congealed mass of energy—with the express purpose of providing an avenue for the spirit or God to experience itself. It can be easy to get lost in the complicated processes that take place for "life" to happen. For the purposes of the Energy Matrix Clearing System, applying this information holographically allows us to at least begin to simplify the interpretation of the identified data.

Determining Levels of Health

For purposes of energy testing, we are using a numerical range of seven hundred as the optimal vitality level (OVL) of an organ or gland. A number below seven hundred indicates under energy, and a number over seven hundred indicates over energy. A number that is one hundred or more over and one hundred or more under indicates an organ or gland that is out of balance.

ORGAN/ GLAND	VITALITY LEVEL	AMOUNT OVER	AMOUNT UNDER
LIMBIC SYSTEM			
AMYGDALA			
HIPPOCAMPUS			
FORNIX AND GYRUS			
HYPOTHALAMUS			
CINGULATE GYRUS			
BRAINSTEM			
VENTRAL TEGMENTAL AREA			
SEPTUM			
PREFRONTAL AND NEOCORTEX			
ENDOCRINE SYSTEM			
PITUITARY AND PINEAL			
THYROID AND PARATHYROID			
THYMUS			
HEART			
ADRENAL			
KIDNEY			
STOMACH			
PANCREAS AND SPLEEN			

If several vitality levels are low after checking, notice the interactions or interrelated aspects of the organs/glands. Next, using muscle testing, determine the priority focus for defusion. If muscle testing indicates the pancreas is the priority, remember to consider not only the physical attributes but the emotional ones as well.

The Energy Matrix Clearing System SCRIPT

MT: "For priority issue to defuse."

MT: "You are here and present on all levels and dimensions: body, mind, emotional, essential, etheric, astral, mental, and causal?"

MT: "You are not here and present."

MT: "I have permission to work with you in this way."

MT: "Any reason not to work with you in this way?"

MT: "You commit to taking 100 percent responsibility for noticing, acting on, and benefiting from the positive change on all levels and dimensions without self-punishment."

MT: "Any reason that is not true?"

MT: "Our command is that any miasms, universal subconscious negative prompters, belief systems, life experience, past life experience, genetic imprinting, karmic ties, or any other kind of distorted energy that would in any way cause or support these effects be pulled from your holographic human energy system, canceled on the compass of time, be genetically re-calibrated, extirpated on all dimensions known and unknown, and transformed into the universal law of light, love, and balanced rhythmic interchange."

MT: "You understand the command."

MT: "Any reason you do not understand the command?"

MT: "You have objections to the command."

MT: "You do not have objections to the command."

MT: "Give me an indicator change for the Level of Responsibility: Emotion, Feeling, Thought."

NOTE THE RESPONSE.

MT: "Give me an indicator change for the Negative Emotional Energy."

MT: "Give me an indicator change for the Positive Emotional Energy."

NOTE THE RESPONSE.

MT: "Give me an indicator change for the Avoidance Behavior priority by the number 1 to 26, 1 to 5, etc."

Note response.

MT: "Give me an indicator change for the Universal Fear priority by the number 1 to 24, 1 to 5, etc."

MT: "Give me an indicator change for the five elements: earth, wood, water, fire, metal."

MT: "Give me an indicator change for the Reflective Mirror by the number 1 to 23."

MT: "Give me an indicator change for the level of consciousness: 1 to 17, 1, 2, 3 . . . 17."

Note the response.

MT: "Give me an indicator change for the priority Subtle Energy Body."

MT: "Give me an indicator change for the priority Element: 1 to 5."

MT: "Give me an indicator change for systems corrections: Matrix I, Matrix II, Matrix III."

If Matrix III makes the indicator change:

MT: Subcategory #1—Limbic System

MT: "Give me an indicator change for the priority subcategory or subcategories: 1, 2, 3 . . . 9."

Note the response.

ENDOCRINE SYSTEM MT: "Give me an indicator change for the priority subcategory or subcategories: 1, 2, 3 . . . 8."

Note the response.

MT: "Do we need to correct anything in the present time?"

MT: "Any reason not to correct anything in the present time?"

If the muscle response is "yes," indicating that corrections can be made in the present time, then make the appropriate corrections after going over the data with your test subject.

Make the corrections using the Fifteen Celestial Blends, determining the number of drops and route of administration. Then MT to determine NEE is 0 and PEE is 100. MT test for homework: use the animal representation from the Five Element chart (Chapter Six).

MT: How many days and how many times a day for homework?

Note the response.

If MT indicated not to correct in the present time, then do the following age recession:

MT: "Do I have permission to age recess?"

MT: "Any reason not to age recess?"

Put the gathered and discussed information/energy into the circuitry. With your thumbs on the subject's wrists, simultaneously make the following statement and action:

MT: "I am putting this information into the circuits," as you flick your thumbs on the subject's wrists.

MT: "Do I have this information in the circuits?"

MT: "Any reason I do not?"

If testing indicates the information is loaded into the circuits, then begin the age recession:

MT: "Give me an indicator change to the age of cause or best understanding or the age that is best to correct."

Then, begin with the present age and recess back until the indicator changes. Example: Present age in ten-year increments until the indicator changes.

MT: "50 to 40, 40 to 30, etc."

When the indicator changes (the muscle releases)

MT: "This is the age of cause?"

MT: "Any reason it is not?"

If testing indicates it is not the age of cause, then:

MT: "Is this the age of best understanding or the age that is best to correct?"

MT: "Any reason it is not?"

If testing indicates it is none of the above, then this identified age could also be an age on line. If that is the case:

MT: "This is an age on line."

MT: "Any reason it is not?"

If testing indicates it is an age on line:

MT: "Identify any information at age on line?

If affirmative (muscle holds strong), gather the following information about this age:

MT: Muscle Test to Identify:
- NEE
- PEE
- Level of Responsibility from the Living in Choice Chart
- Level of Consciousness
- Avoidance Behavior
- Five Elements
- Universal Fear
- Matrix Systems

Discuss the above information and make the corrections.

MT: "NEE is 0"

MT: "PEE is 100"

MT: "Any reason it is not?"

If the answer is affirmative:

MT: "We have permission to continue to cause."

MT: "Any reason not?"

Continue testing to the age of cause.

Once the indicator change occurs again:

MT: "This the age of cause."

MT: "Any reason it is not?"

IMT: Muscle test to identify:
- Physical, Etheric, Astral, Mental, or Causal

- Level of Responsibility
- NEE
- Universal Fear
- Avoidance Behavior
- Five Elements
- Matrix Systems

Review the information with your client.

Corrections: Identify the appropriate Living in Choice Gem and Mineral Essence(s)

MT: "Give me an indicator change for the appropriate Celestial Blend: 1 to 15 for corrections:

MT: "Give me an indicator for the number of drops and mode of administration: On the tongue, under the tongue, or in water."

Note response.

MT: "Do I have permission to correct?"

MT: "Any reason not to correct?

Make the corrections.

Read the accompanying Gem and Mineral information.

MT: "Have we completely diffused all causal energies supporting the negative pattern or blockage?"

MT: "Any reason we have not?"

MT: "Is the NEE 0 and the PEE 100 percent on this issue at the age of cause?"

MT: "Any reason it is not?"

MT: "We are infusing the element"

MT: "Any reason not to infuse the element?"

Once that is determined, explain the animal representation of the element to the subject and tell them to close their eyes and focus on that symbol while you infuse their system and bring them back to the present time:

MT: "Do I have permission to bring you back to the present time?"

MT: "Any reason not to bring you back to the present time?"

Remind the subject to get the symbol in mind. Then, starting with the age of cause, bring them back to the present time in increments of five years, anchoring the infusion symbol by pumping their arms gently twice at each increment until they are back to the present time.

MT: "You are right here, right now, grounded in Unity and Oneness at this moment."

MT: "Any reason you are not?"

MT: "The Negative Energy is 0."

MT: "The Positive Energy is 100 percent in the present time."

MT: "Any reason it is not?"

If the response is affirmative, then:

MT: "Will there be any withdrawal or residual from this process today?"

If the muscle response is weak, indicating a "no," then proceed:

MT: "Is there any specific homework?"

MT: "Any reason there is not?"

MT: "Is the homework focusing on the infusion symbol?"

MT: "Any reason not to focus on the infusion symbol?"

MT: "How many days and times a day?"

MT: "Are we complete and finished with this defusion today?"

MT: "Any reason we are not?"

Congratulations, you have finished the defusion!

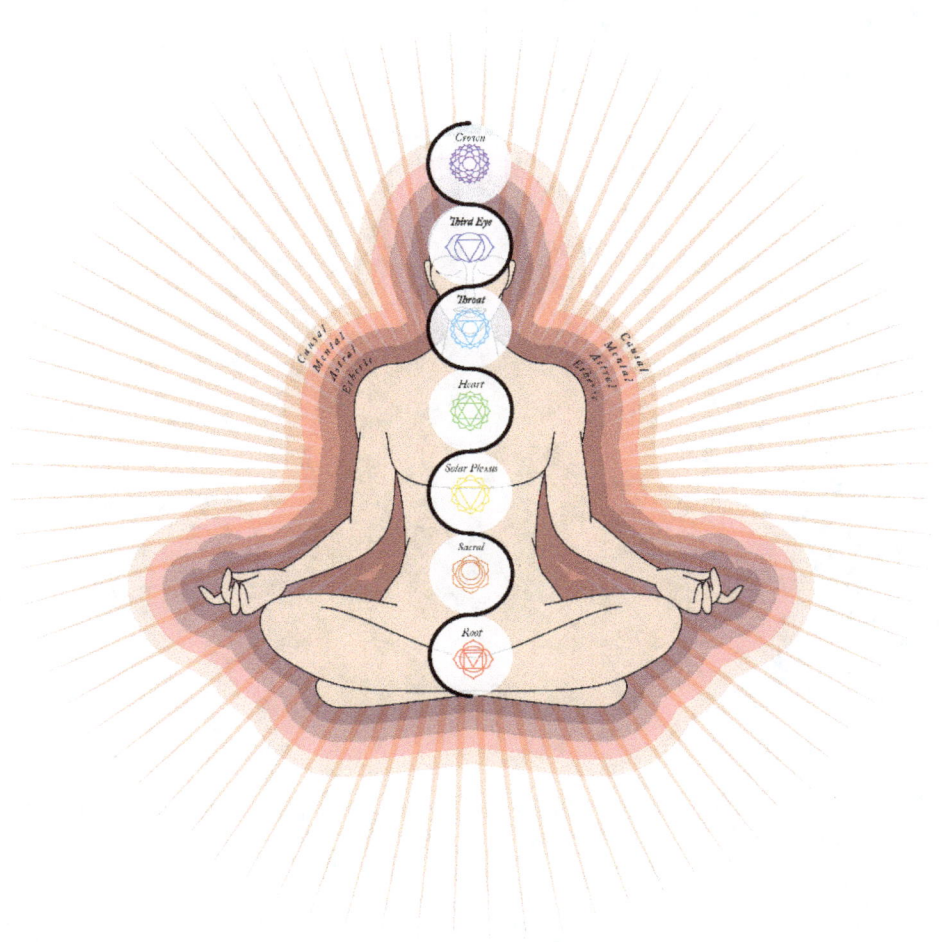

CHAPTER NINE

MATRIX IV

THE CHAKRA SYSTEM

When you step out of your own shadow, you enter the light within. It is then you realize that beneath all your fears, desires, pains, and preconceptions of the ego-self surges the basic drive to remember your essential nature.

—CHARLES BREAUX

The chakra system is EMCS Matrix IV. The study of the chakra system begins with a journey through the maze of subtle energies connecting the inside (physical) and the outside (aura) of the holographic human energy system. We can equate our journey through this maze to the ancient Greek myth of Theseus and his path through the Labyrinth of Crete—a path both crooked and baffling. The labyrinth, built by master architect Daedalus, is at once a road, a prison, and a conundrum. Daedalus built the labyrinth at the request of King Minos of Crete to keep outsiders from entering and to keep the monster who lived there from exiting. The monster, in this case, is the Minotaur, a half-man, a half-bull who feasts on human flesh. Theseus 'goal is to kill the Minotaur and make his way out of the maze, holding the head of the Minotaur as his prize. To assist Theseus in his journey, Ariadne, daughter of King Minos, gives him a ball of thread to unwind as he makes his way through the maze. But this would only help him find his way out. Reaching the Minotaur at the heart of the maze is up to him. Theseus could stop his journey at any time and find his way out, but he chooses to continue despite the danger.

Our personal journey may be just as daunting, but it certainly does not have to be as grim. In his article "The Joy of the Maze," Trebbe Johnson writes, "We like to trudge with our eyes on the goal, praying that our monsters will be small and easily slain . . . Yet, there is joy in the baffling journey. There is wild freedom to be found in the maze."[91]

Let's begin the journey.

The Sanskrit word "chakra" means "wheel" or "disk." It also means a "spinning vortex of energy." For this reason, many authors throughout the ages have referred to chakras as "wheels of light," and we now use the word to refer to those regions of spiritual power that are located throughout the human body. The earliest non-mythological philosophical texts written in India, known as the Upanishads, were written around the eighth century before the Common Era and introduced the idea of a subtle vital life force, which they called prana, and the channels along which it flows, the nadi. The Upanishads speak of the heart as the center of 72,000 nadis or subtle channels and the place into which the senses are withdrawn during sleep. It was not until the second century BCE that the later Upanishads first referenced the chakra system.

Earlier in this text, we explored the limbic and endocrine systems, focusing on an awareness of the interconnection between thoughts, feelings, and emotions along with their chemical and electromagnetic counterparts, including their effect on the health of the physical organs. Further exploration of the interconnectedness of energy systems and the health of the holographic human system must include the chakra system.

The Hindu chakra system is made up of seven major chakras and many minor ones. The seven major chakras are arranged vertically along the spinal column, starting at the base of the coccyx, moving up the spine and ending about the head. In the physical body, these seven major chakras correspond to the nervous system, endocrine system, and numerous bodily processes, such as breathing, digesting, and procreating.

This chapter explores numerous additional vortices of energy, or "minor chakras," located within and surrounding the physical body. Modern and ancient healers have written about these lesser-known chakra centers as well. Ancient Egyptians, for instance, taught a thirteen-chakra system. This system is complicated and cannot be used in conjunction with the eight-chakra system, also used by the Egyptians. Drunvalo Melchizedek, author of the two-volume book *The Ancient Secret of the Flower of Life*, states: "It is a mystery, except to say that the very same thing happens in quantum physics: you can see the Reality as made up of other particles (atoms) or vibration (waveform), but if you try to superimpose both systems at once, neither will work."[92] For the past eighty years or so, the cornerstone of quantum physics has been the "mystery" Melchizedek describes.

In 2004, physicist Shahriar Afshar[93] was able to observe through experimentation the wavelike interference pattern of light while simultaneously measuring the paths of the particular aspect of light called photons. He was able to replicate this experiment in 2006. Other teams of scientists are now attempting to replicate it as well. If Afshar's findings can be verified by other scientists, it would give us a vital clue to understanding how integral reality actualizes. It would mean that quantum waveforms of possibilities do not collapse but become coherent. This would take us a long way down the road toward proving the elegant holographic interconnectedness of the Universe—and, therefore, all things. It would explain how human energy systems like the chakra system, meridian system, and the subtle energy bodies operate on quantum levels.

It is my opinion that the Mayans also used the thirteen-chakra system since the number thirteen plays an important role in their numbering system. Jose Arguelles, in *The Mayan Factor: Path Beyond Technology*, gives credence to this view with his explanation of the 5,200-tun Mayan Great Cycle as a morphogenetic field: "Within the context of morphogenetic fields, the 5,200-tun Great Cycle can be viewed as a galactically activated field of a purposeful resonance divided into thirteen cyclical subfields." Arguelles delves deeply into the meaning of the Mayan thirteen-baktun cycles as an explanation of the "wave-harmonic of history." It is possible to look at these cycles, he says, as a "landscape of morphic resonance divided into seven mountains and six valleys," building to a crescendo of morphic resonance, finally exploding into matter. Similarly, the evolving human chakra system can be described.[94]

Arguelles insightfully explains the progression of the Mayan thirteen-baktun cycles with critical "points of transition" between sub-cycles. Each of the cycles possesses energies or "morphic resonance" represented by a particular archetype or set of archetypal symbols. The point of transition between each cycle called for a change in the archetypal symbols, heralding a new cycle. According to Arguelles, this transition "between" cycles marks an information transfer and imprint that affects and seals the overall memory-bearing quality of the new morphogenetic field." Arguelles suggests that these archetypal symbols are like "resonant capacitors," which, when properly constructed, contain the capacity to evoke the specific frequency at any time or place.[95] Therefore, one set of symbols may carry over from one baktun or one chakra to another. Perhaps this explains the Hindu concept of Karma or the New Age concept of past lives.

In his journey into the consciousness of humankind, the preeminent Swiss psychologist Carl Jung discovered certain universal patterns he termed "archetypes." He believed these archetypal patterns or psychic forces structurally predetermine the anatomy and function of the human psyche, much in the same way that our genetic code predetermines our physical attributes. Jung taught that archetypal energies unless superseded by personal trauma, are the guiding force in the shaping of the individual human experience. He determined archetypal energies appear in all aspects of our lives and experiences, including in art, music, mythology, religion, fantasy, science, and even our dreams.

Ancient teachings from the Bible to the Zohar tell us that consciousness holds within it the record of everything in the universe, even the "number of hairs" on our head. Just as Buddhists speak of the "store of consciousness," or alaya-vijnana, which they perceive to hold within it all human potential and experience, Jung spoke of the "collective unconscious." Can we then surmise that archetypal energies arise from this collective unconscious, providing direction for our individual lives? In addition, do archetypal energies express through the venue of the chakra system? Does each chakra then express different archetypal energies? Unless some trauma alters the course or energy of a particular chakra, are we destined, as Jung suggested, to live out our lives preordained by specific guiding archetypal energies or "consciousness?" My aim is to guide the reader to the answer to these questions.

Since the chakra system forms the matrix upon which each individual body/mind is formed, it defines our various experiences and our reactions to those experiences and records them in our personal unconscious. This information is colored by individual perception and processed as emotion, which surfaces as behavior through the autonomic nervous system. Our memories hold all information concerning everything that has ever happened to us in this lifetime or any other. The Akashic Records are the repository of this information, accessible from the mental and causal subtle energy bodies that make up a portion of the holographic human energy system. This will be discussed more in-depth in a later chapter. This personal record or consciousness tends to play the same song repeatedly, like a phonograph record that is grooved out from playing a particular song too many times, for those of you who remember phonograph records. The constant replay of memories may serve to support the continuance of limiting fears and belief structures, which can obscure the positive expression of personal archetypal energies.

I agree with Charles Breaux that these "seeds" must be uprooted before they bear "bitter fruit." Each chakra holds the potential for its own brand of limiting fears and beliefs. These distorted perceptions of reality may be used by consciousness to construct our inner and outer worlds. Breaux suggests that " . . . the deprogramming and reeducation of the personal unconscious requires much more skill and time, unless this task is successfully accomplished, conscious desires to change will most often prove ineffectual."[96]

The process of deprogramming the unconscious begins with the awareness of our guiding fears and belief structures. The Energy Matrix Cleaning System beautifully and artfully accomplishes that task.

Each chakra holds crystallized emotional and energetic patterns, which can be identified and released through the defusion process. This process of transforming the chasm between the conscious and the repetitive destructive patterns of the unconscious allows for the transformation of the negative aspects of the ego into positive ones. Chakras can have rigid, energetic archetypal patterns, which show up in limiting beliefs and behaviors. In other words, what you may think is a first chakra issue may show up in the heart chakra because it could more easily come to the surface there; thus, the nature of the maze.

Chakras as Information Centers

The entire chakra system, which includes the well-known major ones, the less well-known minor ones, the interface between the chakra systems, and the meridian acupuncture points, are areas where energy flows into and out of the holographic human energy system from the vast ocean of energy surrounding us. This ocean of energy has many names. Some quantum physicists call it the zero point field or unified field. David Bohm calls it the Explicate Order. Still others call it the "sea of consciousness." I like the term zero point field and will use it here.

Whatever the name, we interact with this energy through our thoughts, feelings, emotions, senses, and intuition—all of which we translate into experience. We also may call this life. It stands to reason, then, that the more open we are to receiving energy-information from the zero-point field, the more energy we metabolize through our chakra and meridian systems. The term "openness," in this case, means that we receive an optimum amount of energy-information from which our hard drive, the subtle energy bodies and software, chakras, and meridians must make decisions concerning every moment. This may seem daunting at first glance. However, it makes perfect sense to take a slow and even approach when working with the chakra system so that the least amount of physical, mental, emotional, and spiritual stress is generated.

Barbara Brennan teaches that the chakra system has three main functions:

1. The vitalization of the subtle energy bodies, or the aura as it is sometimes called, leads to the vitalization of the physical.
2. Through the development of the chakra system, different aspects of self-consciousness are also developed. Each specific chakra is specific to different aspects of psychological functioning.
3. The transmission of energy-information between the levels of the subtle energy bodies to the physical. Each level of the subtle body vibrates at succeeding higher frequencies. The chakra system extends concomitantly from the etheric layer to the fullest extension of the causal body. Brennan says the openings of the extensions of the chakra system in the outer bodies are closed in many people. They are opened through spiritual expansion and growth.[97]

First Chakra: Root

Muladhara

The Hindu and Buddhist philosophy of tantra translate Muladhara as "root place" or "root support." In the Taoist tradition, it is called chang qiang. This chakra is located in the area of the coccyx or tailbone at the base of the spine. Muladhara is the first of the yang or ascending energy centers, and its role is to transform and refine sexual energy and universal earth or yin chi before it enters the higher chakras.

This chakra is often confused with a secondary chakra called in Taoism hui yin, located at the perineum, which is the piece of skin located between the anus and the scrotum in men and the anus and vagina in women. The hui yin constitutes the lowest of the yin or descending energy chakras and is the lower meeting point of the governor meridian (yang) and the function of the conception vessel (yin) channels. The conception vessel is also called the central meridian (Western terminology). Through the legs and feet, it is the main link with the earth's chi or yin energy. It also connects to the central channel that is said to connect the human being to the center of the galaxy as well as to the center of the earth, and it runs through the center of the human body.

Hindu traditions and nineteenth-century Theosophists attribute four petals or divisions to the base or root chakra. Tantra teaching colors these petals crimson and the Theosophists red-orange. Vast and varied symbolism, myth, and archetypal representations are assigned to each of the chakras. The Muladhara is the seat of the kundalini, according to the Hindus, and is attributed to the earth element. The white elephant is a symbol of this chakra and represents the vehicle for transporting the ancient deity, Indra. According to the Theosophists, kundalini or serpent fire can be "loosed" from its seat in the base chakra and deflected to the brain by persistently yielding to the lower animalistic nature.

The primary function of the base chakra is to use the life force for survival needs and physical organism processes, such as supporting the skeletal system, the spine, the feet and legs, and the rectum, as well as regulating the immune system. When the base chakra is well-founded and supported, we feel secure in the physical world and trust in its workings. Without safety and security, deep-seated fears may develop that undermine all other levels of experience or consciousness. Manifestations of these survival energy patterns result in the archetypes of the bully, dominator, or aggressor and often show up in violent behavior. Brennan says an underdeveloped base chakra expresses symptoms such as a lack of physical power, coordination, avoidance of physical activity, and a weak or sickly constitution.[98] The base chakra represents the foundation upon which all other chakras rest. It is the manifestation of consciousness into matter in its most solid and dense form.

Past life experiences and genetic and ancestral archetypal patterns may be held within the base chakra as information that colors experience. In addition, prenatal, birth, and first-year life experiences all form the foundation for our later worldview. When first-year life experiences are filled with love, security, and plentiful food, a trusting worldview is imminent. On the other hand, if the first year of life is spent in disdainful, disruptive, and emotionally cold environments, we are likely to develop a threatening and unsupportive worldview. Evidence of these feelings might be heard in such statements as " I feel like an alien," "I don't belong here," or "The world is not a safe place for me."

The base chakra archetypal patterns have their roots in our most instinctual and primitive psyche. Because of this, the mother and father archetypes play an important role as imprinting factors of the base chakra. If these archetypes are distorted ones, we may spend our lives looking for the "fantasy" mother or father. This may become an obstacle to our developing a higher consciousness. Locked into an eternal search for a fantasy that can never be fulfilled, the seeker unknowingly lives in a state of survival and blames their lack of supportive parenting on their inability to thrive.

Other specific aspects originating from information and patterns held in the base chakra include the motivation to care for our physical body, the path taken to earn a living, the maintenance of our home, our attitude toward money, and the way in which we relate to the sensual and material world. A well-developed base chakra ensures an increased ability to trust and feel safe in one's environment. An underdeveloped base chakra expresses just the opposite.

The base chakra must be balanced, or progression into the higher chakras will suffer because the base chakra is the foundation upon which the other chakras are built—it is the very foundation of our material world. An underdeveloped base chakra cannot support further development—any attempt at growth will be easily thwarted. Even a small step taken toward higher consciousness will be quickly sabotaged by fear arising out of a weak foundation. Survival messages from the "survival mind"—"I can't do it!" or "I don't deserve this!"—will win out.

Therapist Anodea Judith, author of *Wheels of Light*, points out that until recently, the focus in spiritual healing has been on sending energy up the chakra channels toward enlightenment and less on grounding or sending energy downward.[99] Without grounding through Mother Earth, we lose our nourishment, power, stability and ability to grow. We all know what happens to a tree when its root system has been severed. To reach for the sky, we must have a solid foundation.

Without a well-developed base chakra, constant health problems and financial crises may be the norm as well. Trapped at this level, one may experience panic attacks, low self-esteem, and constant safety issues. Until the distorting energies are released, advancement to higher consciousness is thwarted.

The physical body represents our foundation in this physical world, and the ability to be present in the body shows a balanced, well-developed base chakra. Clients have reported to me that they find it difficult to stay in their bodies, or they say that they find themselves checked out much of the time. This lack of body awareness spills over into the food one eats and the way in which one takes care of the physical body. Eating "on the run" and not getting sufficient rest are all symptomatic of being "checked out" and are signs that indicate an unbalanced, underdeveloped base chakra. Meats and proteins are foods that ground the base chakra, but too much of them tend to weigh the physical body down and prevent or inhibit movement into higher chakra energy. Though it is not necessary to eat meat to be grounded, it is the protein that is important for the structural tissue of the first chakra. A vegetarian diet with sufficient amounts of protein, such as tofu, beans, nuts, eggs, etc. can also provide the necessary food for the first chakra.

Traumas that most affect this chakra include birth traumas, abandonment, neglect, poor bonding, feeding difficulties, major illness or surgery, physical abuse, and inherited family patterns. Symptoms that indicate this chakra is depleted include chronic fatigue, disconnection from the physical (being checked out), difficulty concentrating, disorganization, generalized fearfulness, financial difficulties, poor boundaries, and being under weight. Symptoms of over activity include obesity, overeating, hoarding, greed, fear of change, addiction to security, and rigidity. Other physical problems often associated with an underdeveloped base chakra include eating disorders, weakness, and chronic health issues associated with hips, legs, feet, knees, bones, teeth, and the lower bowels.

I conclude this discussion of the base or Muladhara with these words from Caroline Myss: "The merging of the first or Tribal Chakra [Muladhara], the sacrament of Baptism, and the sefirah [sefirot plural] of Shekhinah. The power created by these three archetypal forces transmits into our energy and biological systems into the sacred truth, All is One."[100]

Second Chakra: Svadhisthana

In Hindu tantrism, svadhisthana (a Sanskrit word) means "One's own abode, her special abode, place of pleasure."[101] It is the second chakra, the reproductive chakra, and is located on or just above the pubic bone. Hindu tradition shows this chakra has six vermillion petals, or sections. Taoism calls this chakra *wei lu* and places it just a little above the tip of the coccyx. In reality, they are two chakras closely positioned; together, they are called the "sacral center." When studying these, you may focus on them independently or as one. Spiritual teacher Mantak Chia, founder of the Universal Healing Tao, suggests that in the practice of the microcosmic orbit, it is not necessary to focus on each one separately. Either approach is effective.

The sacral center functions to pump spinal fluid up to the brain, which keeps it nourished and young. It is also related to the quantity of sexual energy a person possesses. A developed sacral chakra generates increased sexual energy and power. An underdeveloped or closed sexual chakra expresses weak sexual sensations. People who have negative sexual images based on religious programming may believe that sex is sinful and dirty and that there is something wrong with their desires. They may become psychologically imbalanced, guilt-ridden, or express their suppressed sexual appetites in destructive ways. The Theosophists, whose ideas concerning the chakra system and subtle energy bodies A.E. Powell has compiled, deviate from the traditional Hindu chakra placement by moving svadhisthana from the pubic area to above and behind the solar plexus at the location of the spleen. Theosophists give it the distinction of absorbing "Vitality Globules from the atmosphere, disintegrating them, and distributing the component atoms charged with the specialized and transmuted Prana, to the various parts of the body."[102] Powell indicates this "sun" force is broken up into seven colors or seven different kinds of prana: violet, blue, green, yellow, orange, dark red, and rose red. This primary force of energy or prana is soaked up by the astral body and delivered to the spleen or svadhisthana for distribution to other parts of the body. Yellow and rose pink to the heart center, green to the abdomen and solar plexus center, dark red and some dark purple to the base of the spine center in one channel, and orange from another channel to the base chakra. Two different channels flow toward the throat center, one carrying blue and one violet, that come together, joining into one upward-moving stream. Rose pink is also delivered to the whole of the nervous system by this chakra. Powell suggests that the development of the spleen chakra brings to consciousness the ability to remember astral journeys and has the function of vitalizing the whole astral body. I point out this distinction to avoid any misunderstanding regarding the spleen chakra and its path of functioning.

Modern advances in technology have made it possible to see, as well as read, frequencies emanating from the chakra vortices. This technology, not available to the Theosophists in the late eighteen hundreds, confirms the validity of their intuitive placement of the sacral, second, or svadhisthana at the spleen. Cyndi Dale, in *New Chakra Healing*, discusses the twelfth chakra or secondary chakra system, which includes thirty-two points located throughout the physical body and among them is the spleen chakra. I will cover this secondary chakra system later in the text.

Ancient yogis associated the serpent goddess with the second chakra and attributed to her many aspects of the archetypal Great Mother. She was portrayed with amorous, generative, dominating, and ruthless qualities. Hindu mythological representations of sexual orgies and fertility cults are second-chakra archetypes.

World mythology throughout the ages has attributed youthful, playful, naïve gods who were not yet capable of heroic deeds to the second chakra. These mythological gods, while searching for power, fall victim to the Great Mother and her pleasure palace. According to Jung, fertility cults that sacrificed the ritual male are typical dramas of the second chakra psyche. The opening of the second chakra, therefore, may originate confrontation with deep-seated fears and distorted sexual feelings as the archaic elements of our mutual history, resulting in the collective unconscious becoming apparent in our own lives.

Through the development of the second chakra, we begin to separate ourselves from our mothers and our environment. Once this happens, we become aware of our vulnerability, helplessness, and powerlessness. We realize just how dependent we are on our mother or "mothering" parent, and with this realization, we begin to associate personal survival with this dependence. In this case, "survival" means the need to be loved and to be seen as lovable. It is easy to "see" the underlying foundation of the incredible fear and anxiety in romantic relationships that is generated because we already have internalized a "belief" based on our separation from our mothers or mothering parents that we will be rejected and unloved. This is a devastating feeling and engenders the kind of deep insecurity that immobilizes one's desire to be emotionally available.

The primary focus of the second chakra is fun, pleasure, and excitement; when that is not present, the focus is on the pain involved in *not* having fun. This is known as the pleasure-pain cycle. It is through this cycle that addictions flourish. Svadhisthana sense of self is defined by the totality of objects, persons, and circumstances that create a sense of security based on their association with pleasure or, on the opposite side of the spectrum, connected with pain and suffering.

The seductive, sensuous, treacherous world of the sexual chakra led many early teachers to suggest complete avoidance of pleasure and pain, especially sexual. In addition, the mistaken idea that sex is evil and to be avoided at all costs is the foundation of our current misguided attitudes toward sexual things. These deeply repressed unresolved sexual feelings, infused with shame and guilt, have led us into a twenty-first-century world rife with sexual abuse and addiction to pornography.

Hindu teachings agree with the Theosophists that the second chakra has a unique relationship with the etheric body. The etheric body is the interface between the outer subtle energy bodies and the physical body. The currents of chi, prana, or life force run through it and into the physical body into the meridian system. This life force is vitalizing and has a nurturing and cleansing effect on the nervous system, spleen, lymph system, and urinary tract. The harmonious flow of this energy is vital to the health of the physical system. Since the etheric body receives and transmits energy-information from the astral or emotional body, it reverberates in response to the emotion of the astral world. Because of the relationship between the etheric and the second chakra, it plays a primary role in the processing of energy-information received from the astral.

The second chakra not only receives and interprets emotional information relative to one's own feelings but also receives emotional forces, or impressions and sensations, from environmental situations. Most of this information is unconscious and can be confusing for that reason. These unconscious, painful feelings may be overwhelming because the rational mind is uncomfortable with pain or powerful feelings. The unconscious painful feelings can out-picture in the second chakra as distorted sexual feelings and romantic desires. Sexual addiction can rear its ugly head. Loneliness, feelings of insecurity and vulnerability, depression and anger arise from the lack of the inherent need for love, safety, and security.

With this pain comes the opportunity to identify the deprivation as a second chakra issue. To create security and safety, a person often attempts to control the unconscious. In so doing, jealousy, rage, and possessiveness result. Anodea Judith suggests that if the second chakra is too open, a person can become overwhelmed with unconscious emotions.[103] The "too open" second chakra can also result in being ruled by one's own emotions, characterized by frequent chaotic, dramatic episodes.

Svadhisthana is a place of polarities: male and female, sun and moon, positive and negative, yin and yang. Also attributed to svadhisthana is the desire for more—emotion, sensation, movement, and nurturance. It is here that Hindu tradition speaks of the Ida and Pingala, two alternate channels, which twist in a figure-eight pattern around each of the chakras, causing them to spin. Ida represents lunar aspects and Pingala represents solar.

In conclusion, Judith says:

> The main aspect of the second chakra, however, is sexuality. Sexuality is a life force. The water softens the hard Earth and readies it for change. It is a force too often denied or perverted, and being robbed of our pleasure, we are robbed of our power. When we lose our desire, we lose our will. Power and will are attributes of the next chakra, and pleasure and desire are their seed. Sexuality is the flower of that seed. Power and will are its fruits.[104]

Third Chakra: Manipura

Manipura means "shining like a jewel" in Sanskrit. This chakra is like a ten-petalled flower and is associated with the color yellow because the shining jewel is as bright as the sun. Tantra traditions use an inverted red triangle, symbolizing the fire element associated with Agni, the Hindu god of fire, with a ram inside the triangle demonstrating the obnoxious qualities of the rational mind gone mad with desire. Fire is also the spark of life that calls will into action. The power of the third chakra is the power of life, vitality, and connection with others.

Earth and water symbols of the first and second chakra lead to the fire of the third chakra. The foundation of the first and the emotion of the second chakras leads us in the ever-evolving dance toward enlightenment; this energy is called "will and power." It rises from our center, the solar plexus, and descends from our visions; it releases joyously through the heart. The lighting of the fire element ignites the passion of consciousness that brings us into the light from the depths of the unconscious. The combination of unconscious emotion and psyche wills us into action. When our power activates, we seek a higher purpose.

The manipura, or third chakra, is located at the solar plexus and is sometimes called the solar plexus chakra. It provides vital energy to the liver and the pancreas, which govern the assimilation of the foods we eat, the thoughts we contemplate, and the nourishment of our systems. Besides the purpose of digestion, the third chakra also fires desire and the power of emotions. During the clearing of the third chakra, digestive problems may be accompanied by emotional instability as long-held emotions are released. Issues related to a fired-up ego, such as power trips or ego trips, are signs of an underdeveloped third chakra.

Jung associated the third chakra with the mythological stage of the hero and the development of ego-consciousness. In *The Hero Within*, Carol Pearson writes of this hero archetype, "Heroes—in myth, literature, and real-life—take journeys, confront dragons (i.e., problems), and discover the treasure of their true selves. Although they may feel very alone during the quest, at its end, their reward is a sense of community: with themselves, with other people, and with the earth."[105]

An absence of the hero's journey seems to inhibit the willingness to explore new options and the personal courage to breathe fully of all that life offers. Avoidance of the hero's journey prevents us from giving ourselves permission to make mistakes, thus creating fears that result in anxiety or shallow breathing. The resultant fear of living represented in limited breathing keeps us from firing our passions. Life then becomes a cold, dry, and gray wasteland. Ultimately, there is disconnection from spirit, which provides a spark for the fires of action. Finally, the loss of the personal power center causes one to seek power in sources outside the self.

Codependency and submission become characterized by the archetypal energies of the victim, prostitute, martyr, slave, and coward, i.e., "others" have the power. When others have the power, low self-esteem is the product of those outside influences and results in expressed emotions of inadequacy and inferiority.

Judith writes that the power of the third chakra is dependent upon our ability to connect with the world that surrounds us. By nourishing ourselves through knowledge of our internal power and basic self-confidence, we can direct our lives toward our passion, our natural ability or spirit to seek and take risks. When we are able to access this power, we feel renewed.

David Hawkins, in his revolutionary book *Power vs Force,* defines power as the silent stillness within. In that quiet "ALL that Isness." all potentiality exists. Force represents an attempt to manipulate people, places, and things to reach a desired goal.[106] Anger is force, and so is hostility, resentment, indifference, rage, and fear. As you can see, the energy of force is destructive.

Jung uses the term "shadow" to indicate repressed emotional pain during childhood experiences resulting from harsh criticism, judgments, shaming, and blaming at the hands of family, friends, and classmates. Thus, the statement: "It is our secrets that make us sick." Denial of repressed feelings soon becomes limiting beliefs, according to Jung, and are unconsciously projected, usually onto a person of the same sex. Breaux suggests we must come to terms with our shadow by ceasing to judge and repress it. Eventually, the ego must accept the shadow aspects of "childlike" resentments, needs, aggressions, insecurities, will-to-power, and desires.[107]

Another major issue of the solar plexus chakra is commitment. Commitment is related to responsibility; as we journey our way through the maze of life called the world of work, gaining experience and self-confidence, we come face to face with the need to develop a sense of responsibility and commitment. Success in developing this sense of responsibility and commitment can determine health or illness in the solar plexus chakra and the organs it feeds.

Responsibility and commitment in the areas of love, sex, and power stem from this chakra. Our need for positive self-esteem and a sense of personal power are intricately linked with the need to feel loved, accepted, and worthwhile. Largely, most look to the outside for those feelings to be validated. The greater the need for validation, the greater compromises one makes to get the love and acceptance they need. This breeds resentment and bitterness. This can turn into a power game and is painful. The better plan may be to dig deep into parental and cultural brainwashing and explore questions such as, "How did I get the message that sex is bad?" or "What made me think of my sexual identity as shameful or disgusting?"

There may also be unhealthy parental sexual and emotional bonds that are limiting and insidious. A mother may unconsciously keep her son from appropriate female relationships because of her fear that she will lose him. Alternatively, a father may feel sexually attracted to his daughter and may, while suppressing those feelings, jealously hold on to her, inhibiting her maturation. By freeing ourselves from these dysfunctional patterns, we gain the power of healthy sexual expression. The ability to love through sexual relationships promotes self-esteem and provides the impetus to love more fully.

The struggle within the archetypal third chakra energies of love and power are antagonistic, and the overabundance of one diminishes the other. This double-edged sword of the ego is one that must be resolved at this chakra level. The openness required for love is compromised by the need for power. In our quest to know ourselves through power and love, we must, at some point, surrender our ego-selves to this power and the need to love; in so doing, we can finally reach true power and love. It is as if we build ourselves to a crescendo of pain and suffering through which we finally surrender the ego-self. It is through surrender that we embark upon the path of enlightenment.

To sum up this section on the third chakra, I quote Caroline Myss, "There is nothing simple about developing self-understanding, independence, and self-respect, even though the journey consists of only four stages. The third chakra is filled with the energy of our personal ambitions, our sense of responsibility, and our respect for our strengths and weaknesses, as well as our fears and secrets that we are not yet ready to face."[108]

Fourth Chakra: Heart
Anahata

The Sanskrit name "anahata" literally means "not struck." "It refers to the subtle vibration that is the creative energy of the void," says Breaux.[109] The sacred syllable "om" is the chant associated with anahata. The fourth chakra is located at the heart. It has twelve bright red petals, according to Hindu tradition, which places two smoke-colored interlocking triangles inside the twelve petals. This is representative of a harmonious relationship between the male and female forces of the cosmos, called the Vayu mandala, and represents the element of air. The image of an antelope is the symbol of air in the mandala.

Theosophists attribute the color yellow gold to the heart chakra. Cyndi Dale attributes to it the colors pink, green, and gold, and Anodea Judith gives it the color green. Green is the color most attributed to the heart chakra and sometimes in conjunction with pink and rose. I leave it to you to decide for yourself the color you feel is associated with your own heart chakra—maybe it is a combination of them all.

Lama Anagarika Govinda defines the fire aspect of the heart chakra as psychic fire rather than physical fire. He speaks of the balanced heart expressing as intuitive mind and transmuted feelings or divine love and compassion. The heart chakra is the place of the alchemical fire of religious devotion and compassionate will, which will eventually transform our personal identity. The heart chakra is the place of "Let go and let God."

With an awakened heart chakra, the accelerated vibration alters the astral body, infusing it with the peaceful energy of a mirror-like pool of water. The opened heart awakens the desire for an intimate relationship with the "mystery of life." Living deeply and lovingly in the moment allows for a deeper union with the unknown, the intense beauty and perfection of forgotten divine realms.

Anodea Judith refers to the Hindu mandala associated with the heart chakra when she says, "This symbol [also known as the Star of David] represents the Sacred Marriage: the balanced interpenetration of masculine and feminine. This is the star of radiance that emanates from an open heart chakra."[110]

Physically, the energy connection of the heart chakra relates to the cardiac plexus and rules over the heart muscle, circulatory system, ribs, breasts, lungs, thymus gland, shoulders, arms, hands, and diaphragm.

Caroline Myss says the challenge of the fourth chakra is coming to terms with our internal feelings concerning ourselves. How will we choose to respond emotionally to our own thoughts, ideas, goals, and attitudes? Will we choose wisdom, understanding, and compassion—or judgment, criticism, and hate? What we commit to at this level determines the quality of our personal relationships. Fear of loss, loneliness, inability to protect oneself emotionally, and fear of betrayal are all heart-level considerations.

The power of the heart lies in the ability to love and be compassionate, forgiving, trusting, and, just as importantly, to heal self and others—a function of the heart chakra. To quote Myss on love: "We are not born fluent in love but spend our life learning about it. Its energy is pure power. We are as attracted to love as we are intimidated by it. We are motivated by love, controlled by it, inspired by it, healed by it, and destroyed by it."[111]

We must not forget the importance of the element of air in association with the heart chakra. We all have experienced holding our breath when we are afraid or in pain. Somehow, we think that will stave off the pain or the monster coming to destroy us. When we hold our breath, we limit oxygen intake into the lungs, which limits the oxygenation process of the blood. Our blood, then, cannot be cleansed, and after a while, we could even die. It is through breath that our cells are kept alive. Our breath represents the vital energy or prana through which all life is made. It is the interface between the physical body and the world of the mind. If the mind chooses to take us too far afield, imbalances in the heart occur, which can throw the entire system out of balance. Judith says a balance must occur between the upper and lower chakras and between the mind and the physical body, and this balance must extend "within" and "without" between self and the soul or transcendence.[112]

Love is a choice that the heart can assist in making. Our challenge is to give of our love by taking responsibility for our choices and by making the personal commitment to act with compassion from our heart so that we are expressing states of being that make up the synergy of energy we call love: understanding, intimacy, pleasure, honesty, and humility. A major heart struggle is the loss of "grounding" that happens when the energy of love sweeps you off your feet. You can make sure to say grounded by focusing on gratitude, having respect by setting appropriate boundaries, taking responsibility for your feelings, loving yourself and taking care of your own needs first (and not interfering with those who are doing the same), searching to know oneself, having humility, and acting in a caring manner.

In conclusion, I quote Breaux:

> We might think that opening the heart center brings only peace and love. Aside from our own repressed grief and fear of being vulnerable, there are many difficulties that arise as the heart opens. The heart center invokes intense forces from the soul and inner spiritual realms. The activities, or mere presence, of a person with an enlivened heart center may

stimulate intense defensive reactions in others as the love vibration penetrates barriers and stirs into resonance the love that has been buried beneath untold pain and suffering.[113]

Fifth Chakra: Throat

Vishuddha

Vishuddha (aka vishuddhi) in Sanskrit means "cleansed" or "purified." Ether (otherwise known as spirit or Akasha) is its element, and it has sixteen bright blue petals. Hindu tradition places the akasa (or akashic) mandala here. Represented by an inverted triangle called a yoni, it suggests the feminine powers of creation, and it holds the white elephant with one of seven trunks extended in the air at its center.

The throat chakra functions as a communication center, and it enlivens the throat, thyroid, trachea, esophagus, parathyroid, hypothalamus, neck vertebrae, mouth, jaw, and teeth. The throat chakra is involved in our decision-making processes, and because choice is an integral part of our daily lives, it colors our health and well-being—or lack of it. Caroline Myss says that all illness is associated with the throat chakra because illness is the result of the choices we make.[114] Temporal mandibular joint pain (TMJ), for instance, is a good example of what happens when our throat chakra is affected, as we repeatedly "clamp down" our jaws for fear of making a wrong decision.

The Right Use of Will by Ceanne DeRohan speaks clearly about the issues of the throat chakra. How we use our voice, not only for saying words but also for the energy and vibration behind the words, is important. When we speak from a place of "right use of will," our words and the energy behind our words resonate in a beautiful and harmonious way. The truth rings loud and clear. There is no doubt! The right use of will comes from having cleared and balanced the lower chakras. When we speak from a healed heart chakra, the emanation of our words through the throat chakra is compassionate and understanding.[115]

Sound vibrations can influence the vibrations of the human energy system, and throughout the ages, the voice has played an important role in religious and spiritual ceremonies through chants and singing. Since the right use of will indicates an alignment of one's will with the will of God, our voice represents one method of aligning with the divine energy of the universe. Just chant the mantra om, the great primordial sound, and feel the connection with the Universal All within you.

Vishuddha is the world of vibration. Its element, ether, " . . . can be equated with the all-encompassing and unifying field of subtle vibrations of sound throughout the universe."[116] All vibrations of the universe, no matter their form, interact with other vibrations, each affecting the other like a pebble thrown into a pond, rippling throughout the entire body of water. The essence of the fifth chakra is the world of vibration; it provides the venue through which we attune our consciousness to the subtle energy vibrations that surround us. Cyndi Dale says that without the operational backside of the fifth chakra, we would not be able to communicate, and, more specifically, "No one would know that you exist."[117] The backside of the fifth chakra makes it possible for us to channel thoughts and ideas from others, from the spirit world, from other dimensions, and from aspects of ourselves. As we receive information from the backside of the chakra, we process it, keeping what we want and filtering what we do not want, subsequently sharing it through our voice—our individual vibration.

The divine expression of the self, beautifully and articulately for the entire world to witness, is the realm of the visuddha. Finally, we can share our greatness, the divine wisdom we have intuited from the

"Great Void," and our most fervent desire is to claim our divinity by sharing from the deepest recesses of our being. The human dream is to accomplish this without the voice shaking and quaking, the face turning red, and being overwhelmed by the desire to flee from the room. The quiet expression of our truth without fear of judgment or rejection is the healed realm of the fifth chakra.

According to Caroline Myss, in her discussion of the fifth chakra, "The greatest act of will in which we can invest our spirits is to choose to live according to these rules:

1. Make no judgments.
2. Have no expectations.
3. Give up the need to know why things happen as they do.
4. Trust that the unscheduled events of our lives derive from a spiritual direction.
5. Have the courage to make the choices we need to make, accept what we cannot change, and have the wisdom to know the difference. [118]

Sixth Chakra: Brow or Third Eye

Ajna

Ajna is Sanskrit for "command from above." Ajna, the sixth chakra, is seen as a deep indigo with a silver orb within the indigo field, perhaps representing the indigo night sky surrounding the silvery moon. Light is the element associated with ajna and represents the intertwining of the darkness and the light, which enables us to see. Ajna has only two petals, perhaps representing the light and the dark, manifest and unmanifest—the two worlds of reality, or the ida and the pingala, the intertwining nadis that meet at ajna. The joining of the two worlds allows us to see with clarity that which we chose to manifest. Ramtha, the ancient spiritual teacher channeled by Judy Knight, teaches that the combination of clear intention, the right use of the breath, and the ability to see the concept of our desire on our foreheads make the physical manifestation of that desire a reality.

The sixth chakra, ajna, is located at the center of the forehead. It is related to the cerebral cortex, pineal, and pituitary glands and is therefore associated with the faculty of visual perception. It is often known as the "third eye." We can add the ears, nose, and neurological system to the list of associations as well. Through these physical attributes, the sixth chakra links our mental bodies, intelligence, and psychological characteristics. These characteristics stem from the synergistic combination of knowledge and belief, the records held in our mental bodies, which consist of fear, historical information-memories, facts, and daily activities—all activating emotions. This process assists us in discerning truths.

Through the sixth chakra, it is possible to access memories of past or future events, ordering them so that it is possible to receive the information intuitively. This may come as archetypal symbols, feelings, sounds, or even colors. Many psychics learn to identify the language of the third eye—a rewarding and informative gift—by using symbols to clearly convey the meaning of the message. For instance, I recognize third-eye messages and interpret them according to feelings, vision, and location of the vision. If I see the vision on my internal television screen, the vision concerns present-time information. When I see a vision externally and feel emotions in the lower part of my body, I am referencing information from the past, including past lives. For instance, I may "witness" a scene from some ancient time or other dimension being played out, seemingly in front of me, while I am working with a client. I associate this scene with a message for them relating to the issue we are working on at the present time. This indicates to me that the present-time issue is directly related to a severe trauma, psychic wound, ancestral or past life contract, or curse expressing itself in the present time because the person is ready to release the limiting condition. I perceive I am receiving this information because it is important to the process of clearing this particular destructive pattern.

One psychic whom I consulted uses cars of different colors to order her intuitive information. When the car is near, it means a current event; if the car is in the distance, it refers to something that has already happened or something that will happen. Other psychics, including the well-known John Edwards, "see" pictures that tell the stories that the spirits of the departed want to relay to the living.

Often, people fear sixth chakra information because they were conditioned as children to believe that intuition is "evil" or that only information conveyed by the five senses in the physical world is valid to human experience. But sixth-chakra information tells us that it is possible to experience more than the physical world. This fact calls into question the nature of "reality." This can be uncomfortable and unacceptable in some circles.

Until we learn to free ourselves from our attachment to the physical world and the thoughts and behaviors that keep us solely reliant on that world, it can be difficult to access and use the information conveyed by this sixth sense. When caught only in the physical world, in the consciousness levels below two hundred (or below "courage"), as identified by David Hawkins, truth is illusive.[119]

Caroline Myss teaches that the sacred purpose of the sixth chakra is to "seek only the truth." The truth comes through reaching a level of consciousness where truth can be accessed. The more elevated one is conscious, the greater the ability to move beyond subjective perspectives, which makes it easier to access the idea of non-attachment, and the ability to distinguish between truth and illusion becomes commonplace. Myss relates this idea of non-attachment this way:" It means stilling one's fear-driven voices. One who has attained an inner posture of detachment has a sense of self so complete that external influences have no authority within his or her consciousness."[120]

By way of conclusion, Anodea Judith tells us that:

> Clairvoyance, then, is a matter of seeing the inner relationships of things—the fitting of the part into the whole. It is done by searching for the cross-point or interference pattern between our question (the reference beam) and the piece of information that best fits the space we have created for it. The potency of the image that clicks into place sets it apart from the infinite number of other possible answers. Through meditation, visualization, and training, we can develop our abilities to perceive the subtle difference between the information we request and the countless other possibilities.[121]

Seventh Chakra: Crown

Sahasrara

Sahasrara is Sanskrit for "lotus of the thousand petals." The petals are said to hang downward to cover the "Gate of Being" (the anterior fontanel, or soft spot on a baby's head). In addition, ancient yogis believed this to be the gate of death through which, if opened during life, one could consciously leave the body, propelled by the last breath, thereby liberating oneself from the cycle of death and involuntary rebirth. The Egyptian Left Eye of Horus Mystery School termed this the "Gate of Being," and according to Drunvalo Melchizidec it was the focus of initiation of the Egyptian thirteenth chakra. The initiation focus was the demonstration by the initiate to consciously leave the physical, enter the upper dimensions, and return to the physical. Melchizidec suggests that the design of the Kings Chamber of the Great Pyramid at Giza purposefully included the Gate of Being initiation. The idea that humans could consciously ascend the physical and descend again is present in many religions of the world and in some ancient cosmologies, like those of the Sumerian people.

The crown chakra, from a psychological perspective, contains ideas related to the spiritual realms or God and our relationship to God. This concept that humans are more than physical, that we do have a direct relationship to something greater than ourselves or those things that we can only witness with the five senses, has come down to the present through scriptural teaching, by word of mouth through indigenous tribal shamans, and by ceremony. Even though the original intent may have been to introduce humanity to its divine inheritance, the avenue through which the message has been delivered may, as Charles Breaux says, "Blind us to the intuitive awareness of the crown chakra."[122]

Sacred beliefs, archetypal in nature, held in the crown chakra can lead one to ever-greater awareness of one's divine nature. On the other hand, they can also be limiting; therefore, it is imperative that one question these sacred beliefs rather than blindly continuing to adhere to them. In reality, the original creators of the belief may have misunderstood the message. Remember, beliefs are only stories we repeatedly tell ourselves are true until they become self-fulfilling prophecies. That does not mean our beliefs are necessarily true. It only means they have become a habit—and maybe a destructive one. We can only gain a clear understanding of the great mystery of the universe and the true nature of ourselves by being open to every possibility.

The primary purpose of the crown chakra is to integrate the spiritual with the physical, mental, and emotional. Physically, this chakra is connected to the pituitary gland, cerebral cortex, and the chakras above the seventh level. All ancient traditions indicate that currents of energy from the universal source flow into the seventh chakra and are taken into the body and distributed to the lower chakras. Therefore, it is known as the center for higher knowing, and through it, we receive spiritual information necessary to make active guiding our life purpose. It is from this seventh chakra perspective that we may know the Divine Source, as well as be able to recognize other spiritual beings. When the crown chakra is underdeveloped, physical symptoms may include disorders of the immune system, cellular distortion or cancer, bone weakness, nervous system disorders, and hormonal irregularities that originate in the pineal gland.

The element associated with the crown chakra is thought. The divine intelligence and source of all manifestation resides here. Judith says that the element of thought associated with this chakra is "a fundamentally distinct and unmeasurable entity that is the first and barest manifestation of the greater field of consciousness around us." She goes on to write that our experience of the mind is associated with the seventh chakra. Awareness of our thoughts and their interplay inside our head is like a theatrical production, one that so enamors us that we think we are the characters in the play. It is through our mind watching a play that it assimilates the experience into the meaning and constructs of our beliefs.[123]

In conclusion, I quote Breaux:

. . . the crown chakra level of consciousness is the central point from which the spider web of our individual identity originates. It is, therefore, the place where it is gathered back in, untangling the network of images which have composed our notion of self. Beyond form, beyond thought, beyond concepts of being or non-being, consciousness plunges into the fathomless sea of the Clear Light of the Void through the Gate of Being in the crown chakra. As we integrate this peak experience, we begin to identify with the whole-living-through-its-myriad-parts; the individual body-mind becomes a conscious hologram of the universe.[124]

The Minor and Secondary Chakra System

Secondary chakras are described by Theosophists and New Age practitioners, as well as individual spiritual healers like Cyndi Dale, Barbara Brennan, and Christopher Hills. Secondary chakras differ from the archetypal seven major chakras of the Hindu system in that they are etheric and pertain to the subtle energy bodies that surround the physical. Their function affects not only ordinary, everyday consciousness but also psychic, mystic, and transpersonal states.

I have included in EMCS portions of Cyndi Dales 'model of the secondary chakra system because it also incorporates points from the Egyptian chakra model. Dales 'model includes five additional out-of-body chakras. She designates the twelfth chakra as being secondary, which incorporates thirty-two in-body minor chakra points. Included in these thirty-two points are the eleventh, twelfth, and thirteenth Egyptian chakra points.

I agree with Dale, who describes the eighth chakra as a portal into and out of this space-time continuum. My clients report, as do hers, experiencing a sense of space and having visions around planetary and stellar images when working in the energy of the eighth chakra, which is located one-and-a-half inches above the head and, when intuitively "felt," feels like a floating flat disk. Intuitively, the energy of this chakra reads as silver or ultraviolet. Dale describes its characteristics as being feminine-based with a masculine core. When connecting with the energy-information of this chakra, one can expect to access all past knowledge and karmic memory. In addition, it provides access to other dimensions.

Being a student of the Maya calendar code,[125] I associate activation of the eighth chakra with the approach of the final and ninth levels of consciousness, which Calleman calls the Universal Cycle. The Mayan prophecy seems to indicate this level is where and when humanity reaches the beginning of the full expression of its divine nature. Years ago, I prophesized that this activation would come with the culmination of the Mayan concept of 16.4 billion years of the evolution of consciousness—December 21, 2012, or earlier on October 28, 2011, if the Classical Mayan chronology is used. My perception is that we are now in this eighth level of the evolution of consciousness, the level of ethics, or learning to live fully in harmony with the laws of nature and the cosmos. Activation of the eighth chakra aligns us holographically as "One."

The Incan Pukios System[126] calls the eighth chakra the soul chakra, and they see it as having a gold essence. They teach aspects of the eighth chakra that include the ideas that it instinctually leads one to transcendence, that it is the architect of the body, that it seeds timelessness, and that its negative aspect holds templates of disease. It directly communicates with the thymus gland, certain aspects of the central nervous system, and the right eye, and it involves memory retrieval functions. Cyndi Dale indicates that the eighth chakra develops between the ages of twenty-one and twenty-eight.[127]

Jude Currivan says of the eighth chakra, "The [eighth] chakra of the universal heart is the bridge between our ego-based perception and our higher awareness. On a collective level, we are now experiencing our resonance with this chakra as an increasingly global compassion."[128]

Ninth Chakra: The Soul Chakra

The soul chakra, according to Dale, is located approximately an arm's length above the head. It is most often "seen" as gold and infrared or a combination of the two. "Mushroom" in shape holds a masculine appearance with a feminine overlay. I agree with Cyndi Dale that its language and operation are through a matrix of symbols, patterns, and archetypes specific to each individual's life purpose. The symbols operate in the same way chromosomes operate in the physical body. Each symbol holds a blueprint that molds the physical body into a particular design, allowing the soul's purpose to unfold. The ninth chakra holds the yin ability to channel energy from the zero-point field, which changes the expression of the soul blueprint itself.

The energy of the ninth chakra is radioactive. It originates from the soul's genes and imprints. It communicates to the physical body by assisting in the selection of sperm and egg for this lifetime and regulates the physical and emotional programming functions. All chakra symbols, imprints, and archetypes available to the ninth chakra form the basic beliefs about self.

Since all programming for this incarnation is in the ninth chakra, it makes sense that all changes must occur in the ninth chakra for those changes to be permanent.

Jude Currivan has an alternative view of the ninth chakra, which she says is located a hand's length below our feet. She calls this chakra "earthstar" (Earth Star) and says it offers us a greater connection with the Earth than the personal root chakra. Her perception is that this chakra allows us to "commune at ever more profound levels with the device and elemental realms of the living earth."[129]

I perceive both views correct based on universal principles of "as above, so below," and if there is a front, there must be a back. Currivan speaks to the back of the ninth chakra while Dale speaks to the front.

In the Energy Matrix Clearing System, I use gem and mineral essences to effect changes in the blueprint of the ninth chakra. Muscle testing determines the geometric pattern required for clearing the old symbol, pattern, or archetype and the introduction of a new one. I let the body determine which of the five Platonic Solids, gems, and mineral essences will recalibrate the ninth chakra.[130]

Tenth Chakra

The tenth chakra is located one and a half to four feet below the soles of the feet. Its frequency or color consists of earth tones similar to the colors attributed to the Kabbalistic sefirot (the channels through which God makes himself known) called Malkuth. They include citrine, russet, olive, and indigo or black. The four elements of earth, fire, water, and air are foundational to this chakra. The yang function relates to the elimination of waste energy and the introduction of energy for physical life manifestation. The yin function allows for the reception of vital earth energy to support the entire physical system. Issues related to an "out of balance" tenth chakra affect the feet, legs, weight, and adrenal system. They result in avoidance issues characterized as being "spacey" or "out to lunch" and issues of paranoia, neurosis, or psychosis affiliated with disorientation.

Cyndi Dale calls this chakra the "grounding chakra" because it anchors a person in the everyday world of form. It connects one, through the feet, to the healing energy held in the earth. It feels good to squish one's toes in the mud or to walk on a sandy beach. This chakra also holds programs generated by human interaction with the earth, including earth disturbances, since humanity is a part of nature. Reprogramming of these long-held patterns occurs in the tenth chakra. Dale says this chakra develops or becomes active between the ages of thirty-five and forty-two.

Jude Currivan that the 10th chakra is located energetically about a hand's breath above our head and connects us with the matrix of the group soul that is the consciousness of our entire solar system.[131]

Again, they are speaking to the same chakra—one above and one below.

Eleventh Chakra: The Transmutation Chakra

The eleventh chakra is located at both hands and both feet. Its primary purpose is to transmute negative energy, perceptions, and diseased energies and reflect them back into the universe as positive energy. It is pink in color, and its energy type is etheric. It reads "between the lines" or "below the surface" energies coming into the subtle energy bodies, such as covert anger, hate, or prejudice. This chakra then interprets this energy so that a person can respond to the truth of the situation rather than to its outward appearance. Issues related to this chakra show up in the hands and the feet and are related to reaching out for one's desire or holding on to one's desire as well as moving forward toward that which one desires.

Eleventh chakra energy can be used to command instant change within and outside the body; this energy can also be projected and directed for good. Others in the field of energy work say the eleventh chakra is located above the head and holds the place where the upper point of the energy known as *merkaba* (meaning light, body, and spirit) ends on the human body, and they describe it as having creative, nurturing energy akin to kwan yin or the Mother Earth[132]. It is described as indigo in color, and generates energy that radiates outward to encompass all things around the human body. It is also associated with compassion. From my studies, I conclude that it is the same energy; some people just see it above the head because of its association with the upward movement of the chakra system. In my personal experiences with the eleventh chakra, it originates at the hands, is projected around the entire body, and connects each person with the "will" of all life.

Twelfth Chakra: The Secondary Chakra System

There are several different perceptions of the twelfth chakra. Cyndi Dale delineates this chakra into a thirty-two-point system, as do several other writers. In EMCS, the twelfth chakra takes a secondary role in the overall system. The thirty-two points identify specific minor chakra vortices within the physical body and outside the physical. Each of these points or vortices of energy supports the major chakras, and, like the major chakras, they can be found to connect with the spinal column. The study of the twelfth chakra will start with the unusual and move to the more accepted model of the chakra.

A series of articles published on the *Wisdom's Door* website covers various aspects of the twelfth chakra.[133] This site states that it is a source of an individual's strength and power and the ability to change both the physical and nonphysical dimensions. According to the unknown author of these articles, the twelfth chakra contains ascension energies and causes the chakras below the twelfth, which is "three steps above the crown chakra," to accelerate faster than light. Some say it is a cousin to the base chakra because the base holds the kundalini energy, the seed energy, far from the twelfth chakra. The purpose of kundalini energy is to accelerate individuals into the first phase of spiritual enlightenment. The second phase or stage comes as the ascension energies held in the Twelfth Chakra are released and propel the individual into a new experience beyond time and space.

According to some students of the human energy system, the twelfth chakra is composed of 777,777 spokes and rotates at 768,167 rotations per minute. The energy of the twelfth chakra is masculine, manifesting, vibrant, and gross. Because of the "quantum" movement of this chakra, it lends itself to being what some call the "doorway to the cosmos and beyond." Some writers associate the placement of this chakra with the bottom point of the upper merkaba where it meets the upper point of the human merkaba. Some call it "Father Sky" and color it turquoise.

Problems associated with the Twelfth Chakra include blocked ascension energies, which may show up as spontaneous, uncontrolled, out-of-body experiences; uncontrolled and spontaneous telekinesis; spontaneous inner visions that interrupt daily activities; and uncontrolled healing abilities. As a healer, you may not meet with these types of problems on a daily basis, and you may, in fact, have never had anyone present with these issues. However, it is essential to understand that clearing and healing of the twelfth chakra is possible through the very high vibrational energy of the person doing the healing or the medium through which the healing and balance of the twelfth chakra are accomplished. Some healers suggest using the Enochian mantra pronounced na-el-ee-el, which means "From the highest river flows life."[134]

The more accepted description associated with the twelfth chakra system is that it is a collection of thirty-two points located on the body and in the surrounding aura. The only point located outside the body is point thirty-two, which is situated at the center of the Earth and is called the Earth Star. This is the same point Currivan refers to as the Earth Star, but from a different connection point in the secondary chakra system. The Earth Star is included because our physical survival is contingent upon our ability to tap into Earth elements. Ancient teachers from the Sumerians to the Mayans understood that humans must connect with the Earth for health and well-being. The Essenes, more than two thousand years ago, delineated this philosophy in their poems to Mother Earth.

The standard thirty-two points associated with the twelfth chakra, according to Cyndi Dale, are:[135]

1 Legs	18 Large and small intestines
2 Buttocks	19 Pancreas
3 Coccyx	20 Liver
4 Sacral vertebrae	21 Gall Bladder
5 Lumbar vertebrae	22 Spleen
6 Thoracic (dorsal) vertebrae	23 Stomach
7 Cervical vertebrae	24 Diaphragm and lungs
8 Cranium	25 Arms
9 Silver Cord to the Soul (joins the physical body to the astral body)	26 Bubbling springs in palms
10 Bubbling springs in the feet	27 Wrists
11 Ankles	28 Elbows
12 Knees	29 Clavicle

13 Thighs

14 Hip bones

15 Navel and Sexual organs

16 Appendix

17 Kidneys and adrenals

30 Throat (including larynx, thyroid, and tongue)

31 Upper brain (spiritually oriented functions involving cerebrum, pineal, pituitary, hypothalamus, and thalamus glands)

32 Center of the earth

The EMCS Clearing Technique for the Twelfth Chakra

When working with a client using the EMCS system to clear the holographic human energy system, identify the following:

- Appropriate point(s) of the thirty-two above points using muscle testing
- Appropriate homeopathic gem or mineral essence for balancing and correcting or making active these energies. There are four categories of Living in Choice Gem and Mineral Essences from which to choose. You will find the list of gems and essences in the appendix.

The Egyptian Thirteen-Chakra System

I first learned about the thirteenth chakra in volume two of Drunvalo Melchizedek's book *The Ancient Secret of the Flower of Life.* Since then, I have found information about the thirteenth chakra in other sources as well. All writers who mention the thirteenth chakra do so in conjunction with the chakra system as taught by ancient Egyptians in their Left Eye of Horus Mystery School. Because this is a very complicated system, I refer you to Melchizedek's work.

Other information concerning the thirteenth chakra comes from several websites, one of which says this:

> The 13th chakra is often symbolized by the image of a rose. Its energy is that of Unconditional Love. The truth contained in the awareness of the 13th chakra is simply happiness. Often attributed to Buddha as his last words, "There is no Way to Peace and Happiness - Peace and Happiness is the Way."
>
> The chakra acts on the pituitary gland and inspires creativity to serve another or others unconditionally. When the thirteenth chakra makes the indicator change in EMCS the Celestial Blend Transformation is the correction. Muscle test for number of drops and route of administration.

Fourteenth Chakra

According to Carl Johan Calleman, the Mayan name for the Universal World Tree is Hunab Ku, meaning "giver of measure and movement" or "source of limits and energy," and it is the creative energy emanating from the Central Sun.[136] Calleman states, "As mentioned, the Universal Hunab Ku is beyond the range of our perception, but the galactic and earthly microcosms are within it, and each one of us is an individual expression of Hunab Ku."[137]

While studying the Maya calendar and gaining an understanding of the Mayan perception that consciousness is disseminated through the Galactic Central Sun by way of the Universal World Tree to the earth and finally to the human brain, the thought occurred to me that humans must also have a chakra that aligns with the Hunab Ku in the brain. If so, it must facilitate shifting of human consciousness just as the Galactic Central Sun shifts universal consciousness. To this end, muscle testing indicated that the soul star, located nine feet above the crown chakra, is the location of the fourteenth chakra. My personal work with this chakra indicates it is iridescent white in color and is a spiraling figure eight or infinity symbol. It is constantly accessing and processing information and energies from the Hunab Ku for our use. One purpose of the fourteenth chakra is to transduce consciousness in such a way that it is usable by the human brain. This chakra aligns with the Earth Star of the twelfth chakra to channel consciousness throughout the entire holographic human energy system. The website Ascension Glossary says this of the fourteenth chakra: "This Golden Chakra is about three feet above the head and connects to the Universal Sun and is the Founders Pale Gold Ray. This Chakra acts as the top lid of the 12D Shield and, when activated, creates an additional gold buffer field called the Golden Fleece Buffer."[138]

The three gem and mineral essences tested as being energetically harmonious with the fourteenth chakra are gold, monatomic gold, and a combination of essences that I named Ascendance, which is dark pearl, moonstone, gold, and monatomic gold. These can be used to work with the fourteenth chakra. Remember to muscle test to determine which is more effective for the client's personal work.

THE HUMAN ENERGY SYSTEM

Central Channel
Physical Body
Etheric Body
Astral Body
Mental Body
Causal Body

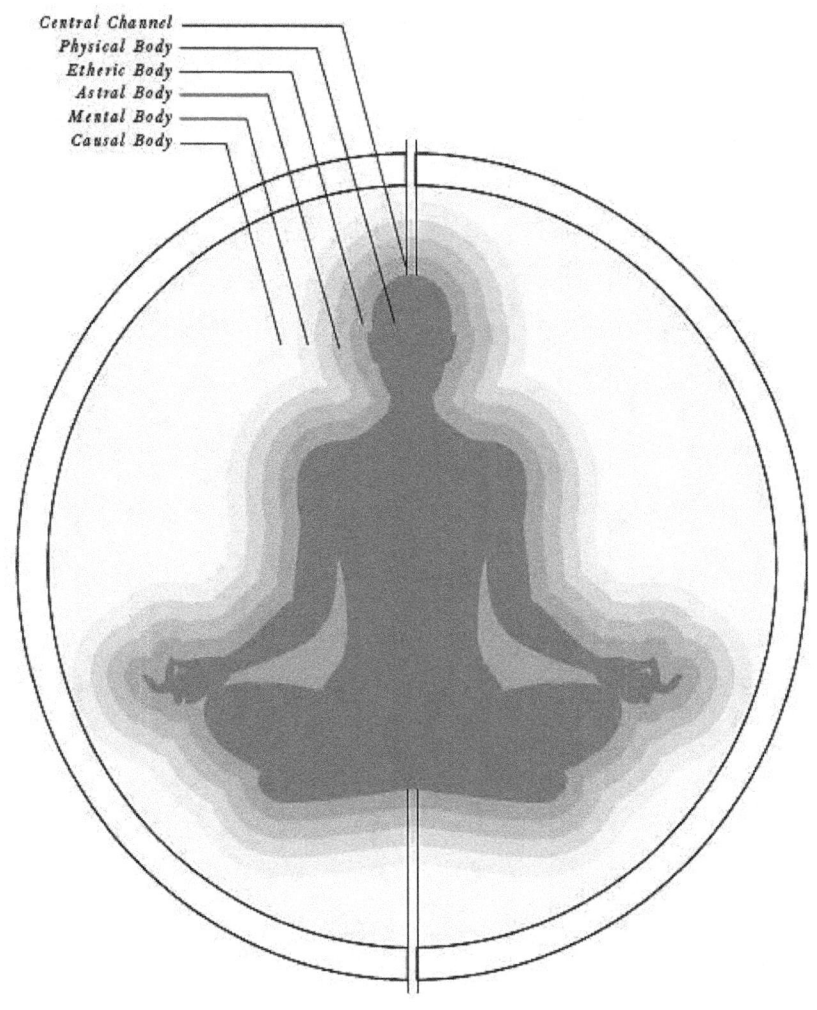

CHAPTER TEN

MATRIX V

SUBTLE ENERGY BODY ANATOMY

If happiness, peace, success, and all that is good is attainable only by obeying the law of balance, the more we comprehend that principle, the more we will be able to keep the human family in orbits which balance with one another as God keeps His solar family in balance.

—LAO RUSSELL

It is in the study of subtle energy anatomy that the transition from the material world of the physical to the emotional, mental, and spiritual world of the quantum takes place. The physical world is the manifestation of energies placed in motion in the subtle energy bodies. In other words, the form of the physical body and our individual material worlds is the effect of causal thought, feeling, and emotion established in the subtle energy bodies.

Paracelsus, a brilliant fifteenth-century vitalist physician, describes the subtle energy anatomy in this way:

> Astral Light—The same as Archaeus. A universal and living ethereal element, still more ethereal and highly organized than A'kasa. The former is universal, the latter only cosmic-viz., pertaining to our solar system. It is, at the same time, an element and a power containing the character of all things. It is the storehouse of memory for the great world (the Macrocosm), whose contents may become embodied and reincarnated in objective forms; it is the storehouse of memory of the little world, the Microcosm of man, from which he may recollect past events.[139]

In previous chapters, we explored the Chinese meridian system and the Hindu chakra system as interconnecting energy sources delivering energy and information from the subtle energy bodies to the physical system. Distortion or blockage of subtle energies manifests as illness, disease, pain, and suffering in the material world, all of which can be summed up as a mentality of lack. Given that fact, the reordering of the material or physical world begins in the subtle energy bodies.

The first or last subtle energy body, depending on which view one takes relative to the subtle energy bodies, is the etheric body. The etheric body is derived from ether and is defined as the state between energy and matter; sometimes called the etheric double because it surrounds the physical as well as interpenetrates it. It is the template or blueprint for the physical. This template consists of an energy matrix upon which cells of the physical body are shaped, anchored, and organized. The physical exists because of the etheric, not the other way around. Understanding the function of the etheric body in the holographic matrix system is imperative to the energician for clarity of the energetic clearing process. To this end, we will identify its nature, appearance, function, and its relationship to the physical and other subtle energy bodies.

The etheric and the physical are inseparable. As a result, the etheric dies with the physical. The etheric possesses a chakra system that receives and distributes vital life force, making it intimately connected with physical health. Structurally, the etheric body resembles a constantly moving web, with sparks of bluish-white light emanating from it. The chakra system of the etheric body is concomitant with the chakra system of the astral or emotional body, according to the Hindu system. All the chakras of the etheric body are the same bluish-gray color as the etheric body itself. Rather than the traditional colors of the astral chakras, the etheric chakras are vortices made of a bluish-gray net of light. With clairvoyant sight, the template of all organs of the physical body can be seen in the matrix of the etheric system.

The etheric body, according to the Theosophists, consists of four grades of matter:

1. Etheric matter: consists of ordinary electricity and sound waves
2. Super etheric: medium of light
3. Subatomic: finer forms of electricity
4. Atomic: medium for the transmission of thought forms from system to system[140]

During the nineteen forties, Harold Burr, a neuroanatomist at Yale University, established the connection of an "electrical axis" aligned with the brain and spinal cord. This was a giant step in Western medical arenas toward acceptance of the validity of the Chinese meridian system. The idea that the human body might be more than what it appeared to be became, at least, a possibility.

The development of Kirlian photography, a process of electrical photography, enabled researchers to graphically record energy as emanations from the physical body, indicating "footprints" of disease. Along with this development, kinesiologist George Goodheart's subsequent discovery of the method to identify weak muscle responses to negative stimuli scientifically proved that the etheric body is a reality of the holographic human energy system. More recently, quantum physics has made it possible for technological imaging techniques such as magnetic resonant imaging, resonant field imaging, the harmonic translation system, and polychrome interference photography to be used in conjunction with computer technology to verify that the human body is composed of matter and energy. These devices are major developments in the authentication of the field of energy work because they "give detailed scientific information and objective interpretations for all Auras and bioenergy fields . . . "[141]

Etheric frequencies represent the first level of energies moving at a velocity faster than light. This identifies the etheric as a vehicle of consciousness to the degree that it has the capacity to access higher frequencies of consciousness. The etheric body is a self-organizing, holographic energy template demonstrating negative entropic properties. Negative entropy is the tendency of a system toward decreasing disorder.

The higher the frequency or consciousness of the etheric body, the greater the balance between the cosmic "rhythmic balanced interchange"[142] and the physical world. The more balanced the intercommunication between the etheric holographic magnetic grid, the grid to electrically based matter, and the cells of the physical body by way of the chakra and the meridian systems, the greater the health of the physical body, the world of matter.

The energy medicines that are most effective in the etheric realm include magnetic therapies, color, sound, selected homeopathic remedies, gem and mineral essences, essential oils, and chelation. Chelation is a term used by Barbara Brennan to describe a method of running energy through hands-on work in the etheric field. This method of healing is taught at the Barbara Brennan School of Healing. The health of the etheric body is negatively affected when the physical body is abused. It is, therefore, important to maintain a healthy physical body through exercise, nutrition, positive thoughts, feeling, and emotions. An unhealthy physical body, attitude, or action sabotages etheric body healing work and healing work on any other level of the holographic human energy system.

Theosophists of the late nineteenth and early twentieth centuries taught a method of "psychic" surgery. A. E. Powell describes the process of "psychic" healing in *The Etheric Double*: "A still more thorough method is to create the organ in mental matter: then to build into it astral matter: then to densify it with etheric matter: and finally to build into the mould gases, liquids and solids, utilising material available in the body and supplying from outside any deficiencies."[143] In other words, consciousness in the etheric body expresses itself as sensation and feeling. When we believe the feelings about our world and ourselves to be the "truth," we can become a slave to physical compulsions.

Astral Body

As Paracelsus says, the astral body is the doppelganger of man, his conscious ethereal counterpart, which watches over him and warns of the approach of danger and death. Furthermore, he writes, "The more the physical body is active and conscious of external things, the more is the Astral body stupefied; the sleep of the body is the awakening of the Evestrum. During that state, it may communicate with the Evestra of other persons or with those of the dead. It may go to certain distances from the physical body for a short time, but if its connection with that body is broken, the latter dies."[144]

In addition, the astral body provides the power through which thought expresses as effective action and manifests itself. The astral or emotional body provides the ability to desire and to have emotions, imagination, and psychic abilities.

Astral body consciousness includes the full range of emotions: fear, hate, sorrow, love, happiness, and bliss. It holds the space for the full spectrum of human behaviors, from selfish and destructive desires to common personal desires to high spiritual aspirations for selfless and service-full desires.

Theosophical literature states that the astral body is the manifestation of the "kama-rupa," which means desire-form or desire-body and that it is life manifesting in the astral body. In its rudimentary form or undeveloped state, sensation is the feeling attribute. Its evolved form is complex and expresses emotions. The astral body acts as a magnet attracting that which is like itself; in other words, pain attracts pain, and pleasure attracts pleasure. Kama-rupa is the brute in us, that which keeps us bound to earth, stifling all higher desires sabotaged by the illusion created by the senses. Kama-rupa, when combined with prana, is termed "the breath of life." The liver and spleen are specifically associated with the astral body or kama-rupa.

The astral body serves as a bridge between the mental body and the etheric and physical bodies. It acts like a transmitter of energy-information (senses) by way of prana and delivers the information to the chakra and meridian systems to the physical system. Without this information exchange there would not be a connection between the external world and the divine mind and no connection between physical affect and the perception of the impact by the mind.

The evolution of the astral body underwent three developmental stages. The first stage was the transmitter of energy information. The second stage of evolution was the astral body as an independent body, and the third stage gave the independent body the vehicle, consciousness coupled with the ability to act.

Along with senses and emotions, the astral body is also concerned with the production of thought forms, which are the product of both the astral and mental bodies. For instance, a very impersonal thought, such as mathematics or geometry, is specific to the mental body. A thought-form concerning feelings or emotions is an astral thought-form. No matter the origin of the thought-form, it produces two effects. First, it creates a radiating vibration and second, a floating form.

Since thought forms of the mental and astral body are intricately linked, it is necessary for clarity to delineate the difference between the two. In the mental body, thought form radiance expressed as vivid and intense color. The radiating vibration of the mental thought form tends to reproduce its own frequency in any mental body with which it comes in contact. Therefore, it tends to entrain the mental body of another to produce thoughts of the same type. An example of this would be a town meeting turning into a riot. It is important to point out that the thought and intention or character of that thought determines the power or integrity of the vibration. A less determined, intentioned vibration quickly dissipates in the ethers.

The floating aspect of a mental thought form is caused by the mental body releasing an aspect of itself, frequency-geometrically shaped, by the nature of the thought and draws to itself matter that corresponds to its order of frequency from the surrounding elemental essence of the mental plane. The higher the frequency or vibration of the matter, the greater the power or effect of the thought-form. When it is combined with the direction of emotion from the astral body, it manifests powerfully and purely in the material world. There are three principles that underlie all thought forms:

1. Color determined by the quality of the thought or emotion
2. Form or geometry determined by the nature of the thought or emotion
3. Clarity of focus determined by the definitive quality of the thought or emotion[145]

The initial intensity and continued reinforcement of repetitious thought determine its lifespan. There are three kinds of thought forms:

1. Those connected solely with the originator of the thought
2. Those connected with another person
3. Those manifested as impersonal[146]

Continuous focus on the same subject creates a thought form of great power. A.E. Powell states: "[Thought forms] remain in his aura, increasing in number and intensity until certain kinds of them so dominate his mental and emotional life that the man rather answers to their impulse than decides anew: thus are habits, the outer expression of his stored up force, created, and thus is character built."[147]

The astral body, though a component of the holographic human energy system, is a vehicle that has the capacity to separate from the physical and other subtle energy bodies without harming the system. In the dream state, we all experience astral mobility. The astral body begins about four to eight inches outside the physical body, just beyond the boundaries of the etheric. The astral is also known as the double of the physical. When a person develops a mastery of the astral body it becomes possible to be in two places at one time. The doctrine of a spirit form or the mobile astral body suggests the astral may survive the death of the physical. This doctrine exists in the lore of all indigenous peoples; the Egyptian Ba and the Greek Eidolon are examples.

The astral body is developed according to choices made by an individual during the physical life as a human being. In other words, a person who takes good care of the physical body—physically, emotionally, intellectually, and spiritually—is at the same time developing the astral body. If the opposite occurs, where the lower passions or "animal appetites" are fostered, a spiritually inferior psyche is developed. The spiritually inferior psyche has been identified over time by many cultures. Some names include the irrational soul of neoplatonism, the p'o soul of Chinese psychology, the Islamic *nafs* ("the soul that commands evil"), the passionate and sensual lower ego of Suffism, the *nefesh behemis* (animal soul) of Kabbalah, the id of Freud, the Undersoul of Ann Ree Colton's Niscience system, the Vital soul described by yogi Sri Aurobindo, and the subconscious or unconscious of popular psychology.

The Theosophists were concerned with the development of the subtle bodies for the purposes of enlightenment and clairvoyant, psychic, clairaudient, and automatic writing abilities. They taught that purity of the physical body is imperative to mastery. H.P. Blavatsky and C.W. Ledbeater, leaders in the Theosophical movement in the late 1800s and early 1900s, expanded their interest in the teachings of the yogis of India, specifically with interest in learning their purification techniques. From this study, Theosophical leaders determined that certain foods and substances have a detrimental effect on the subtle energy bodies and, therefore, made taboo the use of alcohol, tobacco, and red meat. (Neither Blavatsky nor Ledbeater followed their own teachings. Blavatsky was obese and a heavy smoker, and Ledbeater used alcohol and tobacco.)

Nonetheless, Theosophists taught that tobacco numbs or deadens the sensibility of the body while it adds impure particles to the system that are so gross they can be detected by the sense of smell. The use of alcohol, from the point of view of both the astral and mental bodies, is always "evil." The intake of alcohol, tobacco, and flesh foods compromises the function of the pituitary gland. In addition, Theosophists claim that the use of these substances and foods attracts negative entities to the subtle energy bodies.

The idea that "inharmonious" sounds negatively affect the astral body was the subject of a research project by Dr. David Hawkins. In a follow-up study with a group of teens who had completed a drug and alcohol treatment program, he determined that the teens who continued to listen to heavy metal music relapsed into further drug and alcohol use. This is a compelling example of the activation of the lower animal quality of the astral body. There was no relapse in the teens who did not continue to listen to heavy metal music.[148]

Talismans have the ability to affect the astral body, as witnessed in their use by healers, shamans, and even religious leaders, past and present, in their healing and other rites. Healers, for instance, will "program" the talisman with intentional astral body energies specific to their purpose. Talismans, being neutral energy, can be programmed for either good or "evil." The intention of the talisman must be known to all concerned, so "the good" is all that is infused.

As Paracelsus suggests:

> The Nectromanticus [seer] must know these spirits, for without that knowledge, he will not find their true character. By his art, he may sense them, and having perceived them with his inner sense he will find their corpus. Such spirits may be perceived in crystals; they may guide the divining-rod and attract it as a magnet attracts iron; it may turn the sieve and the key and draw the flame of a light away from the wick. By the art of Nectromancy, we may look into the interior of rocks; closed letters may be read without being opened, hidden things be found, and all the secrets of men be brought to light.[149]

As we have seen, the astral body is a powerful force of manifestation that produces the manifestation of desire. It is the instantaneous mirror reflecting every feeling in which every thought form, focused on the personal self, must express. The astral body, originally designed to identify danger before the danger comes too close for escape, has evolved along with human consciousness, expanding its ability to include astral travel and the interpretation of energy from levels other than the five senses. When only used in the survival mode, the astral body becomes part of the problem rather than the solution. The more we understand the characteristics of the astral body and its function and use, the more empowered we become through conscious activation of these life-enhancing energies.

Israel Regardie, Walter Russell, Edmond Bordeaux Szekely, Annie Besant, Ernest Holmes, and countless other nineteenth- and early-to-middle-twentieth-century healers and philosophers devoted their lives and writings to the development of the spiritual self. Their legacy is a rich one, and in your own journey as a student of self-development, I highly recommend you give yourself the gift of their wisdom.

It is impossible to leave the astral body discussion without mentioning dreams and archetypal energies. The brilliant work of the imminent Swiss psychologist Carl Jung concerning dreams and archetypal energies holds a veritable wealth of information about the astral world. According to Jung, highly developed individuals can access pure energy information from the higher self that resides in the dream world and use that wisdom in the physical or material world. This wisdom can be translated into inventions, writing, teaching, future predictions, original art and music, or provide answers to physical-world questions. According to Russell, genius is self-bestowed, not happenstance. Nicola Tesla, Walter Russell, Edwin Markham, Albert Einstein, and other great inventors and writers have shared their own experiences with the astral world in their writings.

Each aspect of the system—the physical brain, the etheric part of the brain, the astral body, and the ego of the causal body —are all factors to consider in the production of dreams. Dreams of the physical brain or the infantile, semiconscious brain express in picture forms. The etheric part of the brain produces a continuous procession of picture fragments. Dreams filled with desire and emotions characterize astral body dreams. The ego—or causal body, as the Theosophists define it—may be in any state of consciousness, from complete insensibility to perfect mastership of all bodies.

Jung, a contemporary of the Theosophists, determined that dreams and myths are constellations of archetypal images. Some suggest archetypal images represent one way in which humans can receive messages from the divine. The ancients called them "gods" and "goddesses." Jung discovered that humans have a "preconscious psychic disposition that enables them to react in a human manner."[150] These potentials for creation actualize when they enter consciousness as images or archetypes. The archetype may emerge into consciousness in a myriad of variations. There are a few basic archetypes or patterns at the unconscious level, but there are an infinite variety of patterns or archetypes pointing back to these few patterns.

In his early work, Jung associated archetypes with heredity and regarded them as instinctual. He determined that humans are born with inherited patterns that structure our imagination and make it distinctly human. Jung later stated that archetypes are "psychoid," meaning they shape matter or nature as well as the psyche or mind. They are elemental forces playing a vital role in the creation of the world and of the human mind itself. He found archetypal patterns in every culture and every period of human history. Jung postulated that all archetypes, no matter their cultural origin, operate according to the same laws. He called this the "collective unconscious." He suggested humans do not have separate, personal, unconscious minds but, rather, share a single "Universal Unconscious."

Jung divided the psyche into three parts: the ego-conscious mind, the personal unconscious (includes anything not presently conscious but can be triggered into consciousness through sights, sounds, smells, etc.), and the collective unconscious, or universal unconscious, also called the "psychic inheritance." The psyche is a reservoir of our experiences as a species, a kind of knowledge with which we are all born. Archetypes are the contents of this collective unconscious. As a result, they have the unlearned tendency to experience things in a certain way. They have no form of their own, but they act as an "organizing principle," for example, the principle of "The Hundredth Monkey."[151] Archetypes are like black holes; their presence can be known only by the way they draw matter and light to themselves.

The astral body can be the avenue of access to unconscious core beliefs, which in some way guide and direct our daily lives. Unless we identify these beliefs, they may carry us to places we do not want to go. These energies are detectable through the ways in which our physical bodies react to them. For instance, when making a statement such as "I am loved," the body may experience a weakening effect because the "system" recognizes that the belief one holds is, in essence, "I am not loved" and is not in harmony with the rhythmic, balanced interchange of greater universal energies. As a result, it registers as a lie, which weakens the system.

An easy method for accessing the system is through muscle testing or kinesiology. Another method of assessment is to stand facing magnetic north and then determine an appropriate "yes" and "no" response. Begin by stating your name and check which way your body moves: forward (north) for a true statement and back (south) for a false statement. If your body moves back on a statement that you know is true, i.e., your name, you may be dehydrated. In this case, drink some water to hydrate your system, then repeat the process until you get a clear response based on known facts. Next, make the statement, "I am loved." Notice the direction your body moves; this will indicate any unconscious archetypal energy guiding your personal system. You may be surprised at what you discover. Other examples of core beliefs include "rich people cannot get into heaven," "God loves poor people more," "I am a failure," "Life is suffering," "I can never have what I want," and "I can never be good enough no matter what I do."

Beliefs are not the truth. They are, as Yasuhiko Kimura of the University of Science and Philosophy says, "poor substitutes for genuine knowledge." Furthermore, he says, "A belief is an assumption that is elevated to the status of a conclusion or a truth without an examination and verification through observation and thinking."[152] When humans accept beliefs as truth and act upon them as truths, it supports their validity because what they believe becomes their experience. This collective unconscious pool of lies then becomes the director of present-day activities and decision-making processes. Our parents did not question their beliefs, nor did their parents before them. As a result, we inherited a set of beliefs based on lies rather than on Universal Laws. Adopting a life-supporting paradigm comes only after elucidating the lies we believed to be true. In the EMCS process we have discovered that beliefs may be held on any level, including the ancestrally inherited, the genetically inherited, the karmic, the past lives, and the soul level. I found reading *The Right Use of Will* series by Ceanne DeRohan helpful for a greater understanding of the soul level.

Changing Beliefs

The process of identifying and changing negative belief systems is one component of EMCS. It uses the language of commanding the universe to release the following from the holographic human energy system: miasms, universal subconscious negative prompters, life experiences, past life experiences, karmic ties, genetic imprinting, and any other distorted energies that support or manifest negative beliefs or patterns. These released beliefs are then transformed into balanced, rhythmic interchange. Additionally, they are released into the universe with peace, love, and light and are replaced with the truth of the divinity of the individual.

For this clearing work, five new categories have been added to the defusion sheet for muscle testing: core negative (see the full list at the end of chapter eleven) and shadow beliefs (see the full list in Appendix III), genetic level, historical level, soul level, and dimensional level (see chapter fourteen).

The core negative belief level speaks to generational programming, for example, "You are not good enough." This message is unconscious, whereas the shadow belief is manifest during the first six years of life and does not have to be a verbal message. It may have been an attitude a parent held toward a child who interpreted the message in that way. After a while, it became a "truth" through which the child viewed itself. Eventually, the perceived truth of that statement translated into self-condemnation and judgement.

The term "shadow" was coined by Jung to indicate repressed, unresolved pain from childhood experiences. He suggested these shadows become powerful "drivers" of human behavior and are subconscious or relatively unknown to the individual. Therefore, in EMCS, these "shadow beliefs" are created and repressed by the time we are six years old. They continue to create a systemic lack of mentality, limitation, and emotional pain in our lives until we become aware that they are actually lies.

When releasing beliefs from the holographic human energy system, intentionally align your energy with the power of the Universal One through desire, as described by Walter Russell as "rhythmically written into the universal heartbeat." Then, state the clearing to be accomplished: "I command the core negative belief or shadow belief of 'I hate myself' to be extirpated from [say client's name]. I command the belief to be released into the Universe with love and light and replaced with the truth of his divine inheritance as a Child of Light, or 'I Love Myself.'" Finally, state, "It is done, it is done, it is done," or, if you prefer, "Thank you, God, it is done." Finish with," Thank you." (Note: You may do this silently or speak with the client if you and the client are comfortable with that—set that up as part of the criteria before every session.)

Then, proceed with the normal defusion process.

Beliefs are often genetically inherited and passed from generation to generation. Perhaps this explains the "Sins of the Father" message from the Christian Bible. When working with a client and muscle testing identifies an issue as genetic, use your skill to determine with the client the exact genetic message ("Money is bad," "I can never succeed," "God loves poor people more," etc.). Use the process outlined above to call upon the Universal One in a cooperative effort to extract the genetic belief, releasing it into the universe and replacing it with the truth. Genetic programming involves DNA blueprinting. This blueprinting comprises several components, including a record of the emotion recorded in the "originator" of the blueprint, the memory of the event causing the emotion, the physical cellular electromagnet structuring to accommodate the memory, and the emotion and the mechanism of the DNA required to pass the blueprint on to the next generation. It is necessary to address each of these components in the defusion of a genetic issue at the time of cause.

Many of you will remember Gregg Braden's video "Beyond Zero Point," in which he films Chinese healers treating a woman with bladder cancer. I was struck by the fact that the healers constantly repeat a Chinese phrase that translates as "It is done" while they work. Since the process was videotaped, we can see the healing taking place on the sonogram monitor. It is completed in just over two minutes. Each of the healers, when questioned about what they were doing during the two minutes, stated that they were visualizing, feeling, and experiencing a completely healthy organ.

All great healers, ancient and modern, teach the importance of visualizing the change happening in the healing process. "It is done" is a command, and knowing the truth for the person and witnessing the change happen is a recognition of the healing power of the Universal One. I have found it a powerful process to direct the client to "witness" the change themselves; this may be through visualization, imagination, or sensation. You, as the energician, must also witness the change in your own intuitive way.

The importance of witnessing the healing process is punctuated by Gregg Braden when he asks this question of the Chinese healers: "What if the patient did not believe the healing had occurred?" One of them answers, "The healing would not last. The cells would revert to the old pattern, and the cancer would return." I always remind clients at the end of each session to be aware of any changes that occur following an EMCS session. I suggest they keep a journal to record what they have noticed as they go through the process. I find if they make that effort, change happens more quickly. As a bonus, it helps them to provide me with information that is helpful for the next session.

In working with clients over the years, I have found that connecting with unresolved past life trauma is a very important aspect of the revitalization process. Often, clients say to me, "I just know this pain or pattern is something I brought in from a past life because it doesn't fit with my life now." Moreover, muscle testing has taken us to a past life for resolving the pattern, and surprisingly, the pattern resolves almost immediately, and the limitation goes away. To incorporate this possibility into the EMCS system, I have added "historical" as an option, along with core beliefs, etc. The historical level, then, refers to past life memories. Whether that past life occurred in a physical form or spiritual form, patterns were set up that affect life today. I also suspect archetypal energies are components of the historical level. Archetypes such as the victim, martyr, hero, nun, priest, hierophant, or fool are examples. This level of discovery might reveal an oath of poverty or martyrdom taken in a past life, or it might be a component of the nun or monk archetype.

In working with this energy, it is important to command that the pattern be resolved on every level, known and unknown, on the continuum of "time" from the origin of the pattern through all eternity. Command that the pattern be replaced with the truth of divinity or something more concrete, such as "money is just energy." Use your intuitive abilities and kinesiological prowess to determine the ultimate Highest Truth for the client. Witness with them the change at the age of cause once you have administered the corrections that came up during the defusion. Then, bring them back to the present time, infusing the new program by way of the identified infusion symbol. Usually, the symbol of the element, white light for instance, is the infusion symbol, but muscle test to be clear.

I have included the soul level as an option for causal programming in this section of the defusion sheet. To understand the soul level, let me define the soul for our purposes in EMCS defusions. A soul is the differential essence of the Universal One. When the One Soul individuated, the individual souls created by the individuation of the One fused with an appropriate form. Elements and systems drawn from nature were used to make up the original form that received the individuated One. We call these created forms or combined elements and systems the human body. The human body is the appropriate system through which the soul can best operate, experience, and express. The soul creates a structure and foundation through which it can operate no matter the level, state, or dimension the soul chooses to participate in. The soul may be operating on levels other than the Earth plane. Soul and body work in partnership through every soul experience, regardless of the level. Individuated souls operate beyond time and space. Although time and space are form structures, they are not the criteria for the definition of form. Form is any reality that has order, organization, life vitality, and consciousness. Time and space are but two kinds of order and organization. A study of the Theory of Enformed Systems, a paradigm developed by David Watson, Gary Schwartz, and Linda Russek and outlined in their paper "A Comprehensive Theory of Consciousness: The Theory of Enformed Systems," might help students understand the quantum levels of human experience. They contend that any theory of consciousness must explain not only the traditional elements attributed to human consciousness but also must explain every phenomenon radically related to these elements. If the theory does not explain all the phenomena, then it cannot explain any of them. Their Theory of Enformed Systems attempts to do just that. [153]

As quantum physics proves, experience happens simultaneously on all levels. Therefore, every experience occurs beyond time and space. Thus, the experience can be said to be holographic. This being true, it means the experience we call lifetimes or even our personal experience in the now can be said to be the illusion we think of as reality.

The soul level indicates patterns developed beyond space and time in this dimension or any other in which the soul chooses to have its experience. That is the reason planetary lifetimes sometimes show up in defusion work. "Alien" races may be a part of the information one determines from muscle testing in planetary past life defusions.

The process of defusion on the soul level is the same as on any other level. Make sure you check each level to ensure that the pattern is successfully released on all levels that apply. Recheck to make certain you have not missed a level. In other words, a pattern that shows up as genetic may also have a soul-level component.

Mental Body

The mental body is the aspect of the holographic human energy system through which the self manifests as concrete intellect.[154] Additionally, within this self or mental body are developed powers of the mind, including memory and imagination, which make it possible for the mental body to act as a separate and distinct vehicle of consciousness. In this developmental stage, one can live and function apart from the physical and astral bodies.

The mental body, according to some metaphysicians, has seven layers. The first four layers or lower subdivisions correspond to the four lower subdivisions of the astral body and to the solid, liquid, gaseous, and etheric matter of the physical plane. According to Theosophists, "The three higher grades of mental matter are used to build the Causal or Higher Mental body . . . "[155]. The mental body has an ovoid shape and surrounds the lower subtle bodies and the physical body.

The mental body is the vehicle through which the self or soul manifests and expresses as the concrete intellect. The mind is the reflection of the self as a "knower," and the mind is the self-working in the mental body. The soul, according to Dr. Bruce Fisher, who has written three volumes on studies in occult anatomy, has three aspects—knowing, willing, and expressing or energizing. From these three aspects develops thought, emotion, and action. Therefore, the act of concrete thinking sets in vibration the matter of the mental body to the grosser matter of the astral. The astral, in turn, sends the vibration to the etheric particles of the brain, resulting in a physical response.[156]

The sympathetic nervous system communicates with the astral body, and the cerebrospinal fluid system communicates with the mental body. Thus, the mental body acts on the astral, which acts on the etheric and physical and is, in turn, delivered to the chakra system, meridian system, and, finally, the nervous system. This process results in electrical and magnetic discharges, causing intricate intercommunication throughout the physical body.

Walter Russell, in *A Course in Cosmic Consciousness,* defines mind and matter this way: "Mind is spiritual and constitutes the invisible universe of Cause. Matter is physical and constitutes the visible universe of effect. Mind has but one Idea: the Idea of Creation as a whole. Mind expresses its desire electrically by thinking and imagining. Matter is the expression of Mind's whole creative Idea through Mind's electric thinking and imagining, which is sensed or Experienced of itself."[157]

Simply put, the mind conceives thought forms and ideas and gives them form in images through imagination. The astral body contributes the senses and passion to create the image in physical form. The individual uses intellect and training to produce the product. A musician receives an idea for a musical composition, hears it in the mind, feels the rhythm through emotion, and uses musical training to produce it in the three-dimensional world. The result is more than training and intellect could produce alone. The result is magical— a masterpiece.

Meditation is the sustenance of the Mind or the spiritual Self. Meditation is necessary for human development. Through meditation, one can knowingly commune with the "Universal Mind of God." Russell says meditation "is communing with God for the purpose of knowingly work with God."[158]

A.E. Powell, in *The Mental Body,* defines meditation as "sustained attention of the concentrated mind in the face of an object of devotion."[159] Meditation consists of the endeavor to bring into the waking consciousness realization of the super conscious. The first step in meditation, says Russell, is to forget the physical body and stop thinking about anything. He suggests becoming a vacuum as far as the senses are concerned. Next, "desire" the light without using words; this process is a realization of light more than a "thinking" of light. The goal of meditation is to be alone with and commune with God. It is the human being calling a conference between his or her soul and the Universal Soul.

The soul, alone, can give out love. Since meditation is the tool for accessing the soul, it is the soul that bestows genius and re-gives the love of God to self and, thus, to humanity. In the meditative process, communication with God is possible only from this soul level. During the meditation, ask questions and be open to receiving the answers given in the silence of the Universal Soul.

Russell states, "Meditation is a communion with God for the purpose of acquiring knowledge and power to manifest God as the CO-Creator of His universe. Meditation is intercommunication between your immortal Mind and the electric senses of your mortal body. Meditation is a conference between your immortal Mind self, who knows; your thinking, which builds images of your knowing; and your body, which acts in obedience to the will of your Mind. Mediation is an expression of desire for knowledge of perfect Cause for the purpose of producing perfect Effect."[160]

In summation, the mental body is the body of manifestation. It is through the proper use of this subtle energy body that we, as human beings, have the potential for greatness and genius. Meditation is one tool for realizing divinity.

Causal Body

Once again, the wisdom of A.E. Powell is worth considering:

> When we come to study the causal body of man, we enter upon a new phase of our work and must take a far wider sweep in our purview of man's evolution. The reason for this is that whilst the etheric, astral and mental bodies exist for one human incarnation only, i.e. ..., are distinctly mortal, the causal body persists throughout the whole of man's evolution, through many incarnations and is, therefore relatively immortal. We say relatively immortal advisedly because, as will be seen in due course, there is a point where a man, having completed his purely normal human evolution, commences his supernormal human evolution and actually loses the causal body in which he has lived and evolved during the past ages of his growth.[161]

Let me begin this discussion by saying that a study not only of Powell's later compiled works but also those of the Theosophists, C.W. Leadbeater, Madame H.P. Blavatsky, and Alice Bailey concerning the causal body is highly recommended. Even after one hundred years of technological advances, the work of the Theosophists is still cited as authoritative knowledge among today's authors when discussing the subtle energies of the human aura.

The causal body is the originating source of each personality. The Theosophists teach that the causal body persists throughout the whole of the evolution of humankind. Thus, it continues from lifetime to lifetime. It is relatively immortal, according to A.E. Powell, in that there is a point in the evolution of humanity when humanity has completed its normal course of progression and makes the quantum leap into supernormal human growth. At this point, says Powell, the causal body is no longer needed and is discarded much as the physical, etheric, astral, and mental bodies are discarded from lifetime to lifetime. If the causal body has an end, it must also have a beginning. According to the Theosophists, this beginning has its origins in a level of consciousness called group-souls. Theosophists traced group-soul origins to "Three Great Outpourings of the Divine Life from which all forms of manifested life arise"[162] He describes eons of time in which group souls evolved and developed to a point where individualization was reached, and the causal body appeared for the first time. Theosophists called the world of matter in which evolution is to take place the "field of evolution." And it materializes as opposite poles of one noumenon or one intellectual blueprint. From this noumenon is created the seven planes or worlds of our solar system. These seven worlds make up three groups.

The first of these is the field of logoic manifestation, meaning the matter of space symbolized by points upon which the next step of the matrix will be added or the lines representing energy manifestation of the One Intellect's individual life or "all-ensouling consciousness." A similar description of the origins of the universe can be found in the writing of the Sumerians over nine thousand years ago, in the Zend Avesta of Zarathrustra (six thousand years ago), and through the teaching of the mystical Kabbalah. The logoic is also called Kether by Kabbalists, or the one divided into two on the Tree of Life as Binah and Chokma; in Sanskrit, the Adi and Anupadaka; and in the Western World, Alpha and Beta or A and B.

The second level of the field of evolution is called the Atma and Buddhi, or Spirit and Intuition, and Geburah and Chesed on the Tree of Life, or intuition and objective archetypes of the supernormal human. The third level is composed of manas (mind), kama (emotion) and sthula (physical activity), or the level of normal human, animal, vegetable, mineral, and elemental entities. In the Kabbalah, this level includes the sephirah of tifereth and the four lower sephirot that make up the "world of formation."[163]

I mention these exoteric and esoteric traditions to establish the long-held foundation of knowledge concerning the process of the evolution of the human being and its subtle energy bodies. The course of human evolution is a long and sacred one, one we are called upon to respect and honor; therefore, any small attempt on my part to fully encapsulate in these pages this evolutionary process is impossible. However, not to include at least an outline of it would be unfathomable.

According to tradition, the causal body has two main functions. The first is to act as a vehicle for the ego. The causal body, according to Powell, is the "body of Manas," the true man, Rodin's *The Thinker*. The second function is to act as a record, a "hard drive" or depository for the essence of human experience in each incarnation. This information could be described as "all information which endures and holds fast," in much the same way universal laws always operate the same way in every situation. Since there could not be an individual human being without the causal body, everyone has as a component of their subtle energy anatomy a causal body.[164]

The causal body is the divine spark in each of us. This divine spark is what animates our physical body, it is the light in our eyes, the flame that draws us into the future, ever exploring, always seeking the greater light. It is the vehicle through which our soul seeks expression in the world of matter, the third-dimensional world of materiality. Our physical body represents the temporary expression of our soul for its purpose in this particular space and time. In that sense, all action is determined—there is no life expression by chance. The soul has a "plan" for our lives. That plan is to express the energies of love and wisdom with ever-increasing intensity until all humankind becomes one in love.

The causal body is constructed from the collective conscious wisdom gained throughout the many lifetimes lived in time and space by the soul. Though the soul is not the causal body, the causal body is an energetic field of resonance capable of being a vehicle for the soul. This matrix functions as abstract thought, while the mental body functions as concrete thought. The powers inherent in the causal body include attention, memory, reasoning by induction and deduction, and imagination. Therefore, the causal body focuses on the essence of a thing rather than on specific details. Powell states, "Again the student may be reminded that, in spite of external differences of function between the higher and the lower mind, yet Manas, the Thinker, is one, the Self in the Causal body."[165]

Even though the causal body is the storehouse of enduring positive knowledge, it can be affected over time by the practice of negative thought or that which is termed "evil" in some traditions. This can dim the luster or luminosity of the causal body. The "I" cannot assimilate this negativity because evil or negativity cannot reach this level of consciousness; however, long continued expression of negative energies over many lifetimes can cause a kind of paralysis of the energy of the causal sheath, resulting in an unconscious state.

Activation and development of the causal body are reached through meditation, a constant connection with the divine. This constant process of living "in the light" expresses a genius in the material world. Someone whose actions are expressed through the light of love manifests as the mastery of life.

In conclusion, I quote Powell:

> The causal body is known also as the Augoeides, the glorified man; it is not an image of any one of his past vehicles but contains within itself the essence of all that was best in each of them. It thus indicates, more or less perfectly, as through experience it grows, what the Deity means that man shall be. For, as we have seen, by observation of the causal vehicle it is possible to see the stage of evolution which the man has reached. Not only can his past history be seen, but also, to a considerable extent, the future that lies before him.[166]

Energy Matrix Clearing System

CASE NOTES

_____
DATE

_____
ISSUE

_____
LEVEL OF RESPONSIBILITY

NEE_____
PEE_____

FlorAlive_____

_____Pleiadian Glyph

_____Avoidance Behavior

_____Level of Consciousness

_____Universal Fear

_____Reflective Mirror

_____10 Elements

_____Archetype

_____Gene Key/Hexagram

_____Kabalistic 72 Names of God

_____
NAME

_____
CORE NEGATIVE BELIVE
Shadow Belief_____
Historial_____
Genetic, Lost Will, All Soul
LEVELS, ANCESTRAL, DIVINE SPIRIT, LEVELS, DIMENSIONS

_____
SUBTLE ENERGY BODIES
__P   __E   __A   __M   __C
MIASM_____   DRAINER_____   ENTITY_____
CURSES_____   NEGATIVE ENERGETIC CORDS_____

MATRIX SYSTEM EFEECTED

_____

_____

_____

_____

_____

_____

_____

_____

_____Casual Age

_____Age on Line

_____NEE

_____Level of Responsibility

_____Avoidant Behavior

_____Universal Fear

_____Reflective Mirror

_____10 Elements

_____Archetype

Miasm____   Drainer____   Entity____
SEB: __P   __E   __A   __M   __C

MATRIX SYSTEM EFFECTED

HOMEWORK:

NOTES:

CHAPTER ELEVEN

ENERGETIC MEDICINES

True knowledge is obtained by participation and fusion of the knower with the object of study— and the scientist is required to become higher in order to understand higher things. We cannot remain separate and detached if we wish to understand. We need to participate in and be one with what we wish to understand. Unfortunately, even when the idea of transformation has an appeal, one generally wishes to be transformed without changing.

—R. RAVINDRA

At the turn of the nineteenth century, there was a departure from the use of homeopathic remedies made from plants, animals, and minerals as healing methods, when previously, they had been a primary source of healing used by physicians in their medical practices. Before embarking on an explanation of "energetic medicines," we will take a cursory look into the reason for this departure from healing methods used since recorded history.

In the first chapter, I presented the idea that humans are essentially energetic beings; therefore, energetic processes for healing should logically follow. Since writing that chapter, I read Carl Johan Calleman's incredible book, *The Purposeful Universe: How Quantum Theory and Mayan Cosmology Explain the Origin and Evolution of Life.* He made astounding conclusions that have ramifications concerning current scientific stances on evolution, biology, and all science. These conclusions are based on the central generating energy that the Maya call Hunab Ku or Tree of Life. Calleman says of the Tree of Life Theory:

> An important rule in this model of the evolution of the universe is that the higher levels of organization of life are senior to the lower, and the latter always need to function within the frameworks provided by the higher levels. This rule also applies to the relationship between a multicellular organism, such as an animal, a plant, or a fungus, and its individual cells. Thus, in a healthy organism, the functioning of individual cells is subordinated to the body organs they are part of, which in turn are subordinated to the whole organism.[167]

In my estimation, this hierarchical view is the very basis upon which energetic-medicine modalities stand. Allopathic medicine focuses on the part; energetic medicine focuses on the whole. Calleman's theory explains the whole. He provides convincing evidence that it is in "centriole-based" medicine that we may find access to extraordinary human advances in health. "We may recall," he states, "that the organismic Halos are senior to interactions with energy and matter and hence outside the reach of physical manipulations . . ."[168]

Calleman uses the term "halo" to describe the energy fields around any living entity, from a galaxy to a single cell. It is through this halo that consciousness guides the evolutionary process of each hierarchy in the halographic universe. In other words, ". . . from the smallest aspect of the halographic universe to the largest," according to Calleman, it is the halos surrounding each system that " . . . serve to organize the universe into life-supporting systems at different levels. Each of these systems has autonomy while they are at the same time connected and synchronized with the other levels through halographic resonance."[169] This explains the ancient statement attributed to the great master Thoth, "As above, so below."

Calleman explains how humans are connected to the halographic resonance of the Tree of Life in this way:

> . . . it seems that the ultimate reason that we have a central nervous system around which our bodies are organized in three dimensions, front-back, left-right, and up-down, is that the microtubules of the cytoskeletons of the participating cells at an early state of embryonal development through Halographic resonance were directed in a special way by their centrosomes.[170]

He concludes with this powerful statement: "All development in multicellular organisms, including their anatomy and morphology, ultimately emanates from the centrosomes.[171]

The centriole, says Calleman, "functions perfectly in accordance with what we would expect from a Cellular Tree of Life."[172] The centriole, he explains, "are invariably formed by thirteen filaments made from dimmers of alpha- and beta-tubulin proteins."[173] A cross-section of the centriole shows the "ninefold symmetry of the microtubules, which are triplicated, 9(+2). The component microtubules consist of thirteen filaments."[174]

This numerical ordering of the centriole aligns the human form exactly with the waveforms of energy identified by the prophetic Maya calendar. Perhaps the thirteen filaments play a similar role in the evolution of life processes and consciousness that is portrayed by the thirteen kingdoms in the prophetic Maya calendar. This calendar was divided into nine levels, and each level was further divided into seven days and six nights, or thirteen kingdoms. Each kingdom played an important role in the process of the evolution of consciousness in each cycle, much like the process of a seed. The seed sprout produces leaves, flowers, and fruit and then perpetuates itself by, in turn, making seeds. The centriole alignment is foundational to the sprouting of the seed in that the alignment happens at the very moment of conception when the sperm fertilizes the egg. From the very origin of human experience, the halographic alignment is ordering each individual process of development.

Since it is the halo that provides the informational guidance for each cell in its growth process, it makes sense that any distortion or blockage in the halo system would result in misdirected cellular growth. Since the halo is energy and the source of information on the cellular level, it also makes sense that using energetic processes to communicate with the halo would be the most direct avenue of harmonization on the whole. Research to determine methods of communication or to affect the halo could be valuable in determining the efficacy of energy medicine. Energetic medicine may already be doing that, but as Calleman indicates in his book, the centriole and the part it plays in human development and health have been, until now, overlooked by the scientific community. We can only hope that a new science based on these new discoveries will begin to explode on the scene of health and wellness.

The term energetic medicine refers to a group of approaches and specific energetic frequencies used to positively affect or increase the human life force. Illness or "dis-ease," by definition, is an unstable energy. Illness, then, is simply a disturbance in an otherwise normal, stable condition called health. It is a well-accepted premise in the global energy medicine community that, no matter the distortion—disease or "dis-ease"—and no matter the level—mental, emotional, spiritual, or physical—"sympathetic vibrations" are an effective treatment. This means applying a stronger signal or frequency that introduces an electrical current to initiate a harmonizing function into the halographic system. This energy-information then serves to correct and balance the "dis-ease."

I see the human form not just as a physical form of flesh and bone, blood and sinew, organs and brain, but as a holographic matrix of interacting energy grids. Even though we cannot "see" these fields of energy with the naked eye, they nevertheless make up the totality of what it means to be human. Just because you may not be aware of this matrix does not mean it is not there. Although we are not aware of the cell phone signal coursing through the atmosphere, we hear the voice on our phones and see the text message as it arrives. There is a signal—a ring, vibration, or song—from our phone that alerts us to the fact that we are receiving a transmission: a phone call, text, or email message. In the same way, the energy matrix system that surrounds us and interpenetrates us signals when we are receiving a message. The signals include thoughts, feelings, and emotions that inform us that we are receiving a message about our internal and external worlds.

The first step in becoming your own energy practitioner is awareness of the rhythms inherent in the flow between the energetic systems. Those systems are the physical body, the motor function of the system and the mind, the awareness function, and the interpreter, which determines the value of sensations and impressions from the internal and external worlds. Once valued, the observer (or the "I") questions and investigates to determine the facts and then reports the facts to the "X" factor of the system or life force that activates the biological function, determining the physical body's response or reaction to the information delivered. The type of information delivered to X, either factual (reality) or perceived (fight or flight), determines whether the biological information is geared toward survival or toward a proactive process of harmonious living.

The model just presented is the work of Robert Rhondell Gibson, which he called The Way of Intelligence. James and Andrea Steward expanded on Rhondell's work in their Mayan Calendar Code Core Training: Evolution of Consciousness. Their expanded model, The Human Source Code or Four Functions of Man, is, for me, a beautiful representation of how the human system operates.

I mention their work here to punctuate that the "X" factor or life force, the biological factor of the human operating system, generates human health. According to the Stewards, when given the facts by the observer or "I" concerning health status, the life force appropriately generates energy-information revitalizing the human system. Therefore, because "X" is one function of the human system and not a separate entity, avenues of healing the system from within the system are always present.

"X" just may be the human connection to Calleman's "Halographic Universe." He says, "The Halos all serve to organize the universe into life-supporting systems at different levels. Each of these systems has autonomy while they are at the same time connected and synchronized with the other levels through Halographic resonance."[175]

I suspect homeopathic remedies communicate "halo graphically," causing alignment of frequencies within the halographic human system, ultimately ordering the balancing or realignment with those frequencies within the human organism that are "dis-eased" and thereby returning them to a healthy stasis, or eliminating them altogether and ordering a new, healthy structure to replace it.

This kind of research is out of my educational purview; however, scientific theory, in particular quantum physics, tells us that when two different objects, each vibrating at their own different frequency, come together, the impact they have on one another is converted into a new form of energy that has its own unique vibratory frequency. That would certainly align with the use of vibrational medicines to affect the health structure of the halographic and holographic human energy systems. This, of course, would be the field of biophysics, which brings together the latest knowledge from the fields of physics and biology.

As I have discussed in earlier chapters, the quantum level of the halographic human energy system, termed the biofield, instructs the biochemical body in perfect functioning. When or if this field provides misinformation to the biochemical body, dis-ease will eventually manifest as physical, mental, emotional, and spiritual discomfort.

The premise from which energy medicine and energy psychology operate is working with the holograph by way of energy processes and energy medicine, thereby restoring the system to its natural state of health.

Let us take a moment and explore the use of gem and mineral essences as viable components of vibrational medicine. The healing properties of gemstones lie in their crystalline structure. These structures are able to maintain a resonance or harmonics that defy permeation by other forms of resonance. This stable element or pattern of molecular activity can act as a frequency resonance capable of amplifying the vibration of other life forms. In other words, their healing ability, based upon the transference of their stable form of molecular structure, permeates all energetic levels where there is a sympathetic resonance.

Gurudas, as channeled through Kevin Ryerson, says it this way:

> Based upon these principles, disease within the body physical, although it may first seem to be on the anatomical level, has been traced by [the] scientist to the cellular level and eventually to the level of the biomolecular system, contained perhaps within the very genetic structure in its own right. In the final analysis, the body physical is healed through energy, energy upon the biomolecular level, not even upon the level of chemical reactions but more so upon molecular structures. Real healing extends from the biomolecular to the cellular level, and eventually to the anatomical level, where it is brought into harmony with other levels of the body physical. This is because the biochemical properties of the body physical in their final element are based upon vibration.[176]

He goes on to explain that:

The cellular level refers to the physical body, on the level of each individual cell such as the individual muscle cells. The cellular level has similar properties to the DNA and RNA, but they are still different levels. The entire cellular level constitutes the DNA and RNA in their singular, united functions, but when divided, they become a specific level within their own patterns. The terms molecular and biomolecular refer to chemical activity on the subatomic level within each cell that organizes into structures such as DNA and RNA to become genetic tissue.[177]

This explains how gem and mineral essences can effect change from the biomolecular to the cellular levels of the holographic human energy system.

He also points out that gemstones can amplify thoughts. He compares the process of thought amplification to light passing through a system of filters that shapes the thoughts by way of the frequency of the gemstone filtering it. In my own Living in Choice Gem and Mineral selection, I have provided text suggesting an intended thought focus with each combination of gem and mineral essences used in the combination. During the production process for each essence, I used the intention to infuse each gem and mineral essence with celestial spirit energy to enhance and strengthen the inherent quality of each essence.

Each essence, imbued with a specific intention, promotes natural vitality and optimum functioning at all levels of the halographic and holographic human energy system. Records of homeopathic preparation of gemstones for healing purposes have existed since ancient times. The literature identifies salts of calcium and graphite and diamond and pyrite dust as combinations used for healing purposes. The difference between a homeopathic remedy or gem elixir and a gem-mineral essence is that the homeopathic remedy has some of the gem-mineral in the mixture, whereas the essence only has the vibration of the gem-mineral.

Traditionally, homeopathic remedies are prepared by taking nine drops of alcohol to one drop of the mother tincture (these are the undiluted essences) and mixing them together to get "one time," which is traditionally written as 1x. This dilution can be repeated any number of times, with each repetition termed the number plus the x, representing the number of times the dilution has occurred. The more diluted the solution, the more powerful it becomes.

In the United States, the Food and Drug Administration (FDA) regulates homeopathic remedies. Only gems, minerals, or flower and herb remedies and essences listed in the *U.S. Homeopathic Pharmacopoeia* are approved for public consumption. Any new remedy must undergo strict guidelines for testing before the FDA will approve it.

When used clinically, vibrational remedies affect the halographic and holographic human energy systems by following a specific path of assimilation. First, they travel through the circulatory system and settle midway between the circulatory and nervous systems in anticipation of the next process of assimilation. That process takes place via an electromagnetic current that creates a polarity of these two systems in which the vibration/information of the remedy can be utilized. The biosciences are beginning to investigate the intimate connection between these two systems and life force and consciousness. Life force seems to influence the blood, while consciousness seems to influence the brain and nervous system. Both systems contain quartz-like or crystalline properties and electromagnetic current. These properties hold the key for life force and consciousness to enter and stimulate the cellular structure of the physical body. Through the crystalline and electromagnetic currents, the gem and mineral essence is carried by the nervous system and circulatory system to the meridian system, which delivers it to the chakra system and then to the subtle energy bodies. The life force within the essence returns to the physical body by three main portals: the etheric body, the chakras, and the skin. As the life force returns to the physical system on a molecular level, it seeks out the imbalanced areas of the physical body. This process takes place in an instant. The crystalline properties of the lymphatic system also play a part in the process by assisting in the removal of the toxins resulting from system imbalances.

When administering gem and mineral essences, employ muscle testing to determine the number of drops necessary for the correction of the imbalance. In the EMCS process, there are four routes of administration for essences:

1. On the tongue
2. Sublingual
3. Topical
4. In water

Each of these methods speaks to a different process of communication with the issue. On the tongue speaks to the issue of "right use of will," integrity, and speaking and acting on one's inner truth. Sublingual administration relates to a cellular and perhaps unconsciously held belief. Topical refers to the skin and its connection with the nadi of the meridian system. In water is a cleansing correction, i.e., to release toxins from the system, especially the lymphatic system.

As in any system of healing, the medication can only assist in the healing process; each individual must attune to their own spiritual illumination and higher consciousness for the best harmonizing results. Energetic medicines cannot override free will. We are all responsible for the choices we make. Any unhappiness in life is the result of a choice made, and, of itself, a gem essence cannot change the individual choice. It can, through its vibratory process, illicit insight, vision, and access to higher levels of consciousness through which an individual finds the courage to make better choices. It is the responsibility of each individual to notice internal changes and act upon them.

As stated earlier in this section, the utilization of homeopathic remedies in the healing arts is a centuries-old practice. Dr. Samuel Hahnemann, a German homeopathic physician of the eighteenth century, believed that a miasm was at the core of all chronic diseases. He noticed in his practice that sometimes an herbal remedy known to affect the healing process did not work with a particular client or that the illness would clear up and then return. He began to suspect some underlying cause of the illness. He called this "derangement" a miasm, from the Greek "taint" or "fault" (indeed, Hippocrates, the father of medicine, postulated that certain infectious diseases were transmitted to humans by air and water tainted by miasms). Hahnemann saw miasms as the vibrational foundation of genetically inherited diseases in the physical body. He felt these vibrations included viruses and bacteria that lie dormant in the subtle energy system. He also determined that miasms could lie dormant for centuries in what he termed a "delicately balanced symbiosis."[178]

David V. Tansley, in his book *Chakras: Rays and Radionics*, published in 1972, states, "In homeopathy, miasm denotes a transcending and predisposing condition that causes illness." Like

Hahnemann, Tansley views miasms as a "four-dimensional dynamic encompassing the vital force, the mind (psyche), the body (soma), and the species. . . ."[179] If disease is regarded as an imbalance in life force, meaning that somewhere in the holographic human energy system, something is distorting or blocking the flow of life force, disturbances show up in the physiological and anatomical health of an individual.

Some conditions or situations disturbing the delicately balanced symbiosis of a miasm are stress, trauma, or illness. Along with these, the process of aging, which can weaken the human energy system, may also activate a miasm. Underlying miasms may contribute to or affect a chronic illness. Treating the symptoms may be ineffectual because of the miasmic frequency. Gurudas makes the point that "It is essential that holistic health practitioners understand the profound impact [miasms] have on chronic diseases. Underlying [miasms] contribute to making one susceptible to various acute illnesses."[180]

It was generally accepted by early homeopaths and vitalist physicians that miasms played an important role in the root of disease. They accepted that miasms were stored in the cells of the physical body and were present in the subtle energy bodies of the holographic human energy system, especially in the etheric, emotional, and mental bodies, but to a lesser degree in the astral body. Gurudas says, "Some [miasms] are passed on to the next generation genetically by inhabiting the molecular level of the physical body, which is the genetic code."[181]

A miasm is a disease signature held in the system, but that does not necessarily mean that the disease will be made active. As Gurudas says, "Indeed, [miasms] are a crystallized pattern of karma."[182] I see a miasm as an encapsulated pattern or void held in the subtle energy bodies. It may be seen as a lack of light or life force. When the soul expresses itself in the physical realm, the pattern, void, or miasm is activated and reveals the essence of the void or blockage as disease or lack of life force. The specific miasm conveys information about the lack of light or the void. Recognizing the manifested disease as an opportunity to heal the void that created it by bringing in source light to enter into the void brings the system into harmony. Once the void it is illuminated with source light no longer exists, its disease symptom likewise cannot exist.

Research reveals that there are four types of miasms: planetary, inherited, acquired, and stellar. Planetary miasms, according to Gurudas, are found in the collective consciousness of the planet as well as the ethers surrounding it.[183] Alice Bailey first discussed planetary miasm in her 1953 work, *Esoteric Healing*, in which she identified the three planetary miasms of cancer, syphilis, and tuberculosis. Only syphilis and tuberculosis have settled in the cellular level of individuals and so are also included in the inherited miasm category, but Gurudas does not include cancer in the inherited category. Inherited miasms become a part of the memory of the physical cells. Hahnemann identified three forms of inherited miasms as psora, syphilitic, and sycotic. Today, most homeopaths include tuberculosis and cancer in the inherited miasm group, with cancer being a combination of them all. Acquired miasms present as infectious diseases, or they may be acquired from exposure to toxic chemicals over time.

Machaelle Small Wright, in an article published on her website, the Perelandra Center for Nature Research, defines miasms as ". . . energy realities that exist independently of and within life systems. A miasm within a life system may be viewed as a localized pocket or concentration of energies composed of elements that do not enhance, stabilize or maintain the balance and well-being of the larger life system." In addition," A miasm is, therefore, a smaller energy reality that is part of a larger life system but is out of time and place with the overall direction and purpose of that larger system. Within a life system, the [miasm] may be dormant or active." Furthermore, she states that once a miasm becomes a part of a life system, it will remain in that larger system until the larger system becomes strong enough to eliminate the miasm or transform it in such a way that it changes form and becomes a harmonious addition to the larger system.[184]

Homeopaths have determined there are five types of miasms. We will take them in order as determined by Hahnemann.

Psora

Psora, known as the oldest "contagion" of the life force, is the fundamental miasm affecting the vital life force. Tansley states:

> Once the [miasm] has affected the vital force it has a stationary period with a localized manifestation which, more often than not, gets suppressed. Then the [miasm] affects deeper spheres, and multiple symptoms begin, which can give a false appearance of being unconnected with the [miasm]. From that moment on, the vital force becomes a tributary to the [miasm], bearing its seal whilst retaining its own individuality.[185]

He suggests there is a heredity factor of the miasm and concludes there is the development of a stable energetic framework or matrix in the holographic energy system upon which the miasm is found.

Tansley lists ten aspects of miasms:

1. They constitute the basis of every chronic condition, always being determined by the constitution and temperament of the individual.
2. They spread out among the generations of the species.
3. Being of an infectious, contagious nature, they are dynamic and can only be extinguished dynamically.
4. The most important miasm is psora, which lies beneath an illness and lends foundation to it.
5. In treatment, the last miasm to disappear is psora.
6. When the morbid framework is a complex of three miasms, its cure can become impossible when we find, in addition, some other "miasm" of medical origin (here "miasm" is used academically) such as vaccinosis, toxins, poisons, viruses, etc.
7. Syphilis and psychosis take root in psoric terrain.
8. Miasmatic contagion is of a dynamic nature, i.e., there would be acarus in a psoricskin, neisseria in a psychotic mucous, and treponema in a syphilitic mucous. There are sufficient foundations to presume that miasms are contagious.
9. The miasm has its seat in the dynamic, expressed in the body, and transcends the psychic sphere.
10. In practice, one should not forget that a miasm is a constitutional state resulting from anti-natural suppressions.

The psora miasm is found in both superficial and deep levels of the human being, and symptoms include everything from skin irritations and blisters to anxiety and epilepsy. It is the most widespread of the miasms affecting humanity, as well as the most contagious and the most versatile. In earlier times, the miasm was strengthened and worsened by the unenlightened use of thermal waters and the abuse of metals and metalloids and is likewise exacerbated today by antibiotics, X-rays, alkaloids, antihistamines, hormones, and other pharmaceuticals.

David Little, who has done an in-depth study of Hahnemann's Paris casebooks, suggests that the potentially harmful chemical toxins released into our environment by our "massive industrial complex" create the need for compulsory immunization, which in turn results in the vaccinosis miasm. Additionally, he says, the great number of new medicines produced by the pharmaceutical industry has led to a second category of chronic disease. "Illnesses that involve all three factors of causation (continual stress, drugs, toxins, vaccinosis, and natural miasms) are the most difficult to treat because all these factors intermingle to form complex layers."[186]

According to Hahnemann, the psora miasm manifests in the skin as itching, redness, and blisters. He prescribed homeopathic solutions of sulfur as a psoric remedy and recognized the pathologic process of the psora miasm as a deficiency. Gurudas suggests certain gem and mineral essences are effective in releasing and transforming miasms. Wright also outlines a method of using the Perelandra rose and garden essences to effect the release and transformation of miasms. The Bach Flower essences are valuable in releasing and transforming miasms as well. In EMCS, all energetic medicines are included as options for the body to choose in the process of releasing miasms. At the end of this chapter, you will find the EMCS corrective process to follow during the client's session.

Sycosis

The word "sycosis" comes from the Greek "sycon," meaning a wart or excrescence. Tansley states, "Psychosis is a clinical reality and expresses itself in hyper functions such as catarrhal and eliminative eruptions of the skin, the mucous membranes, the digestive system, the respiratory and urinary systems."[187]

Sycosis, according to Hahnemann, produces disorders of the mucous membranes, the linings of the passageways that lead into the body. Symptoms include sinusitis, bronchitis, mucous colitis, vaginitis, gonorrhea, and middle-ear congestion—but gonorrhea is the foundation of the miasm. In more recent times, HIV/AIDS and herpes have been placed in the sycosis category.

Tansley identifies a person operating out of the psychosis miasm as anxious, harried, fearful, nervous, and suffering from feelings of inadequacy and low self-esteem. They are often slow, careless, and introverted. In stressful situations, the psychotic hesitates, withdraws, and then thinks after the fact that they really could have handled the problem. Psychotics are rude, irascible, and ill-mannered, though they quickly apologize. The psychotic is sensual and often participates in sexual excesses and boasts about them. The psychotic tends to "overdo" everything: over worry, overeat, overwork, overthink, overspend, etc. Hahnemann treated the Sycosis miasm with Thuja and medorrhinum; the latter made from the urethral discharge of a patient with gonorrhea.

Syphilitic

Syphilitic

Syphilis is, of course, the major symptom of the syphilitic miasm. This miasm shows up in the erosion of the physical structure, but perhaps more so in the mind. Alcoholism, heart disease, strokes, ulcers, and insanity are also symptoms of the syphilitic miasm.

Behavioral symptoms include cruelty, hostility, sexual voyeurism, mental lapses, hateful attitudes, and jealousy. People suffering the syphilitic miasm are easily upset and antagonistic, and suicidal ideation is another common expression.

Hahnemann used mercury (mercurius), known to have an affinity with the nervous system but with a profound toxic effect, as the treatment for syphilitic miasm. Other heavy metals such as lead (plumbum) and gold (aurum) were used in the treatment of this deeply held miasm. Eventually, a potentized preparation called lueticum or syphilinum was developed from the chancre or initial ulcer of syphilis, and it is now the common treatment for this miasmatic state.

Besides these three miasms identified by Hahnemann, two more have been identified to make five known miasms in total. These are tuberculosis and cancer, with cancer being a combination of them all.

EMCS Miasm Correction Method

Identify by muscle checking to determine if the person you are working with holds a miasm in their holographic human energy system. If checking indicates the affirmative, muscle check determines which of the miasms are present in the system. If more than the psora miasm is present in the system, clear the psora miasm last. Should all five miasms be present, muscle check to clarify which of the miasms are presently operating. In other words, are they active or inactive? If dormant, clarify by muscle checking whether that miasm needs to be disturbed. After determining through muscle checking which miasm will be released and transformed, first, identify the basic information normally outlined in your defusion sheets. This gives information concerning the effect the particular miasm has on thoughts and behaviors. This is a present-time observation. Explore with the client any symptoms they may be aware of that are associated with the identified miasm.

Once this information has been explored, muscle test to the age when the miasm became a part of the person's holographic/halographic energy system. Age recession will likely take you to a generational age of cause or even a past life experience, so do not be surprised when muscle checking takes you beyond conception.

While on your way to the age of cause, also make sure to test for any ages on line where additional symptoms of the miasm may have occurred. The miasm may have mutated in some way since its inception. If ages on line show up, muscle check to see if you need to make any corrections at that age, or simply put the age on line into the circuitry and continue to age of cause. Once you reach the age of cause, muscle check for the number of symptoms associated with this particular miasm. Make a note of them by numbering the symptoms on your defusion sheet. Once you have gathered all the information at the age of cause, identify through muscle checking the corrective energy medicine for each symptom.

You may discover that there are multiple energy medicines you can use to release and transform each symptom. For instance, the possibility for more than one gem-mineral essence may be identified, or both a gem essence and a flower essence may be determined for clearing. If ten symptoms are identified, you will identify ten or more energy medicines for correction purposes. Once you have identified them all you can begin correcting one at a time until all symptoms have been corrected. The client will take the essence according to the number of drops and route of administration identified by muscle checking.

Finally, muscle check for permission to correct the miasm itself. Remember, you have just been releasing the symptoms associated with the miasm. Next, muscle check for verification that symptoms identified as ages on line have been released through corrections made at the age of cause. If they have not been cleared, then muscle checks to verify if you can combine them into one correction. Alternatively, muscle check to see if there is one specific age on line not cleared and correct that one. (Correction always means identifying the method of clearing and administering to the client the identified essence in the dosage amount and place of administration.)

Once you have identified the information, muscle check for the corrective energetic medicine and make the correction. Once that is accomplished and you are certain all the symptoms, at every age, have been cleared, continue with clearing the miasm. Make the corrections and verify by muscle checking that the miasm and its attendant symptoms have been absolutely canceled, resolved, and released. If yes, identify an infusion symbol and return to the present time.

When back to the present time, re-verify that all symptoms and the specific miasm are cleared from the holographic/halographic energy system. Muscle check to determine if there will be any withdrawal or residual from the releases and if there is any ongoing homework. If muscle checking identifies the affirmative for homework, then the next step is to muscle check for what, how much, and how long to do the homework.

If multiple miasms were identified at the outset, muscle check to determine if continuing with the next miasm is appropriate. Repeat the process outlined above. The last miasm released will be the psora because it is the foundation of them all.

Essence Oils as Energy Medicine

The definition of essential oils, according to *Essential Oils Desk Reference,* is ". . . subtle, volatile liquids distilled from shrubs, flowers, trees, roots, bushes, and seeds."[188] Chemically, essential oils are very complex; they are composed of hundreds of highly concentrated chemical compounds and are more potent than dried or fresh herbal decoctions, infusions, or macerations, which are phytomedicine or herbal medicine preparations. Essential oils have played a major role in healing throughout the ages. Essential oils are similar to gem, mineral, and flower essences in the way they affect the frequency at which the holographic/halographic human energy system vibrates. They cross the body/brain barrier, flowing through every cell of the body in a matter of minutes, thus affecting the vibration of the entire system.

There are several methods of administering essential oils but use caution because applying essential oils topically is much like administering pharmaceuticals. Energicians have the advantage over typical Western practitioners in that muscle testing can advise which oil to administer, where to administer it, and whether the client can tolerate the essential oil. Because many people are sensitive to essential oils, it is imperative that you take time to gather the medical history of the individual, including any medications the person might be using and their sensitivities. I strongly suggest you become well-informed about the pharmacology of each essential oil and plant from which it originates; do not apply essential oils topically or internally until you have knowledge of possible reactions and sensitivities to the oils!

There are many excellent essential oil reference books available for purchase, and they provide the energician with a greater awareness of the effects of essential oils on the human system.

Since an exhaustive study on the use of essential oils would take volumes, I will concentrate this discussion on the German inhalation model. This model is based on the principle that a fragrance exerts strong effects on the brain through the olfactory system. In doing so, it affects brain oxygenation and activity. Essential oils that are high in sesquiterpenes[189], such as myrrh and frankincense, are examples of oils that affect the limbic system, known to be the seat of emotions, and the hypothalamus, which regulates hormones. Located at the base of the forebrain, the hypothalamus contains nerve centers that regulate certain of the body's vital processes, including the metabolism of fat and carbohydrates, sleep, temperature, and sex drive. It also plays an important role in emotional response, sensations of pleasure and pain, and, through the pituitary-hypothalamus connection, in the maintenance of the homeostatic levels of growth hormones.

Hypothalamus receptors monitor blood levels of thyroid hormones, thus, they have the ability to, as stated in the *Essential Oils Desk Reference*, detect low blood levels of the thyroid stimulating hormone and trigger the negative feedback process involving the anterior pituitary.[190] As such, "In some cases, inhalation of essential oils might be preferred over topical application if the goal is to increase growth hormone secretion, induce weight loss, or balance mood and emotions."[191] The reference continues by suggesting sandalwood, lavender, and fir oil as excellent examples of essential oils used for the above purposes. Alternative medicine supports this view:

> Aromatic molecules, that interact with the top of the nasal cavity, give off signals that are modified by various biological processes before traveling to the limbic system, the emotional switchboard of the brain. There, they create impressions associated with previous experiences and emotions. Because the limbic system is directly connected to the parts of the brain that control heart rate, blood pressure, breathing, memory, and balance, scientists have learned that oil fragrances may be one of the pathways to achieve physiological or psychological effects.[192]

It bears repeating that the fragrance of an essential oil can be emotionally and physically very stimulating. The same oil may affect two people in very different ways and to different degrees. It may be calming to one and stimulating to another, so exercise caution and common sense when using essential oils.

Although the focus of this work is on inhalation as the method for administering essential oils (and, in fact, the inhalation of essential oils is an option for EMCS corrections when clearing in Matrices IV, VI, VII, XI), the two most effective applications of essential oils are cold-air diffusing and undiluted topical application, referred to as "neat." The topical application of essential oils, when used with the Vita Flex or meridian points massage technique, is very effective in combination with acupressure or reflexology. There are charts available online to help you identify these points. The beauty of EMCS is that any energy medicine product can be added to the matrix system as a system harmonizing option. The method of use, as well as the product option, is chosen through muscle checking. I have tried many essential oil companies in my quest to obtain the best oils for use in my practice, and I strongly recommend only purchasing from companies that manufacture therapeutic-grade essential oils. An oil advertised as "pure essential" does not necessarily mean it is a therapeutic-grade oil.

On her website, chiropractor Carolyn Mein provides a list of essential oils and the ways in which each corresponds to emotions and body alarm points. These points are traditional Chinese medicine meridian acupuncture points, reflexology vita-flex points, neuro-emotional, and lymphatic points, all of which are discussed in earlier chapters of this text.

EMCS Core Negative Beliefs

In EMCS, the term "core negative beliefs" refers to beliefs that are either inherited through generational patterns that have become "facts" and are therefore seemingly unchangeable, or they have been carried over from unresolved past life experiences. Core Negative Beliefs are unconscious or unknown to us except through the realization that we keep repeating the same destructive patterns again and again.

The following is a list of core negative beliefs identified through working with many clients over the years. You may find you have similar ones.

1. I have to be strong.
2. I do not deserve love.
3. I am not creative.
4. I am wrong for being a boy.
5. I am wrong for being a girl.
6. I am wrong for not being a boy.
7. I am wrong for not being a girl.
8. There is something wrong with me.
9. I am not appreciated.
10. I have nothing of value to offer.
11. I am not good enough.
12. I don't know what to think.
13. I can't do anything right.
14. I have to be perfect.
15. I never have enough time.
16. I do not deserve success.
17. I do not deserve happiness.
18. I do not matter.
19. I do not deserve to live.
20. I have to prove myself.
21. I am not wanted.
22. I do not know what to do.
23. I am not ready.
24. Nobody cares about me.
25. God is punishing me.
26. God does not love me; I am not worthy.
27. Nobody listens to me.
28. I was not wanted.
29. I am not wanted.
30. I owe my parents.
31. I should be able to do it all myself.
32. Men get all the breaks in life.
33. Women get all the breaks in life.
34. It is difficult to be successful, no matter how intelligent I am.
35. I never have any luck.
36. It is safer not to confront anyone because then you can't get hurt.
37. Everyone is out to get me.
38. I always get taken advantage of.
39. I can never get ahead.
40. You have to work very hard to get ahead.
41. Life is not fair.
42. I need someone special to make me happy.
43. I am the only one who can get the job done.
44. I will never change.
45. I am better than everybody else.
46. Nothing is worth doing.

47. Nobody loves me.
48. Nobody takes care of me.
49. All men are insensitive.
50. All women are insensitive.
51. I am not worthy of love.
52. I am not worthy of health.
53. I am not worthy of friends.
54. I never have enough money.
55. I am not worthy of having money.
56. Even if I get or make money, I will just abuse it or lose it.
57. Life is hostile.
58. People are out to get me.
59. I need the pain to survive.
60. Somebody is trying to kill me.
61. Women hurt me.
62. Men hurt me.
63. People hurt me.
64. I hate God for putting me here.
65. I have to fight to get what I need or want.
66. I do not want to be here if this is it.
67. It is not safe for me to express my emotions.
68. People do not like to see my emotions.
69. I am afraid of my emotions.
70. It is not safe for me to express my distrust.
71. I cannot trust men.
72. I cannot trust women.
73. There is never enough love to go around.
74. I will get even forever for this pain.
75. I was conceived in original sin.
76. I should never have been born.
77. I am not the man I want to be.
78. I am not the woman I want to be.
79. I will suffer even more than I do.
80. I am bad/no good.
81. I am helpless, powerless.
82. I am insane.
83. I am dirty.
84. I am ugly.
85. I am scary.

86. I can get you to listen or pay attention to me only if I scream, rant, rage, or have a tantrum.
87. When I abuse or use violence, I am strong.
88. Who I am and what I want does not matter.
89. I do not count.
90. I am not appreciated.
91. I am not ready yet.
92. I can never get ahead.
93. I am not worthy of health.
94. There is no help for people like me, people with my problems.
95. No one can save me.
96. This will never stop.
97. It makes no sense.
98. I must be making all this up.
99. I have to be strong.
100. I have to be perfect.
101. I have to prove myself.
102. I have nothing of value to offer.
103. I cannot get what I want.
104. I cannot do anything right.
105. I can trust no one but myself.
106. People "use" me.
107. Life is hell.
108. People do not like me.
109. I always get taken advantage of.
110. It is safer not to confront anyone because then you cannot get hurt.
111. It is not safe for me to express my distrust.
112. I do not know what to think.
113. I don't know what I trust.
114. I don't know who I trust.
115. It is difficult to be successful, no matter how intelligent I am.
116. I should have known.
117. I can't let people down; they depend on me.
118. I'm better than everybody else.
119. I'll get even forever for this pain.

120. I cause people pain.
121. I must be in control.
122. I must be right, or else.

123. I must "get even" to have value and worth so that you will respect me.
124. Being needy is repulsive.

THE HUMAN SKELETAL SYSTEM

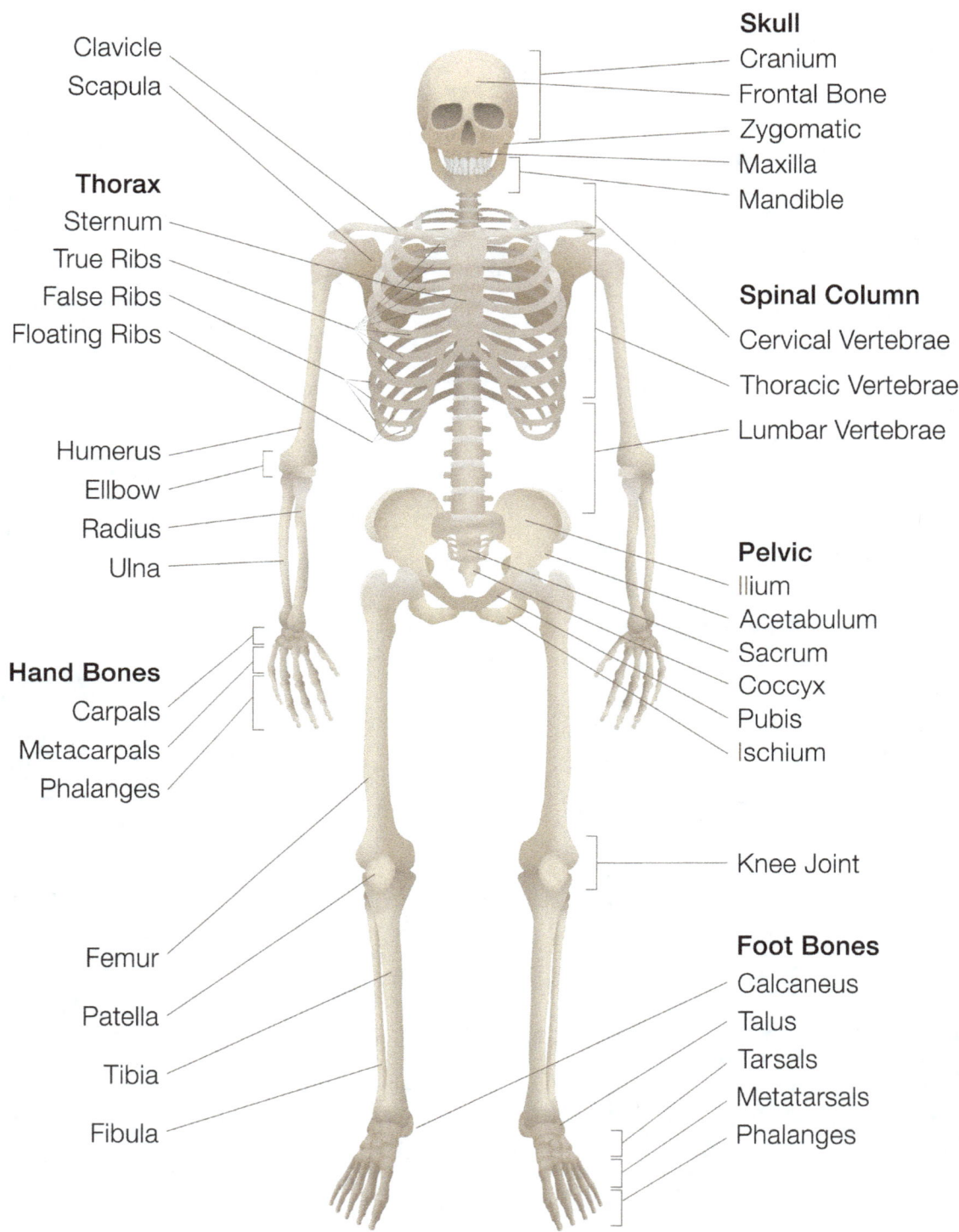

Clavicle
Scapula

Thorax
Sternum
True Ribs
False Ribs
Floating Ribs

Humerus
Ellbow
Radius
Ulna

Hand Bones
Carpals
Metacarpals
Phalanges

Femur
Patella
Tibia
Fibula

Skull
Cranium
Frontal Bone
Zygomatic
Maxilla
Mandible

Spinal Column
Cervical Vertebrae
Thoracic Vertebrae
Lumbar Vertebrae

Pelvic
Ilium
Acetabulum
Sacrum
Coccyx
Pubis
Ischium

Knee Joint

Foot Bones
Calcaneus
Talus
Tarsals
Metatarsals
Phalanges

CHAPTER TWELVE

MATRIX VI

SKELETON, MUSCLES, AND MUSCLE CIRCUITS

The skeletal system represents the structural foundation of our physical body; therefore, when working with an issue and the skeletal-muscular system makes the indicator change, holding the blockage for that issue, you have accessed the "core" or causal blockage. The concept of muscle *circuits,* as developed by Gordon Stokes and Daniel Whiteside in their Three in One Concepts, gives new insight into how the body works as a whole.[193]

When discussing the emotional meaning of a particular bone or muscle group, remember the role it plays in the operation of the whole system. As an example, Karol Kuhn Truman, in her book *Feelings Buried Alive Never Die*, associates the pelvis with being "unable to remain grounded or focused in emotional activity" and "holding on to sexual feelings."[194] Another volume defining the emotional components of the physical structure is Michael Lincoln's *Messages From the Body: Their Psychological Meaning*.[195] As a whole, the skeletal system speaks to issues of separation, abandonment, rigid mindsets or beliefs, resisting authority, self-blame, and perfection.

Matrix VI includes the skeletal system and muscles of the human body. When this category is identified by way of muscle checking during an EMCS session, identify the specific muscle or muscle group holding the blockage by muscle checking for the appropriate page number (list of skeletal components and muscles) and then check for the exact bone or muscle "by the number" as they are listed on the page. To correct energy blockages associated with the skeletal-muscular system, use all EMCS matrix systems to identify the correction. The correction may come from any of them or all of them.

Muscle Circuits

Muscles work together to perform such physical activities as walking, running, sitting, standing up, bending, and stretching. Sometimes, these "circuits" are involved in movement at the moment of a shock or trauma, everything from twisting your ankle while running to the jolts suffered during a car accident to the protective reflexes that come into play during a life-threatening situation. These circuits record and hold the "memory" of that incident or emotionally overcharged event. The body remembers. So, when muscle circuits make the indicator change in a defusion process, explore the "story" of what happened with your client. Moreover, as outlined in Three in One Concepts, "Clearing muscle circuits release blockages that relate to heavy issues of Left Brain over-control, Right Brain issues of 'creativity denied,' or issues that speak to the 'wounded spirit.' All these relate to the avoidance of responsibility for clearing such issues, an avoidance that results in "physical symptoms that have no clear clinical cause."[196]

The following is a list of muscles and their supportive circuit:

CIRCUIT 1: pectoralis major clavicular – quadriceps (left), gluteus maximus (right), gluteus medius (right), psoas (left), neck flexor (left), lower abdominals (right), pectineus (right)

CIRCUIT 2: pectoralis major clavicular – quadriceps (right), gluteus maximus (left; prone), gluteus medius (left), psoas (right), neck flexor (right), lower abdominals (left), pectineus (left)

CIRCUIT 3: neck flexor (right) – psoas (left), gluteus minimus (right), anterior deltoid (right), latissimus dorsi (right)

CIRCUIT 4: neck flexor (left) – psoas (right), gluteus minimus (left), anterior deltoid (left), latissimus dorsi (left)

CIRCUIT 5: anterior deltoid (right) – pectineus (left), piriformis (right), quadriceps (right)

CIRCUIT 6: anterior deltoid (left) – pectineus (right), piriformis (left), quadriceps (left)

CIRCUIT 7: pectoralis major sternal (right) – anterior deltoid (left), teres major (right; prone), teres minor (right; prone), teres minor (right, supine), psoas (left), gluteus minimus (right)

CIRCUIT 8: pectoralis major sternal (left) – anterior deltoid (right), teres major (left; prone), teres minor (left; supine), psoas (right), lateral hamstrings (both sides; prone)

CIRCUIT 9: middle deltoid (right) – rhomboids (left), facia lata (left), gracilis (right; prone), iliacus (left; prone)

CIRCUIT 10: middle deltoid (left) – rhomboids (right), facia lata (right), gracilis (left; prone), iliacus (right; prone)

CIRCUIT 11: rectus abdominals (right; sitting) – upper sacrospinalis (left; prone), gluteus maximus (left; prone), quadratus lumborum (right; prone/supine)

CIRCUIT 12: rectus abdominals (left; sitting) – upper sacrospinalis (right; prone), gluteus maximus (right; prone), quadratus lumborum (left; prone/supine)

CIRCUIT 13: lower abdominals (right; supine) – gluteus maximus (left; prone), lower sacrospinalis (right; prone), anterior serratus (left; supine)

CIRCUIT 14: piriformis (right) – iliacus (left; prone), gluteus maximus (left, prone), pectineus (right; supine)

CIRCUIT 15: piriformis (left) – iliacus (right; prone), gluteus maximus (right; prone), pectineus (right)

CIRCUIT 16: Iliacus (right; prone) – piriformis (left), adductor (left), anterior serratus (left)

CIRCUIT 17: Iliacus (left; prone) – piriformis (right), adductor (right), anterior serratus (right)

CIRCUIT 18: Psoas (right) – gluteus minimus (left), neck flexor (left), neck extensor (right; prone), coracobrachialis (right)

CIRCUIT 19: Psoas (left) – gluteus minimus (right), neck flexor (right), neck extensor (left; prone), coracobrachialis (left)

CIRCUIT 20: peroneus (right) – posterior tibial (left), gluteus maximus (left; prone), lower abdominals (right), psoas (right)

CIRCUIT 21: peroneus (left) – posterior tibial (right), gluteus maximus (right; prone), lower abdominals (left), psoas (left)

CIRCUIT 22: upper sacrospinalis (right; prone) – posterior tibial (right), gluteus maximus (right; prone), lower abdominals (left), psoas (left), medial hamstrings (right; prone)

CIRCUIT 23: gluteus maximus (right; prone) – lower abdominals (left), gracilis (left; prone), pectineus (left). peroneus (right), posterior tibial (left)

CIRCUIT 24: gluteus maximus (left; prone) – lower abdominals (right), gracilis (right; prone), pectineus (right), pectineus (right), peroneus (left), posterior tibial (right)

CIRCUIT 25: medial hamstring (right; prone) – lower sacrospinalis (right; prone), middle deltoid (right), pectineus (right)

CIRCUIT 26: medial hamstring (left; prone) – lower sacrospinalis (left; prone), middle deltoid (left), pectineus (left)

CIRCUIT 27: latissimus dorsi (right) – middle deltoid (left), gluteus maximus (left; prone), gluteus minimus (left), adductor (right), pectoralis major sternal (right), pectoralis major clavicular (left)

CIRCUIT 28: latissimus dorsi (left) – middle deltoid (right), gluteus maximus (right; prone), gluteus minimus (right), adductor

(left), pectoralis major sternal (left), pectoralis major clavicular (right)

CIRCUIT 30: gracilis (right; prone) – anterior tibial (right), gluteus maximus (left; prone), iliacus (right; prone)

CIRCUIT 31: gracilis (left; prone) – anterior tibial (left), gluteus maximus (right; prone), iliacus (left; prone)

CIRCUIT 32: sartorius (right) – piriformis (left), gracilis (left; prone), neck flexor (left), psoas (left), lower abdominals (right)

CIRCUIT 33: sartorius (left) – piriformis (right), gracilis (right, prone), neck flexor (right), psoas (right), lower abdominals (left)

CIRCUIT 34: quadriceps (right) – adductor (left), piriformis (left), medial hamstrings (left; prone), lateral hamstrings (left; prone)

CIRCUIT 35: quadriceps (left) – adductor (right), piriformis (right), medial hamstrings (right; prone), lateral hamstrings (right; prone)

Muscles and their emotional correspondences

1. Abdominis (rectus): willing/indifferent (small intestine meridian)
2. Abdominis (oblique): peace/separation/guilt (small intestine meridian)
3. Abdominis (transverse): love/grief (small intestine meridian)
4. Abdominals (lower): reason/fear (small intestine meridian)
5. Adductors: courage/indifference (pericardium meridian)
6. Brachioradialis: love/grief (stomach meridian)
7. Coracobrachialis: courage/indifference (lung meridian)
8. Deltoid (anterior): acceptance/desire/hostility (gall bladder meridian)
9. Deltoid (middle): joy/shame (lung meridian)
10. Fascia lata: neutral/anger/resentment (large intestine)
11. Gastrocnemius: willing/pride/indifference (triple warmer meridian)
12. Gluteus maximus: reason/fear (pericardium meridian)
13. Gluteus minimus: joy/shame (pericardium meridian)
14. Gluteus medius: peace/separation/guilt (pericardium meridian)

15. Gracilis: courage/antagonism (triple warmer meridian)

16. Hamstrings (lateral): courage/antagonism (large intestine meridian)

17. Iliacus: acceptance/desire/hostility (kidney meridian)

18. Infraspinatus: joy/shame (triple warmer meridian)

19. Latissimus dorsi: neutral/anger/resentment (spleen meridian)

20. Levator scapulae: courage/antagonism (stomach meridian)

21. Neck flexors: Acceptance/Desire/Hostility (Stomach Meridian)

22. Neck extensors (posterior): acceptance/desire/hostility (stomach meridian)

23. Opponens pollicis: love/grief (spleen meridian)

24. Pectineus: enlightenment/apathy (pericardium meridian)

25. Pectoralis Major clavicular: peace/separation/guilt (stomach meridian)

26. Pectoralis Major sternal: enlightenment/apathy (liver meridian)

27. Peroneus: willing/pride/indifference (bladder)

28. Piriformis: acceptance/desire/hostility (pericardium meridian)

29. Popliteus: courage/antagonism (gall bladder meridian)

30. Psoas: willing/pride/indifference (kidney meridian)

31. Quadratus lumborum: acceptance/desire/hostility (large intestine meridian)

32. Quadriceps: neutral/anger/resentment (small intestine meridian)

33. Rhomboids: reason/fear (liver meridian)

34. Upper sacrospinalis: acceptance/desire/hostility (bladder meridian)

35. Lower sacrospinalis: acceptance/desire/hostility (bladder meridian)

36. Sartorius: enlightenment/apathy (triple warmer meridian)

37. Serratus (anterior): neutral/anger/resentment (lung meridian)

38. Soleus: acceptance/desire/hostility (triple warmer meridian)

39. Subclavius: "There is no choice in this situation; I am totally blocked." (heart meridian)

40. Subscapularis: peace/separation/guilt (heart meridian)

41. Supraspinatus: enlightenment/apathy (central meridian)

42. Teres major: reason/fear (governing meridian)

43. Teres minor: enlightenment/apathy (triple warmer meridian)

44. Tibial (anterior): courage/antagonism (bladder meridian)

45. Tibial (posterior): courage/antagonism (bladder meridian)

46. Trapezius (middle): neutral/anger/resentment (spleen meridian)

47. Trapezius (upper): love/grief (kidney meridian)

48. Trapezius (lower): enlightenment/apathy (spleen meridian)

49. Triceps: enlightenment/apathy (spleen meridian)

Note: When testing muscles, make sure the central and governing meridians are clear before beginning testing for muscles or muscle circuits.

Correction for Central and Governing Meridians:

Place one palm on the navel, use thumb and forefinger to massage the K27 (just below the collar bone on either side of the throat notch), and move fingers up to the mouth, placing the thumb under the lower lip and the forefinger just above the upper lip, and massage. Next, move your hand to the lower back just above the buttock area and massage with four fingers. Then, switch hands and repeat the process.

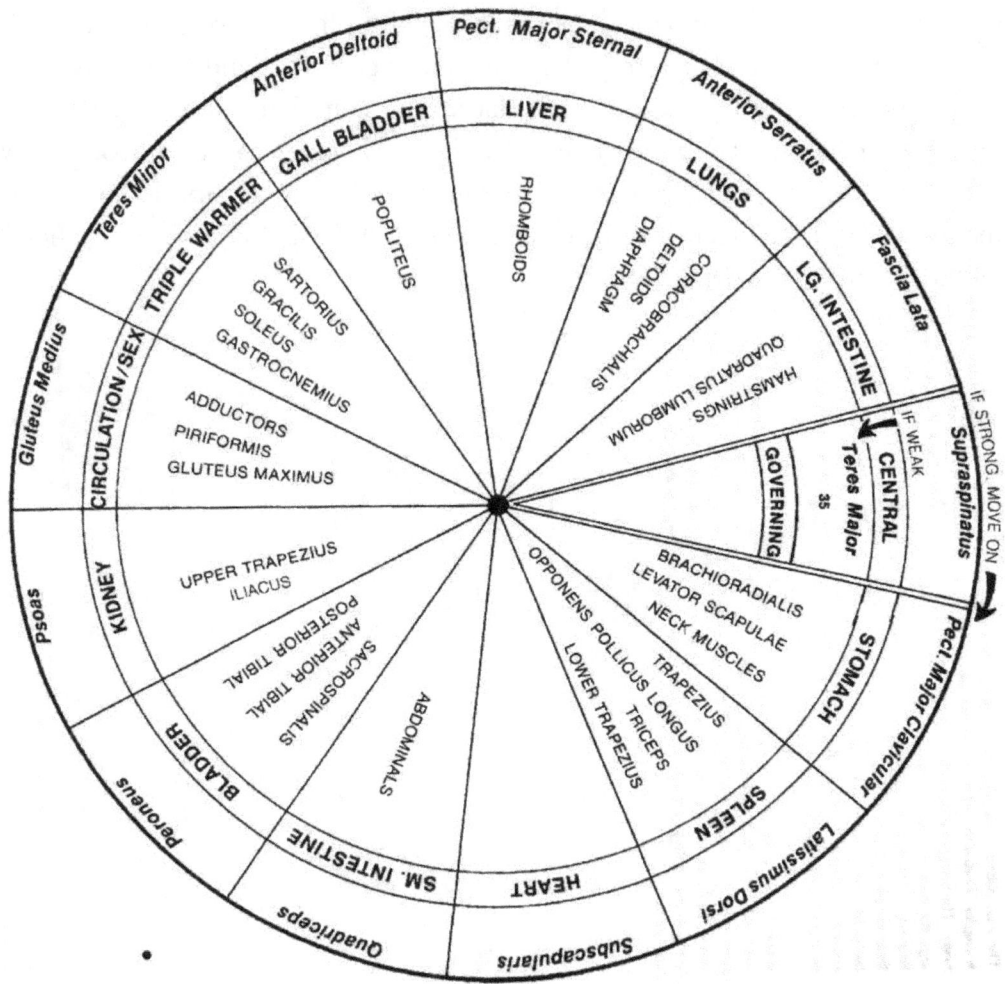

The model above illustrates the flow of meridian energy. The Energy Matrix Clearing System uses this wheel as a tool to muscle test the flow of chi through the entire meridian system. By muscle-checking each meridian in a counterclockwise movement around the wheel for balanced energyfor balanced energy, over-energy, or under-energy, you can easily determine the health of not only the meridian but also see the connection with muscles, muscle circuits, and organs. This model was taken from Robert and Kerri Broe's publication *Advanced Medical Awareness*. They explain the chart in this way:

The lines within the wheel denote subsidiary energy flows among meridians [and] may help you notice the patterns underlying a particular set of muscle weaknesses. If we tested the [fourteen] indicator muscles and found facia lata, pectoralis major clavicular, and latissimus dorsi weak, which muscle shall we strengthen first? Since the meridians are part of one continuous flow, we can look upstream and see where the block is, causing the energy not to flow properly. If we release the block, the energy can resume its unrestricted flow and energize the meridians downstream. If you look at the muscles listed on the meridian wheel, you will see that the three meridians involved lie next to each other. When the flow is resumed, you will find when retesting the pectoralis major clavicular and latissimus dorsi you will find them strong and energized just by working on the facia lata. If another muscle is still weak, you deal with each of them in turn, moving around the wheel of meridians. You test muscles associated with the central and governing meridian first and strengthen these muscles if they are found weak. The central and governing meridians are called exit or storage meridians, and it is helpful to ensure they are unblocked at the start of the balancing process.[197]

CHAPTER THIRTEEN

MATRIX VII: CRANIAL NERVES

For the purposes of this discussion of cranial nerves, EMCS uses both the physical function of each nerve as well as their ". . . reflections of the signs of the Zodiac and the twelve houses or departments of life."[198]

The Twelve Cranial Nerves

1. Olfactory – sensory fibers to the nose
2. Optic – sensory fibers from the eyes
3. Oculomotor – motor fibers controlling the eye muscles
4. Trochlear – motor fibers controlling the eye muscles
5. Trigeminal – sensory fibers from the skin of the head to the teeth
6. Abducens – motor fibers controlling eye muscles
7. Facial – sensory fibers from the taste buds and motor fibers controlling the muscles of facial expression
8. Auditory vestibular nerve – sensory fibers from the ears
9. Glossopharyngeal – sensory fibers from the taste buds and motor fibers of the throat and salivary glands
10. Vagus – sensory fibers from the internal organs. (e.g., gut)
11. Spinal accessory – sensory fibers from tissues of neck and shoulders and motor fibers to neck and shoulder muscles
12. Hypoglossal – motor fibers to muscles of the tongue

Metaphysically, the twelve cranial nerves are associated with the twelve signs of the zodiac and the twelve houses of the astrology chart. Each house represents one aspect of a person's life. The following is a synopsis of the influence of each house:

Twelve Signs of the Zodiac and the Twelve Houses of the Astrology Chart

FIRST HOUSE: AIRES (persona, the face shown to the outside world). Aires is a pioneer archetype and it rules personality, personal affairs, physical appearance, physical make-up, and how the outside world sees you. It is the house of the "I" and includes general health conditions and susceptibility to disease.

SECOND HOUSE: TAURUS (personal ownership). Taurus is often associated with the qualities of fixity, fertility, fruitfulness, security, and sustainability. This house includes your value system, self-esteem, and money and personal possessions gained through your vocation, investments, inheritance, and other means.

THIRD HOUSE: GEMINI (communication of personal will, beliefs, and thoughts expressed to others). It indicates how you relate to your siblings and neighbors and includes messages or news you may receive. It is the first of the human signs, i.e., the Gemini twins of Castor and Pollux and Helen and Clytemnestra. Today, we think of Gemini as a sign of intellect and duality. Its ruling planet, Mercury, has much to do with the symbolism of the intellect associated with it. It also represents the conflict of the ego and the shadow of the personality.

FOURTH HOUSE: CANCER (home, home base, your inner self). This house includes basic security, how you see yourself subjectively, your relationship to the parent you are closest to, family origins (ancestry), end-of-life conditions, unconscious or conditioned responses toward personal interactions with the world, and issues of transportation. It may also represent the more authentic self than the first house, which is the house of the persona or the face one presents to the world.

FIFTH HOUSE: LEO (eros and creativity, including sexuality and your vocation). This is the house of romantic love and self-expression, and it includes all kinds of creative energies, including bearing children. It is also the house of recreation, hobbies, and speculation (gambling, stock market ventures, etc.).

SIXTH HOUSE: VIRGO (work and health, or how you will serve the world). It includes the relationships of servants and employees or you as a servant or an employee. It is the house of health and illness, duties and obligations, the mundane. It is the least free area of the chart.

SEVENTH HOUSE: LIBRA (partnerships of all kinds). The house of marriage, business, enemies, competitors, the public, and those who challenge or assist, and it includes the extent of dependency you have on others. It is the house indicating your audience in life—those who dominate or guide.

EIGHTH HOUSE: SCORPIO (legal and financial). The house of your relationship to other people's money and possessions, and it includes money acquired from partnerships, inheritances, and insurance benefits. It shows important life changes and your response to those changes. It is the house of sexual expression and regeneration. Some call this the house of death.

NINTH HOUSE: SAGITTARIUS (spirituality and wisdom). This house rules your philosophical and religious outlook on life, including the education you pursue to prepare yourself for a vocation or to broaden your perspective. The challenge to reach your higher potential is associated with this house. Dreams, long-distance travel, legal issues, your worldview, and relatives through marriage are a part of this house.

TENTH HOUSE: CAPRICORN (highest potential). This house rules your career and the honors received from that career. It is associated with conscious ambition, material and physical judgments, and recognition. It is the house of "fate" and relates to the more distantly linked parent. It reflects your true profession, behavior on the job, and your public life.

ELEVENTH HOUSE: AQUARIUS (relation to the world). This house includes the ideals toward which you strive, the income from your career, your attitude toward social interactions, and the number and kinds of friends you have.

TWELFTH HOUSE: PISCES (the "collective soul"). The twelfth house is known as "the house of self-undoing" because it holds the secrets you keep hidden from yourself, including secret attitudes held in the subconscious mind that are harmful to you. It is the house where you can abstract the meaning from the past and build a foundation for the future. It is the seat of self-judgment and where you discover your capacity for inner awareness, spirituality, and growth. This is the house of secret enemies to which you are the most subservient. It is your access to the collective unconscious and karma.

EMCS Correction Essences for Cranial Nerves

When a cranial nerve makes the indicator change, it signals a blockage to be cleared.

The following includes the combination of essences used to clear nerve blockages, along with their therapeutic properties. Muscle check for the number of drops and placement of the drops: on the tongue, under the tongue, or in water.

OLFACTORY NERVE – aventurine, purple fluorite, silver: This combination of gem and mineral essences balances male and female energies, enhances creativity, supplements motivation, and augments the pioneering spirit. These essences bring rationality to intuitive qualities and assist one in the precise communication of that which is psychically presented. In combination, these energies are the mirror of the soul, the heart, and the mind. They provide "sight" that is without judgment and serve as "steppingstones" to the "superior human" within.

OPTIC NERVE – amethyst, jade, emerald: This combination balances the energies of the intellectual, emotional, and physical bodies and provides a clear connection between the earthly plane and other worlds. The essences facilitate peace within the physical, emotional, and intellectual structures. They transmute negativity and instill resourcefulness. They activate and stimulate (invigorate) the heart chakra and bring harmony to all areas of a person's life.

OCULOMOTOR NERVE – turquoise, malachite, jamesonite, lapis: This combination serves to strengthen and align all chakras, meridians, and subtle bodies. They raise all energies to a higher level. The energy of these essences is excellent for attuning with the spiritual and healing and cleansing both the energy centers and the physical body. They clarify emotions and allow for the recognition and release of negative experiences that one cannot recall. They facilitate insight into the basic disorder within the body, mind, and spirit. The energy of these essences enables a person to obtain relief from that which is repressed, and it provides objectivity, clarity, and mental endurance during the release of emotional bondage.

TROCHLEAR NERVE – 10 series (all tourmalines): The energy of tourmaline affects the chakra system, acting to clear, maintain, and stimulate each individual chakra center. Use it to attract inspiration, diminish fear by promoting understanding, and encourage self-confidence. Tourmaline balances the male and female energies of both body and mind. In addition, tourmaline aligns the energy centers of the entire auric body and induces alignment of the mental processes and chakras with the ethereal structure. The energies of tourmalines assist in the release of "being a victim" and help one to maintain fortitude and a sense of humor while retaining consciousness.

TRIGEMINAL NERVE – Madagascar rose quartz: This essence emits a calming, cooling energy that stimulates all chakras while gently releasing negativity and reinstating the gentle forces of self-love. It provides the energetic message that there is no need for haste in any situation, brings calm and clarity to emotions, and restores the mind to harmony following a crisis or chaotic situation. It attunes a person to the energy of love. In addition, it balances the yin-yang energy and attunes each chakra to its optimum energy vibration frequency.

ABDUCENS NERVE – beryl, lapis, blue sapphire, gold, limestone: This essence combination delivers the message that there is no obstacle in any circumstance that confidence and conviction cannot resolve; there is only the need to assure that one remains open to and has not withdrawn from the solution. This combination assists in the healing of all parts of the body, stimulates the throat chakra, and provides strength in endeavors of diversification. It balances the energy fields and assists one in the elimination of ego conflicts and the feeling of futility. These essences combat feelings of depression and inferiority.

FACIAL NERVE – gold, silver, copper, amethyst: This combination of essences symbolizes the purity of the spiritual aspect of "All That Is." It is symbolic of spirituality and development in the realm of complete understanding, allowing one to both attain and maintain communion with the Source of All Being. It emits energies that allow beauty to come forth from the inner being as one travels in and through the world of experience. These essences open the base and sacral chakras, advance and stabilize the energies of intuition, sexuality, desire, and vitality, and direct these energies toward the pursuit of one path of evolution.

AUDITORY VESTIBULAR NERVE – diamond, beryl, peridot: This combination of essences supports one's inner composure, creates an atmosphere of love and harmony, and dispels anger. It reminds the user of their goal of achieving spiritual consciousness and imparts trust, confidence, and fidelity to interpersonal associations. This combination cleanses and stimulates the heart and solar plexus chakras, bringing openness and acceptance to the intellectual pursuit of matters of love and relationships. It provides a shield of protection around the physical body.

GLOSSOPHARYNGEAL NERVE – turquoise, malachite, jamesonite: This combination of essences ameliorates volatile energies and helps one achieve emotional clarity. It stimulates thought by augmenting the frequency of brain wave transmissions. It also stimulates grounding energies, which assist in achieving the clarity of thought needed to encourage the practical side of one's nature. This combination stimulates a deep state of meditation and attunes one spiritually for healing and cleansing of both the energy centers and the physical body. It provides protection, heals the spirit, brings peace of mind, and bestows goodness.

VAGUS NERVE –jelly opal, yellow opal, gold: These essences, in combination, produce the ideal state of cooperation within the mind and promote the reprogramming of the mind with positive thoughts, giving access to full response and action potential. They define and refine self-limiting attitudes and beliefs.

SPINAL ACCESSORY NERVE – jelly opal, opal, pearl, quartz, silver: This combination of essences promotes accuracy, effectivity, and practicality, and stimulates clairsentience and clairvoyance. They balance male and female energies and align and balance the chakras. These essences attune one to the ethereal realm and stimulate the proper flow of energy to the physical body while facilitating alignment with the higher self. They provide an energetic foundation that stimulates sincerity, truth, and loyalty.

HYPOGLOSSAL NERVE – ruby, turquoise: This combination brings lucidity to the dream state. It lights the way in the darkness of one's life, giving birth to a spark of light that progresses throughout the body and spirit, conquering darkness on all levels. In combination, they generate energies that can change one's world, promoting creativity and expansiveness in awareness and manifestation, grounding and protecting the user while exploring spiritual realms.

CHAPTER FOURTEEN

MATRIX VIII

EMOTIONAL ENERGY

Archetypal" belongs to all culture, all forms of human activity . . .

—JAMES HILLMAN

I briefly introduced archetypes in a previous chapter in association with the subtle energy bodies and their characteristics. In this chapter, we will look more deeply into archetypes and their interplay with human life expression, *Archetypes,* but first, a brief history of the association of archetypes with human culture.

Carl Jung is recognized as the father of archetypal theories, and he first published on the subject in 1902 in his doctoral dissertation, "On the Psychology and Pathology of So-called Occult Phenomena." which has been included in several collections of his work.[199] From this original idea, Jung developed the theory known as "collective unconscious" and what has since become known as "archetypal psychology." Jung states in *The Archetypes and the Collective Unconscious*:

> A more or less superficial layer of the unconscious is undoubtedly personal. I call it the personal unconscious. However, this personal unconscious rests upon a deeper layer, which does not derive from personal experience and is not a personal acquisition but is inborn. This deeper layer I call the collective unconscious. I have chosen the term "collective" because this part of the unconscious is not individual but universal; in contrast to the personal psyche, it has contents and modes of behavior that are approximately the same everywhere and in all individuals. It is, in other words, identical in all men and thus constitutes a common psychic substrate of a suprapersonal nature which is present in every one of us.[200]

According to Jung, psychic existence is only recognizable or capable of consciousness where there is a presence of content. He determines that the personal unconscious expresses emotional content or "feeling-toned complexes," and that archetypes are collective unconscious contents.

The word archetype, writes Jung, has an extensive history. Research verifies it was used by Philo Judaeus of Alexandria (20 BCE to 50 CE) regarding the *Imago Dei* or "god image in man." The Corpus Hermeticum uses the term *archetypal light* to refer to a universal god-like being. Irenaeus used the term in his work *Dionysius the Aeopagite,* and Jung felt that, even though St. Augustine did not use the term specifically, the archetypal idea is evident in his writings. The significance of finding archetypal ideas in early writings is that, according to Jung, it proves the presence of "primordial" archetypal energies or universal images has been in existence since the earliest of times.[201]

According to Jung, primitive tribal lore indicates archetypes modified to fit and explain the tribes' experiences. This brings the archetype out of the unconscious into the conscious realm of human experience to explain the experience itself. Using archetypal methods at the conscious level to communicate explanations of similar occurrences over time has become a tradition, and it is ultimately the foundation of esoteric teaching. Myths and fairytales, according to Jung, are other expressions of conscious archetypes that have received a "specific stamp" that is passed from one generation to another.

" In this sense," Jung says, "there is a considerable difference between the archetype and the historical formula that has evolved. Especially, on the higher levels of esoteric teaching, the archetypes appear in a form that reveals quite unmistakably the critical and evaluating influence of conscious elaboration. Their immediate manifestation, as we come across it in dreams and visions, is much more individual, less understandable, and more naïve than in myths, for example."[202]

Archetypes have a polarity, or a positive and negative side, like most energy in this three-dimensional world. Jung explains that it is not enough to understand the concept or identify a list of archetypes to reflect upon; rather, they are ". . . complexes of experience that come upon us like fate, and their effects are felt in our most personal life."[203] He explains that when all our survival techniques have failed, and any attempt to shore up the damage also fails, only then is it possible to experience an archetype. Jung calls this experience the "archetype of meaning." He suggests this archetype has been a guiding influence for a long time, waiting for the opportune moment to express itself. He makes the point that there is not a single important thought, idea, or worldview that does not have its origin in history. From Jung's perspective, all have their foundation in primordial archetypal form arising out of a time preceding consciousness's ability to think—a time when "thoughts" were only objects of inner perception and sensed as external phenomena.

Among the many categories of archetypes identified by Jung is the category he termed "archetypes of transformation." Unlike the category of personalities—Mother, Father, Child, etc.—archetypes of transformation include situations, places, ways, and means that symbolize a specific type of transformation at hand. Like the personalities, he says, ". . . archetypes of transformation are true and genuine symbols that cannot be exhaustively interpreted, either as signs or as allegories."[204] Archetypes are both allegorical and paradoxical.

To illustrate, Jung gives the example of "the old man and a youth at once." He also suggests that the Tantric chakra system, the mystical nerve system of Chinese yoga, Tarot cards, and the I-Ching are examples of the paradoxical transformational archetypes. All these systems are chock full of archetypal symbolism—Tarot cards in particular.

Others working in the field concur. Caroline Myss, for instance, echoes Jung when she states that the language of the "gods" is a paradox, and in her book *Sacred Archetypes*, she links the archetypal symbolism present in common religious icons to their origin in the cultural symbolism of the distant past.

I have discovered a paradoxical archetype as well. In my workshop "Living in Choice," I refer to an energy I call "veils," which I write, " . . . can take any form—from what we call good, positive feeling or situations to ones we call bad or negative feelings or situations. Veils are insidious and covert because they are so normal or familiar that we never question them. In fact, we may be so clueless about them that we would never think about them at all."[205] The paradox is that these veils are, at the same time, our best friend and worst enemy. It feels as if we could not survive without them, and yet we cannot be happy without freedom from them. These veils or archetypal energies have a particular language, form, context, feeling, emotional expression, and distinct action. From this understanding, I formed this definition:

Archetypal energies are primary forms or matrix systems holding universal patterns governing human expressions such as language, behaviors, and actions found in all aspects of society, including culture, art, and spirituality. This introduction and discussion of archetypes is to explain my rationale for including in the EMCS format the following archetypal information.

Universal Fears

Many of us live in fear to one degree or another. These fears color our actions and choices and envelop our lives like dense gray smoke. It seems natural when making decisions to think first of what might go wrong, what could be stolen from us, or what we might lose—money, life, health, and relationships. Our first choice, much of the time, is to guard against the manifestation of these fears. But much of this happens at the subconscious level: Societal conditioning has taught us to mask our fears so well that we may even consciously forget they exist.

Discovered among the teachings of the ancient Essenes was their examination of three fears most common in their daily personal inventories. These corresponded to the three periods of Moses's life, described in *From Enoch to the Dead Sea Scrolls* by Edmond Bordeaux Szekely. The first period is of bondage and the darkness of ignorance. The second period is when false values are recognized, and the way ahead is just emptiness. The third period is when the "light" of intuition emerges, but the path out of the abyss of darkness seems long and arduous. These three periods have been synthesized by modern writers into the universal fears of abandonment and separation, self-worth, and surrender and trust.

As a result of my own research into ancient and modern writings, my work with clients, and my personal experience, I have identified a set of archetypal energies that I call "universal fears" for the way in which they transcend culture, borders, and race:

FEAR OF ABANDONMENT AND SEPARATION: From our earliest recorded history, we have been taught that God is out there somewhere in the heavens, and we are on Earth, separated from Him by a great distance. *The Apocalypse of Adam*, a document dating from the first or second century CE, describes this separation, "After those days, the eternal knowledge of the god of Truth withdrew from me and your Mother, Eve. Since that time, we have learned about dead things, like men. Then, we recognized the God who had created us. For we were not strangers to his powers. And we served him in fear and slavery."[206] We are so far removed, in time and awareness, from these early teachings that we no longer have a conscious memory of how they have an impact on the collective unconscious. Nonetheless, they lurk there somewhere in the dark recesses of our psyche as a hidden driving archetypal force behind our thought processes. These shadowy thoughts, nebulous in their character, play out in our relationships, work-related success-failure stories, health or disease manifestations and spiritual limitations.

FEAR OF SELF-WORTH: In almost all religious teaching, as in the example above, we find evidence that we are "less than," and no matter what we do, we cannot reach "good enough." We hold in the collective unconscious the shadowy memory of the achievements of the great masters we never reach. Therefore, the message clearly is, "If we reach any greatness at all, it is only fleeting and perhaps even an accident." We have thoughts such as, "Who do I think I am?" and "Don't get too big for your britches."

FEAR OF SURRENDERING AND TRUSTING: Perhaps the previous two fears set the stage for the third. When we think we cannot trust that the world is a safe place, we are constantly guarding against the "other shoe" that is just about to drop. We have become so convinced of this that we fail to notice the correlation between what we think and the experience that shows up in our lives. The gift of coming through the "dark night of the soul" is the ability to accept the information that our life experience is so eloquently revealing to us, learning from it in such a way that we make the choice to change our thoughts and beliefs to ones that more easily express our true desires.

FEAR OF OUR OWN DIVINITY: Ernest Holmes, in *The Science of Mind,* makes this statement: God Manifests Himself through all individuals. No two people are alike; each has a unique place in the universe of Mind; each lives in mind; each contacts It through his own mentality, in an individual way, drawing from Its unique expression of Its Divine Nature" [207] This universal super-conscious mind that flows through everyone knows no lack or limitation, nothing is impossible in it. Its predominant characteristic is creativeness. Since it does not have to spend time learning, gaining more substance, or getting more power, creating is the only thing it can do. This fear speaks to our holding on to the illusion that we can make it happen in and of ourselves. We cannot. We can only consciously accept a thought, imbue it with intention, conviction, or emotional energy, then release it into the universal super-conscious mind and wait for it to show up in experience.

FEAR THERE IS NO GOD: Our experiences with God over the centuries may not have been very satisfying. A popular perspective is that God is an old man sitting on a throne in heaven who keeps a record of every thought and feeling we have, every action we take. We think there is a scorecard being kept on each of us, but we are not aware of the score; thus, we are in the dark regarding how we are doing. We wonder if we'll be cleared to go to heaven or if we will be sent to burn in hell forever. The pain of this unknown takes a toll on us mentally, emotionally, and spiritually, and as a way to survive, we may have decided that it is just easier to believe God does not exist. This brings up another question, which is the foundation of this fear: "If God does not exist or does not exist in the way I have been taught [the wrathful God], then what?"

FEAR OF DEATH: This fear originates from our birth experience. For the most part, the womb is a place of peace. We are being nurtured in an atmosphere that is warm and safe, where our every need is filled abundantly, and where we are not plagued by bright lights, temperature fluctuations, and loud noises. That is until the contractions begin, and we are violently pushed out of our sanctuary into a world of dualities in every sense. Because of this, we fear that our dying will be just as painful. Inherent in this fear is the fear of aging—of getting old, becoming diseased, and suffering until we finally let go of the death of which we are afraid. This fear supports others 'victimization of us. We would rather suffer the most horrendous abuses—slavery, torture—than die. We could add a whole host of fears, such as poverty, starvation, and cancer, as adjuncts to the fear of death.

FEAR OF NOT UNDERSTANDING WHAT GOD IS TRYING TO TEACH US: This fear is rooted in a statement that comes from the *Right Use of Will* book series by Ceanne DeRohan. Muscle testing identifies this statement as an EMCS universal fear. It is an extension of the fear that there is no God. In other words, there may be a God, but God did not do a very good job teaching His children. Because of that, our life is painful, and we hate God for his inadequacy in teaching us the tools necessary to create a better, more successful life. This is another distorted way in which we unconsciously abdicate our throne of power, resulting in our assuming the role of victim.

FEAR THERE IS NO RECOURSE, SO WE ONLY HAVE OURSELVES TO BLAME: Another extension of the fear of God, which further justifies God's rightness and our stupidity. This is the ultimate victim role because it leads to the hopeless position described in the statement, "There is nothing I can do about my situation." This corresponds to the Apathy position of the EMCS Levels of Responsibility Chart.

FEAR OF BEING UNSAFE AND UNPROTECTED: Another aspect of the ultimate victim role, i.e., "This is not a safe world, and I can never feel safe or protected no matter what I do."

FEAR OF LOVE: Based on our deeply held belief that because we gave up heaven and separated from God, our feelings of extreme guilt for having done so mean that God will ultimately retaliate against us for the sin of rejecting him. Thus, love has become a conditional state.

FEAR OF THE LIGHT: Our ego tells us we are so horrible that if we look within ourselves, the unconscious part of us, we will die. Through the ego's constant fear-mongering, we are afraid of exposure, meaning the Light. In reality, the ego is afraid of the Light because if we choose to see through the lies, the Light will be the death of the ego.

FEAR OF SPLENDOR: Splendor signifies the eighth sephirah (plural, sephirot) of the Kabalistic Tree of Life. Majesty, glory, and feminine and passive action are its nature. It supports the fifth sephirah of the Kabbalah tree of life, Gevurah ("severity"), whose attributes are power and justice. It symbolizes the fifth day of creation when God created the creatures of the air and sea. It also connects us to the higher consciousness available from the upper reaches of the Tree of Life. Without that connection, we lose our ability to access divine thought. Perhaps it is the feared accountability inherent in splendor, should we make misuse of it and our connection to the divine of which we are afraid.

FEAR OF THE DEATH OF THE EGO: This relates to the ego's fear that we will look within and find there is no "sin" within us. The belief that we separated from God and that choice caused God to be angry with us is the foundation upon which the ego has its illusionary existence. If we debunk that lie, then the ego becomes what it is—nothing but illusion.

FEAR OF BEING PUNISHED: This relates to the fear of the death of the ego and our illusory fear that God will get us for having rejected him.

FEAR OF PROPHECY: Prophecy is a movement toward our higher self, a connection the ego does not want us to have because it threatens it with exposure for the illusion that it is.

FEAR OF THE CONSEQUENCES FOR SPEAKING THE TRUTH: Another strategy by the ego is to keep humanity locked in the illusion that its suffering is real and that the ego "protects" us from victimization; thus, the source of the victim role.

FEAR OF SEXUAL POWER: Sexual power is related to our ability to create and propagate the species and is the direct connection to our origin—our Creator. The ego fabricated the Adam and Eve story to make us believe that sex is evil and disconnects us from God rather than the fact that it connects us to God.

FEAR OF CHANGE: Change not happening is an illusion of the ego world. The ego wants us to believe that change either causes pain or is necessary to reach God and, thus, a better life, but we do not have the knowledge to make that change painlessly, so we need to give the power to the ego so it can do it for us. The reality is that God expresses in a dynamically changing universe. Everything in constant change is the nature of the universe. The fear of change—the belief that change is bad—is an ego manipulation and a trap.

FEAR OF THE JUDGMENT OF RIGHT VERSES WRONG: Cultural conditioning fosters the idea that some behaviors fall into the category of "right" and others into the category of "wrong." Choosing behaviors that are "wrong" leads to punishment. Therefore, it is important to always choose the "right" behavior. The problem is that judgment can be life-limiting.

FEAR OF BEING INCAPACITATED: An extension of the fear of judgement, the inherent punishment for behaving "wrongly."

FEAR OF ONENESS: Oneness suggests there are no individuals. The fear is if we are one then that means we are nothing, individually. At least, that is the ego message.

FEAR OF PERFECT FAITH: Using the definition of faith as "making up one's mind," the fear is that we will make up our mind, but it will turn out to be the wrong choice, and we will, therefore, be punished for having not had perfect faith.

FEAR OF JUSTICE: The definition of justice here is the golden rule: "Do not do unto others that which you would not want them to do to you" or "Do not do unto yourself that which you would not want others to do unto you." Embedded in this is the fear that because of original sin, we are not good and, therefore, are incapable of being good to others or ourselves.

FEAR THAT WE ARE NOT READY: Self-sabotage comes from the belief that "If I take action, it will be wrong, and I will fail."

FEAR THAT WE WILL NEVER HAVE A PLACE IN THIS WORLD: Stemming from a belief that "God did not make a place for me here. I don't belong and, therefore, will never be a part of life."

FEAR OF PRESENT TECHNOLOGY: Permanently disconnecting humanity from the source, thereby signaling the extinction of the species.

Reflective Mirrors

"Reflective Mirrors" is the next category of archetypal energies included in the matrix system. This term, taken from ancient Essene scrolls, means that our thoughts, feelings, and actions determine our life experience. When we are consciously aware, what we see reflected to us from "out there" is a direct response to our thoughts, feelings, and emotions, and then we have the advantage of choice. We can choose to continue the same thought expression, or we can change it knowing it will change our experience. The Essenes saw the world around us as a reflection of our intentions put into action through thoughts, feelings, and emotions. In his book *Walking Between the Worlds: The Science of Compassion*, Gregg Braden examines the seven Essene mirrors of relationships, and his writings there serve as an excellent source of further exploration of these concepts. As an Essene minister who has studied their teachings for twenty-five years, I have included my own interpretation of the Essene mirrors below, using the names Braden gives them for consistency.

EMCS Reflective Mirrors

REFLECTIVE MIRROR OF THE MOMENT: I have said for many years that miracles only happen at the moment; that is the only place that life—God—is. It is not in yesterday or tomorrow. Now is all there is! If we focus on what happened yesterday or wait in anticipation for what will happen tomorrow, next month, or next year, we are missing the moment of joy that is now. Eckart Tolle's book *The Power of Now* is a great resource for learning how to live in the moment.

REFLECTIVE MIRROR OF JUDGMENT: Recognizing that we are all one, thinking with the same mind, living the same moments, occupying the same space in the universe, and recognizing that to judge oneself or others as being "right" or "wrong" is to support the illusion generated by the intellect, or as Richard Rudd, in his groundbreaking book, *The Gene Keys*, terms it, the "psychotic mind." Once we understand that every experience is directly related to a thought, that "I" (you) or any other "I's" have projected into the great universal subconscious mind, which just says "yes" to the manifestation of the thought into form, it becomes clear that we are, in fact, manifesting into form that thought which we have initiated, grabbed hold of, and fed with energy. As a result, how could either positive or negative judgment accomplish peace, harmony, and love? It could not. Judgment is the language of the psychotic mind, and it can only support the illusion of separation from God.

REFLECTIVE MIRROR OF LOSS: This mirror reflects what psychology has, for decades, called "codependency." Throughout our lives we make the mistake of projecting our self-hate and fear of not being enough or lovable onto others. The psychosis of the intellect attempts to convince us that what is inside of us is so horrible that no one can ever love us. It has led us to attempt to ingratiate ourselves with others in such a way that they feel they cannot survive without us. When under this illusion, we may also not speak our minds, fearing that doing so might hurt someone else's feelings. This loss of self indicates growing up in an emotionally barren family environment, where patterns of survival were more important than creating the inner peace necessary to hear the small, still voice within. Loss of self, which may have seemed like a bargain at the time, is the manifestation of having lived in an environment that was emotionally, physically, or spiritually unsafe. This conditions us to believe it is dangerous to have feelings or to draw attention to our feelings by expressing them. Therefore, we learned to suppress what we feel.

REFLECTIVE MIRROR OF FORGOTTEN SELF-LOVE: Societal conditioning teaches us that to love yourself is self-centered and selfish. Thus, you may have come to believe that self-love is selfish through your own interpretations of life experiences. No matter what influenced your thinking, the results are the same. To surround oneself and fill oneself with love is a personal responsibility; each of us must do our own work. Those who fail to recognize the importance of self-love will experience the consequences of this belief—addiction being one of them —until until the pain and suffering of those consequences lead to self-forgiveness. This reminder of leaving oneself out of the equation of living and loving results in a path of losing all that one holds dear in life until the pattern is recognized or until, little by little, all is lost, including life itself.

REFLECTIVE MIRROR OF FATHER/MOTHER/CREATOR: Greg Braden effectively explains this mirror, "There is a good chance that the way you have perceived your mother and father in your life has mirrored to you, your belief of how you feel your creator views you."[208] This mirror concerns your relationship with God and your parents, whom you view as God's representative on Earth. Braden suggests that our parents loved us so much they contracted to hold the mirror for us to reflect our issues with God. Their contract is to hold this mirror until you can see the pattern, change it, and move on into freedom. This mirror may reflect your issues of abandonment, feeling not "good enough," and lack of trust. When you resolve these issues with your earthly father and mother, you also resolve the same issues with your Creator. The greatest gift of this mirror is the fact that it is much simpler to resolve the issues with someone you can see as opposed to an entity you cannot see.

REFLECTIVE MIRROR OF DARK NIGHT OF THE SOUL: The gift of this mirror is that it will not show up in your experience unless you have amassed the emotional stamina and the tools to face your quest into the dark night of the soul. The gift of facing it is you will come out on the other side with grace. This mirror, according to Greg Braden, may very well be the mirror of the "death of the ego." Many have said it is impossible to enter the Kingdom of God without first checking your ego at the door. This mirror may be the mirror of your most denied fear; therefore, it becomes manifest in such an unmistakable manner as to be undeniable.

REFLECTIVE MIRROR OF COMPASSION FOR ONESELF: Your greatest act of compassion is the act of coming to know the true cause of all our fears and doubts, the ultimate cause of all fear related to survival, the fear not only of our individual death but also the fear that we, as a species, will not survive. This fear is hardwired into our DNA at a low frequency. Any experience we have ever had in this life is the direct result of the vibration/frequency of this driving thought. Coming to a full realization of this fact, coupled with the knowing we hold within ourselves and our destiny, then and only then can the illusion of separation from self, others, and Source itself collapse. This, quoted from a fragment from the Dead Sea Scrolls and translated by Edmond Bordeaux Szekely, describes the collapse of separation:

"My children in whose hearts is my law;
Ye shall go out with joy and be led forth with peace.
The mountains and the hills
Shall break forth before you into singing,
And all the trees of the field shall clap their hands.
Arise, shine, O Children of Light!
For my Light is come upon thee,
And thou shall make the Glory of the Law
To rise upon the new Earth!

REFLECTIVE MIRROR OF ILLUSION: This mirror refers to the illusion of separation from God revealed through the greed, misuse of power, hatred, victim/perpetrator world in which we are swimming. Readers might want to reference *A Course in Miracles*, a work by Helen Schucman and William Thetford, two professors of medical psychology at Columbia University working in the 1970s. Originally presented as a series of workbooks for students, it was later compiled into book form in 1976. In it, Schucman writes, "Freedom from illusion lies only in not believing them," and, "Nothing real can be threatened. Nothing unreal exists. Herein lies the peace of God."[209]

REFLECTIVE MIRROR OF THE ILLUMINATOR OF DARKNESS: Darkness is the illusion of the ego and its world. Because human beings are the Light, only we can illumine the illusion that is the darkness. *We* are the light in the darkness.

REFLECTIVE MIRROR OF OUR JOURNEY'S PURPOSE: Our purpose is to create experiences that draw from us the strength, wisdom, and compassion to move through our lives with grace. Jesus said to live in the world but not of it. Compassion and forgiveness are the keys to living *in* the world without attachment *to* the world. According to Buddha, attachment to the world is the cause of our pain and suffering.

REFLECTIVE MIRROR OF GUILT: Allowing guilt to convince you that you will never be good enough to get what you want is another ego trap.

REFLECTIVE MIRROR OF THE FEAR OF SPLENDOR/GLORY AND HONOR. *In order to access this 8th Sephira of the Kabbalastic Tree of Life called Hod we must break through the Veil of* *the Profane on the pathway called Shen or Fire leading to Hod*: This is another ego attempt to convince us we do not have perfect intelligence and power.

REFLECTIVE MIRROR OF CREATIVE WORK: Kama Yoga teaches us the difference between doing and being. It suggests that as we express our passion in our work world we have the opportunity to grow and evolve to ever-higher levels of consciousness. The work world provides us the mirror through which we can develop the inward focus and self-reflection by which we recognize it is not the "doing" that is important but the "being." In other words, if we detest our job, the apathy, sloppiness, and negative attitude with which we do it is a reflection of the disconnection from the authentic self that seeks expression through passion.

REFLECTIVE MIRROR OF FREE WILL: We only have free will if we consciously choose to determine whether or not our thoughts align with love. Anything else is a choice to stay in the illusion.

REFLECTIVE MIRROR OF RECOGNIZING THAT WHICH IS HIDDEN: Very often that which is in our sight (the illusion) hides the truth. Gary Renard, who wrote about his spiritual awakening in what has become one of the most popular contemporary books on the subject, describes the nature of this mirror perfectly: "What is everything you see around you anyway, except a series of pictures or images; a movie of your own hatred and guilt?"[210] Yes, you have some seemingly good experiences mixed in that are designed to mask things, but that is just the nature of duality. On this level, the duality that is perceived in the universe simply reflects the duality of your own split mind, symbolized as opposites and counterparts. Therefore, there are innumerable polarities or dual forces, which we term good and bad, life and death, hot and cold, north and south, east and west, inward and outward, up and down, dark and light, left and right, sickness and health, rich and poor, yin and yang, love and hate, wet and dry, male and female, hard and soft, near and far—all of which have nothing to do with God. God is whole and complete and does not create anything that is not the same. All splits are merely symbolic of division and separation, and therefore designed to keep us chasing after supposedly "good things," so that we never find out that the good and bad are equally untrue. This method ensures that our attention is continuously fixed on the psychotic intellect instead of on the inspiration of the higher self.

REFLECTIVE MIRROR OF THE SUBCONSCIOUS: What we suppress into the subconscious mind or hold there from primal archetypal messages becomes the avenue of our destruction. Again, Renard speaks to this: "Never forget the ego is a killer, so it wants you to think [God] is a killer and fear him."[211]

REFLECTIVE MIRROR OF THE OPENED STARGATE: The Opened Stargate represents a moment in time, like a wormhole in the fabric of consciousness itself, in which one can step into a new paradigm, a new way of living. The opportunity is at hand. Now is the time to walk through it. There are no blockages. The only caveat is that you must check the ego/psychotic mind at the door.

REFLECTIVE MIRROR OF TRANSFORMATION: The circumstances present now are reflective of your path of transformation. You are on the path, and all is in divine right order.

REFLECTIVE MIRROR OF THE ILLUSION OF TIME: Time does not exist except in the mind of man. Conditioning supports linear thinking rather than holographic thought. This limitation separates us from living in the present.

REFLECTIVE MIRROR OF ETHICS: This mirror is specific to the last thirteen-year period of the Mayan Calendar—1999 to 2011—when consciousness filtered out unethical behavior, systems, beliefs, or any matter not in alignment with universal and cosmic laws, thus bringing to public awareness political, economic, educational, medical, and legal corruption, as well as the sexual abuse committed by some members of the Catholic Church. When this reflective makes the indicator change in defusion work, it is a reminder to look into one's own unethical behaviors. The external world is just a mirror of our internal worlds.

REFLECTIVE MIRROR OF THE ILLUSION THAT HUMANITY CAN MALFUNCTION: This stems from the conditioning that humans are inherently faulty.

REFLECTIVE MIRROR OF BEING: (*A New Earth* by Eckhart Tolle): This mirror speaks to the perception that it is what we do and accomplish that is important, not who we are. We seem to forget we are the ones taking the action, manifesting our own masterpiece, and giving importance to what we do rather than who we are.

In the context of EMCS, both the Universal Fears and Reflective Mirrors give the energician, as well as the client, direct and life-changing information concerning the beliefs that have directed their lives. We can say that our concept of "survival" is an archetypal energy. I often hear "I am a survivor" stated with great pride. In turn, I ask, "Do you desire to just survive, or would you like to thrive?" Thriving is a completely different ball game. The ego mind and the illusion it creates are dependent on the continuance of fear, guilt, and the belief in separation. The only way it can end is for each of us to see it for the illusion it is and begin the work of waking up from the hypnotic trance inherent in the illusion. Knowledge of archetypal systems allows one to consciously discern the type of energies or belief systems organizing one's life. They are paradoxical clues to the truth. Caroline Myss punctuates this concept when she writes:

> Archetypes are genuinely powerful forces, in fact, and it may not be inaccurate to state that the whole of life is nothing more than an archetypal playground in which we are participating . . . we are all connected to an individual Sacred Contract and that this Contract contains the learning processes we are meant to experience and absorb as a means of expanding the endless realms of consciousness that lies within the nature of our spirits.[212]

Understanding the role your archetypes play in your Sacred Contract as defined by Myss is a powerful tool, a lens through which you may begin to see the symbolic meaning of your life's relationship patterns and your career successes and failures. Myss uses the astrology wheel, which is divided into twelve sections that represent twelve aspects of our lives, on which to play out a Sacred Contract. She identifies twelve major categories of personal archetypes, followed by secondary or private archetypes associated with the twelve major ones. For instance, one of the twelve major archetypal categories is Security, and secondary to that heading is Rescuer. Using the model Myss sets forth, if we place the personal archetype of Security in the first house of the astrology chart (which represents the face one shows to the world, one's personality, personal affairs, physical appearance, i.e., how the world sees you), it becomes clear how "codependency" issues, low self-esteem, and feelings of unimportance can emerge. Opposite tendencies can emerge as well, in other words the "bull in the china shop" mentality or the "I can handle it all" mentality.

For the purposes of EMCS, adapting Myss's model of archetypes and astrology and using them in conjunction with your skills in kinesiology will identify your client's natal Sacred Contract. Begin by muscle testing as you state, "Give me an indicator change for the archetypal energies most influencing your life at conception." Then continue with the list of archetypes provided in the index. Gather first the personal archetypal heading and then the secondary private archetype for each of the twelve houses of the chart. Once you have identified the category, then muscle test for the secondary or private archetype most significant to your client at conception. Under the heading of Security, there are sixteen private archetypes. Muscle test "by the number" for the most significant.

After identifying each archetype significant to your client's conception, explore the definition of each archetype, keeping in mind they provide the framework upon which life experiences developed from the moment of conception to this very moment. I caution you to remember that even archetypes indicate the illusion of separation. To give them meaning, purpose, and validity, or to become attached to them, only supports the illusion. Our mission is not to strengthen the ego world; rather it is to identify the way out of the illusion. To this end, the archetypes can give a perspective on how broad and deep the illusion seems to be. They will show you the paradox of duality, which keeps us tangled in the web of deceit, i.e., the illusion. They provide the seeker with a vision of his/her own brand of ego nonsense and knowledge of the specifics that need to be unraveled through forgiveness. Once you have completed the natal chart contract information, you can repeat the process for a financial, relationship, and present-time career chart.

Originally, I used only the five Chinese elements as archetypal energies based on the five ancient animal symbols used in traditional Chinese medicine. These are specific to the meridian system explained in detail in chapters six and seven. I believe they are important to include, because as a default informational system based on thousands of years of research and practice by Chinese doctors and health care practitioners, identifying the element brought the archetypal energy into the physical world. By that I mean that all the other default information speaks to language, thought, feeling, emotion, and action; the element identifies the physical position in the body holding the trauma, archetypal, or survival pattern. This proves valuable when connecting a feeling or archetype to a "disease."

After reading Cyndi Dales's book, *Advanced Chakra Healing: Energy Mapping on the Four Energy Pathways*, I adapted the five elements she identified in that work as follows:

WHITE LIGHT: the representation of Divine Love in the third dimension.

YELLOW LIGHT: the representation of Divine Power in the third dimension.

ROSE GOLD LIGHT: the coming together in equanimity; the Divine Masculine and Female in the act of manifestation.

ETHER: the energy through which all things manifest.

STONE: As an element, it is representational energy that strengthens the holographic human energy system. It is used as an imaginal tool to build a vessel in which energy can be held to heal, to strengthen the bones, or to wall off destructive energy, isolating it for healing purposes.

STAR: As an elemental energy, it represents the wisdom of the ages. The stars have been in existence for billions of years and, therefore, have witnessed the expansion of the universe from the beginning of time. They are the evidence that there is something greater than humanity driving the show. Meditating upon the stars or spending time outside at night and looking up at the night sky with the intention of receiving the wisdom the stars impart can open you to their wisdom.

I Ching/Gene Keys

The I Ching, as used in the EMCS process, is not a method of divination in the traditional sense. It is, however, a thumbnail sketch of the identified issue. For example, the hexagram number five made the indicator change in muscle testing for the specific issue at hand. This hexagram is called "Waiting" in the book *I Ching for Everyone.* Like the astrology wheel, each hexagram is divided into twelve sections, each of which represents a specific aspect of life expression. In the middle of the wheel, you can see the six changing lines of the hexagram. Each line indicates a particular experience with some guidance in moving through it. The indicated line must be read through the lens of the issue at hand. It does not necessarily pertain to all of life experience, but it is specific to the current issue. Each section of a line corresponds to the twelve sections of the wheel; each line speaks paradoxically of a situation. For example, the "Judgment Statement" from hexagram five, line two states: "A reluctance to come to a decision may be seen as indecisiveness but is correct."[213] When seen in context with the current issue, it suggests there is the need for more information before making a final decision. It is wise to listen to the reluctance and seek more information before taking action. Each line goes on to provide an understanding of action to take or not take in relationship to the issue.

My experience with working with the *I Ching* in this way not only assists the client in gaining valuable insight into the issue but also often helps me "see" the issue in an expanded context. Therefore, using the I Ching in EMCS is a tool for divination because it clearly elucidates that continuing the pattern will generate a certain outcome. Recognizing the pattern and changing it makes it possible to change course.

Since first writing this section, I have been introduced to Richard Rudd's groundbreaking work *The Gene Keys,* a modern understanding of the I Ching and its relationship to the sixty-four codons of the human DNA. In the foreword of *The Gene* Keys, Rudd writes:

> Recent breakthroughs in biology point towards an amazing truth—your DNA, the coiled code that has made you who you are today, is not in control of your destiny. Rather, it is your general attitude to life that tells your DNA what kind of person you want to become. This means that every thought, feeling, word[,] and action that you make in life is imprinted in every single cell of your body. Negative thoughts and emotions cause your

DNA to contract, whereas positive thoughts and emotions cause it to expand and relax. This process is going on all the time, from the moment you come into the world to the moment you leave.[214]

Rudd recognizes the physiology related to each codon of the DNA, including the amino acids, and delineates the three aspects of each codon or gene key or hexagram of the I Ching: the shadow, the gift, and the siddhi.[215] It is a beautiful work and takes the original I Ching and its connection to the codons of our DNA to a whole new level of understanding—the realization that we can change our DNA through positive thoughts, feelings, and actions.

The 72 Names of God

As a set of esoteric teachings established by an ancient sect of Judaism to explain the relationship between God and the physical, mortal universe, the Kabbalah is rich with tradition and insight into human behavior and experience. I have incorporated into my practice Rev. Yehuda Berg's book *The 72 Names of God* as another archetypal tool for explanation and awareness. Again, the particular name of God as identified by muscle testing for a particular issue adds insight and clarity. For the purposes of EMCS, the energician muscle tests for the specific name of God, and when the name is read with the identified issue in mind it can give incredible insight into the origin as well as the healing of the issue. Clearly, the more insight into a limiting energy blockage the more successful will be the transformation!

Lost Will Causal Beliefs

The group of beliefs ascertained from the work of Ceanne DeRohan's *Right Use of Will: Healing and Evolving the Emotional Body* series have proved to be valuable when tracing a limiting pattern of behavior to its origin using EMCS. DeRohan claims to have received the words directly from God, who wants the people of Earth to claim what DeRohan calls Divine Will. "Without Will, the Spirit has no selection process," she writes. "Your Will is your individual magnetic energy field and draws the experiences you are going to have. If you hold something in your Will that is denied and disconnected from your conscious awareness by not being accepted and allowed free movement or free expression, you will then draw a reflection of this to yourself."[216]

I include the group of beliefs here:

1. The Will is not part of God
2. Terror of the Will of falling away from God/Spirit.
3. The Will's guilt for feeling there was no basis for its feelings or complaints.
4. The Will feeling that God/Spirit could not understand.
5. Avoiding manipulation.
6. Denial had the effect of instructing these feelings to disguise themselves and to appear to be something other than what they were because they were not acceptable to us in their true and original form.
7. God's denial of the vividness and reality of the Rainbow Spirits, who felt that they were not parented right and because of that they could not become the white light they felt they needed to be in order to get the attention they needed. The more

they attempted to be the light, the darker they became.

8. Fear and guilt of not helping and being helped out of love.
9. Feeling foolish for having sexual needs.
10. Parental denial of fragmentation
11. Gaps between God/Self and Will.
12. Manifestation's guilt for Spirit's lack of self-acceptance, gaining power that was not their true and original form.
13. The Will's feeling of powerlessness at Its first experiences with God.
14. Spirits feeling like they did not have a proper home.
15. Feeling guilt about giving into desire and ignoring the needs of the Spirit.
16. Time layered conditioning that does not allow Will to move.
17. Fear that God is not God and is not in control of His creation.
18. Fear of feeling anger.
19. Lost Will received this and everything else that was not given acceptance here, including the Mother's (Will's) fear that She really was at fault.
20. Repeated expression of some emotions can indicate emotional habit patterns that may give the appearance of emotional release but are participating in furthering the denials of other emotions.

When Lost Will makes the indicator change, gather present time information as usual. Go over the present time information with your client, then begin the age recession to the age of cause of the Lost Will causal belief by stating while muscle testing, " Give me an indicator to the moment of your conception in this incarnation." When the indicator change occurs, state, " Give me an indicator change when we have reached the moment when this belief was first activated." Wait for the indicator change, then state, "Give me an indicator change for all that apply." Then state the elements from the case notes sheet waiting for an indicator change. Once gathered, make the correction according to the Matrix Systems identified.

Drainers and Entities

The late Byron Gentry, a chiropractor and energy worker as well as a wonderful friend, refers in his book *Miracles of the Mind to drainers as* people "who literally drain the energy and life force away from others"[217] Some energy workers refer to drainers as "energetic parasites" that live in the unseen energy surrounding us and attach to human energy systems for sustenance. It seems the astral body, one of the four energy fields that make up the holographic human energy system, is more susceptible to drainers because of its chaotic nature. The astral body is also known as the emotional body and is greatly affected by negative emotions such as anger and rage. Some drainers feed off this chaotic energy and are therefore attracted to it. This is one reason that maintaining a calm and peaceful state is so important for healthy and creative living. The Energy Matrix Clearing System is especially effective at clearing drainers and returning to a healthy stasis those energy centers that have been blown out or distorted through unhealthy boundaries created through codependency, abuse, and addiction.

Entities are altogether a different matter. These disembodied spirits have not been able to cross to the "other side." They are earthbound and, having lost their physical bodies, need to fuse with a living person in order to move. They often do this at conception, and the influence they have on their host is phenomenal, usurping its body and will and interfering with its its soul path. Evicting the entity can be a challenging process because the entity is not keen on leaving. Some suggest calling on whatever spiritual guide the host has an affinity for, whether that be the White Brotherhood, master teachers, Jesus, or Buddha. In EMCS, in addition to honoring that tradition, we identify a gem and mineral essence whose frequency or combination of frequencies can eject the entity or drainer.

Historical

Sometimes, the issue with which a person is grappling is a carry-over from a past life experience. I also realize that not all people "believe" in past lives. To honor that, I use the term "historical" in EMCS work. If it makes the indicator change and you know the client does not believe in past lives, just refer to "what came before" this life experience and go on. Don't identify a specific past life or any information that pertains to it, just ask that all information pertinent to the defusion is brought forth and loaded in the circuit to be released through the defusion correction. If the client accepts that they may have lived other lifetimes, then muscle check to identify the specific timeline by age recessing to conception, then continue to past life of cause, beginning with most recent past life as number one and continuing until the indicator makes the change. Once identified, muscle check for gender, age of death, cause of death, and time and place of the past life. Remember, the past life could have been lived in any part of the Earth or even on other planets and star systems known or unknown. Once this information is identified, follow the EMCS protocol to complete the defusion process.

Negative Energetic Cords

Vows, Curses, Hexes, and Rituals

We make vows for many reasons, including to get married, to enter a religious order, or to join the military. We also make vows to ourselves. When it comes to the latter type, I always think of Scarlett O'Hara in *Gone with the Wind*, near-starving and standing in the remnants of the vegetable garden at her family home, Tara, shaking her fist at the sky and vowing that she'll never be hungry again. Every action she takes from that point on is in service of that vow, even to the point of betrayal of a sister and the loss of a love.

Vows are often carried over from lifetime to lifetime and can negatively affect success and freedom in the current life experience. When a vow makes the indicator change during the EMCS process, determine what kind of vow—poverty, obedience, or allegiance—then continue with the protocol, age recessing to the age of cause or time when the vow was taken to diffuse or release the vow. When releasing the vow, ask the client to make this statement: "I, _____, completely and totally release from my soul the vow of _____." Ask them to make this statement following any corrections you make at age of cause and before returning the client to present time. Always muscle check to make sure the vow is completely released from their holographic human energy system on all points on the compass of time, from the beginning of time to the end of time and on all points in between.

Curses and hexes are associated with black magic, and they weave themselves throughout popular culture, from the Arthurian legends to Shakespeare, *The Wizard of* Oz to *Snow White and the Seven Dwarfs*. Little do we realize that when we swear in great anger and frustrated condemnation we can bind that negative energy to people or objects. For instance, if your house was foreclosed on by the bank, you might curse that no one will ever live in that house again, causing anyone who walks in to feel that negative energy and leave immediately. We can also curse others who we perceive have hurt us or betrayed us, causing them similar hurt or betrayal, even unhappiness or disease.

When a curse or hex makes the indicator change along with the normal EMCS protocol, ask the client to call in any spiritual guides, master teachers, angels, etc., to assist in the release of this curse or hex.

Rituals are a part of how we operate in our daily lives, and they can govern everything from how we get dressed in the morning to our preparations for bed at night. These are habits that are comfortable and familiar, and we often perform them without noticing.

Rituals are also a part of the sacred rites of some religions or methods of worship. There are rituals in healing practices led by shamans and rituals that are integral to the practice of black magic and satanic worship, rituals that govern initiation into a social group like a fraternity or sorority and rituals to establish membership into a street gang. People who have been involved in rituals—especially dark rituals that involve physical, mental, emotional, spiritual, and sexual abuse—often exhibit symptomatic responses, the two most prevalent being post-traumatic stress and disassociation. If working with a client who exhibits these symptoms, you may find that ritual abuse is a cause of the reaction. If ritual abuse makes the indicator change, the EMCS protocol is the same; however, be aware that it is possible that the process may trigger either of these symptoms. If that happens, you may find that stopping the process and administering the frontal/occipital hold while instructing the client to focus on the breath interrupts the episode. Use all your skills as an energician to clear the energy system so that the work can continue. It is important to know your limitations when you are dealing with ritual abuse. You may want to refer to someone who specializes in this area.

Ancestral Wounds

Unhealed ancestral wounds may be carried forward into the next generation. These wounds can come from trauma of any kind, including the loss of a loved one, dire financial lack or the loss of wealth, power situations, disease, and murder. These traumas get imprinted in the DNA and are passed on. This information may be the source of lack and limitation in future generations. Your client can become the surrogate for that ancestor to clear the trauma for them now.

If ancestral wounds make the indicator change, gather present time information. Age recess to the moment of conception for the client in this incarnation and then recess to the ancestral age of cause. Muscle check to see which ancestor holds the energy block or trauma, identify the gender of the ancestor, the relationship, and which family line (mother or father). Identify the usual age of cause information from the protocol and diffuse for the matrix system identified. For ancestral wounds, I use fifty years for each ancestral age. For instance, if the indicator leads to the fifth ancestral age, the age of cause would be two hundred and fifty years in the past. Sometimes, the client may have some family history to draw from, making it easier to connect with this particular ancestor.

Upon making the corrections for the ancestor, muscle check to make sure the trauma has been cleared from that particular ancestor as well as any DNA imprinting carried on to future generations. If the DNA imprinting has not been cleared, muscle check all EMCS clearing possibilities to clear the imprinting. That would include all gem and mineral essences, flower essences, essential oils, or other methods you have included in your system. When complete, return to the present time, infusing the identified symbol for infusion. It may be the symbol for the element or any other symbol identified through muscle checking.

Divine Spirit Level

According to many traditions, including the Theosophical Eastern System and the Rosicrucian Western System, there are seven levels of worlds.[218] The Cosmic Scale correlation to the two are:

Rosicrucian	Cosmic	Theosophical
World of God	Intergalactic (Scale of Universe)	Logoic
World of Virgin Spirit	Interstellar I (Scale of Galaxy)	Monadic
World of Divine Spirit	Interstellar II (Scale of Zodiac)	Attic
World of Life Spirit	Interplanetary (Solar System)	Buddhic
Thought World	Abstract Thought/Concrete Thought	Manasic
Desire World	Desires, Emotions, and Feelings	Astral
Physical World	Etheric and Chemical Regions	Physical

The Divine Spirit level (or scale of the zodiac/attic) relates on a personal level to willpower or the Spirit of Being. It is the essence of divinity and its utilization in the physical world or not. When Divine Spirit level makes the indicator change, muscle check for which sign of the zodiac is at play and which house of the astrology chart is most affected. Is the issue one of misuse of power? How? Explore all the avenues at your disposal as an energician for this one.

Dimensional Levels

Kabbalists have determined that there are ten dimensions represented by the Kabbalistic Tree of Life and its ten sephirot arranged on three pillars connected by twenty-two pathways.[219] Since the Kabbalah represents a body of knowledge covering wisdom from all ages and traditions, access to a Tree of Life chart is essential to understanding the deeper spiritual underpinning of this particular issue.

Barbara Hand Clow's book *Alchemy of Nine Dimension* is also a good source of information when exploring dimensional information. This resource gives insight and provides sources of information that can be helpful in defusing the issue.

Clow's nine dimensions are:

1. The iron core crystal in the center of the earth
2. The telluric world —the realm between the iron core and the curved crust of the Earth

3. Linear time and space—the level in which we live
4. The world of myths and archetypes
5. Realm of light that generates in the human heart and radiates out to plants, animals, the earth, and each other
6. Sacred geometry and platonia (five platonic solids)
7. Cosmic sound and vibrational resonance.
8. The divine mind
9. The black hole in the center of the Milky Way

When working with dimensions, the questions for defusion may be:

- Does the client connection to this dimension need to be established?

- Is there a blockage to this dimension that needs to be cleared?

- Does the client need a greater understanding of dimensional influence in their present situation?

You may discover it is necessary to access that particular dimension via intention while muscle checking. While doing so, state, "Give me an indicator change when we are fully connected to the dimension in question so that we may work within the appropriate parameters of that dimension." Wait for the indicator to change and then proceed with identifying any gem and mineral essences, platonic solids, or other sacred geometry essences available to work in that dimension.

When complete, muscle check to ensure the connection has been made, the blockage cleared, or the information downloaded into the client's energy system for utilization.

Return to the present time, infusing the appropriate symbol based on muscle checking.

Since dimensions are just one component of the overall defusion schema, muscle check to determine at what point during the process you will work with the dimensional data. Muscle checking may indicate the process needs to be done in present time before age recessing or the EMCS process of clearing the issue at causal age may need to occur. In which case, return to present time and then work with the dimensional information. Let muscle testing be your guide here.

CHAPTER FIFTEEN

MATRIX IX

VENOUS ARTERIAL ENERGY

This matrix speaks to the reality that the holographic human energy system is a system of energy flow. The use of the words "venous" and "arterial" serves to suggest that there is a connection between the source of the energy flow and its extensions. The Energy Matrix Clearing System works with the energy of the system not its corporeal constitution, or physical body. When this system makes the indicator change in a defusion, it indicates that there is a blockage within the flow of energy from its source to its greatest extension. The emotional organ energy (for example, the emotion associated most commonly with the liver is anger) can provide clues instrumental to discovering the cause of the energy blockage.

Correction is determined by identifying, through muscle testing, which Living in Choice gem or mineral essence will clear the blockage. Once you have identified the essence for clearing, identify the number of drops and route for administration.

1. *Liver energy*: emotion - anger; feeling - assertion/will; sense organ - eyes (sight); body parts – ligaments, body fluid, tears; partner organ - gall bladder
2. *Gall bladder energy*: emotion - control issues
3. *Spleen/pancreas energy*: joyless - the fun has gone out of living
4. *Eliminative energy (left and right kidneys)*: emotion - fear; feeling – resolution/willpower; sense organ - ears; body parts - bone marrow, body fluid, urine; partner organ - bladder
5. *Large intestine*: holding on to toxic waste
6. *Small intestine*: assimilation of nutrients; emotion – self-love
7. Bladder: emotion - not feeling safe
8. *Heart, heart muscles and valves*: emotions - excitement and shock; feelings - joy and happiness; sense organ - tongue; body part - vascular system; body fluid - sweat; partner organ - small intestine
9. *Respiratory energy (lungs)*: - emotions - fear, "I can't take life in!"
10. *Adrenal energy*: emotions - grief from being burnt out, overwhelmed with life experiences
11. *Lymphatic System (upper and lower)*: a message that one needs to refocus on the essentials of life, specifically their need for joy and love
12. *Endocrine energy (pituitary, pineal, thyroid)*: emotions - disconnected, stuck, lost, "I can't connect with myself," "I don't know what to do!"
13. *Thymus energy*: emotion - indignant ("nothing I do works")

Remember, if this information comes up in the present time, it is only information to share with the client. It is a correction when it comes up at the age of cause. Occasionally, corrections are made in the present time, but rarely.

Corrections: Living in Choice Gem and Mineral Essences from the entire list of singles, Celestial Blends, Cranial Nerves, and Chakra blends from all subtle energy body levels.

CHAPTER SIXTEEN

MATRIX X

BODY POLARITY

Much like a magnet or a car battery, our body contains negative and positive poles. Therefore, it generates both negative and positive energy, which ebb and flow like waves, creating a harmony, a melody of life itself. The flow of body polarity is both within and without the physical body. Without body polarity, the systems of the physical, mental, emotional, and spiritual (energetic) system could not be. In other words, without polarity, we could not exist.

Body polarity can also be seen in terms of masculine and feminine, the archetypal sacred masculine and sacred feminine conjointly ruling as equals, balancing the flow of life expression within and without. Research indicates that body polarity is an important component in human health because it is related more closely to issues of the "essential" self than either the chakra or meridian energies.

If body polarity makes the indicator change, the essential self is the issue. This suggests that some experience or negative self-perception has caused this person to have such a low sense of self-worth that it "colors" every one of their decisions. Gordon Stokes and Daniel Whiteside term this the "Wounded Spirit."

As mentioned above, when we speak of male-female energy within the scope of the physical body, we are referring to body polarity. The principle of body polarity means that while the body functions as a whole unit, every organ, neuron, cell, muscle, etc., is activated by interchanging positive and negative charges created by sodium and potassium ions. Every part of the physical system is polarized. The body itself is polarized, both front and back. The right front is positive, while the left front is negative. The polarity is reversed on the back side of the body: the right back is negative, while the left-back is positive. The hands are polarized as well. The palm of the right hand is positive, and the left palm is negative. The index and ring fingers on the right hand are positive, and the long and little fingers are negative. The finger polarities of the left hand are reversed: the index and ring fingers are negative; the long and little fingers are positive. The thumbs of both hands are neutral.

There is also polarity within the belly of the muscles. When the muscle is in contraction, it has negative polarity, and the ends of the muscle have positive polarity. When the muscle is in extension, the polarity is the opposite. When a muscle is in contraction, its origin and insertion have a positive polarity and the belly of the muscle has negative polarity, which is the reverse when in extension. When muscle testing a balanced muscle, either in contraction or extension, using neutral touch (two fingers of opposite polarity or the thumb), testing the belly of the muscle will produce a hold-strong muscle response. An indicator change in either position indicates energy imbalance.

If you touch the belly of a balanced muscle with a negatively charged finger, the muscle will go weak. The same happens if you use a positively charged finger. This is because the polarities repel each other like two magnets. The body polarity demonstrates the need for both polarities, male and female, with neither dominating the other.

One simple correction for "Wounded Spirit" is for the client to hold both hands on the forehead while the thumb of each hand touches the top of the nail of the little finger and the first three fingers touch the frontal eminences. As the energician, you then massage the K-27s—right hand massaging the right and left hand massaging the left. Kidney meridian point twenty-seven lies just below the collarbone and to the left and right of the throat soft spot.

You can also flush the energy of the right side of the body of your subject with your right hand (palm toward the body) from the top of the head to the feet and, at the same time, place the left hand with the palm facing the back of the body. Repeat on the left side of the body with left palm facing the front and the right palm facing the back. Always do both sides, or you will create an imbalance. Muscle check to determine if body polarity is now balanced.

The twenty-second gene key/codon/hexagram, called "Grace Under Pressure" by Richard Rudd in *The Gene Keys,* speaks with its shadow of dishonor to the six core wounds of humanity, which are:

- Repression
- Denial
- Shame
- Rejection
- Guilt
- Separation

I noticed that Wounded Spirit kept coming up in certain EMCS sessions, even after testing indicated it had been cleared. After I read gene key twenty-two, I tested to see if the Wounded Spirit and the core wounds of humanity were one and the same—or at least connected in some way, i.e., one triggering in the other—and I got an affirmative answer. When Wounded Spirit makes the indicator change, I muscle test for which of the six sacred human wounds is at play.

In EMCS, using the honey calcite (green infused) Living in Choice Gem and Mineral Essence automatically clears body polarity. Muscle check for the number of drops and method of administration—on the tongue, under the tongue, or in water.

When Wounded Spirit comes up in your EMCS session, always check for a muscle circuit connection triggering the polarity reversal. Muscle test for the muscle circuit, by the number, to see what story the muscle tells regarding the wounded spirit. Then muscle test for the Living in Choice gem and mineral essence to clear the muscle circuit connection to the wounded spirit.

CHAPTER SEVENTEEN

MATRIX XI

SPINAL DISCS AND THIRTY-ONE SPINAL NERVES

Every sensation in the human body—every movement, every thought, every working of a vital organ—is controlled by a complex system of nerves. This system includes the central nervous system, which is composed of the brain and the spinal cord, the latter of which communicates with thirty-one spinal nerves placed along the spinal column; the peripheral nervous system, which carries information to and from the central nervous system; the somatic nervous system, a voluntary system that reacts to outside stimuli affecting the body and serves both the musculoskeletal system and skin; and the autonomic nervous system, which is involuntary and automatically seeks to maintain homeostasis. Affected by internal and external factors, this nervous system receives information from the body and the environment and then initiates an appropriate response by transmitting that data to the brain.

Dr. Bruce Fisher, in volume two of his *Man, Grand Reflection of the Greater Cosmos: Studies in Occult Anatomy,* suggests that the spinal column reflects the "deepest and most hidden meanings in scriptures, legends and rituals."[220] He relates the thirty-three vertebrae of the spinal column to the journey of the thirty-three years of the biblical King David's reign, the thirty-three years of the life of the biblical Jesus, and the thirty-three degrees of Freemasonry.

Mystical teachings suggest that the seven cervical or neck vertebrae reflect the seven "planetary spirits before the throne," a reference to the formation of the solar system from a singular point or "creator." These seven planets—Mercury, Venus, Earth, Mars, Jupiter, Saturn, and Uranus—are said to embody great and exalted spiritual intelligence and exercise a particular influence on the ongoing evolvement of living beings. This concept suggests that the seven neck vertebrae of the spinal column correlate to the influence of those seven planets our individual spiritual growth and make up the intellectually creative zone or the connection between the supreme and superior worlds of humanity. The point being that humans are influenced in particular ways according to the qualities of each planet supporting the concept that human beings are a microcosm of the macrocosm. As the structural foundation of our physical body, the spinal column plays a much greater role in the overall expression of the human species than it appears to if looked at strictly from a physical perspective.

The atlas, or uppermost vertebra of the neck, supports the skull just as Fisher says, "the legendary Titan Atlas supports the heavens upon his shoulders."[221] Perhaps this indicates that the human head/brain has the responsibility of the whole of human endeavor.

Cyndi Dale was inspired to do a deep dive into the spinal column, exploring energy points, as she terms them, from the bottom or tip of the spinal column to the top cervical vertebra.[222] She suggests that each of the energy points serve to move particular types of energy throughout the system. She surmises that each point has a particular purpose, function, energy form, and communication process. As with any other system, she suggests problems may arise in this flow of energy based upon life experience, inherited data, limiting beliefs, etc. She gives each vertebra of the spine a number, beginning with numbers one through eight for the coccyx and sacrum and ending with number ten at the very tip of the coccyx, which she gives the function "groundedness," for example.

For brevity's sake, I will associate the point number with the vertebra.

Second coccyx vertebra: Awareness
Third coccyx vertebra: Feeling
Fourth coccyx vertebra: Love
Point Five apex of the sacrum: Expression
Fused transverse ridges of the sacrum: six (Vision), seven (Divinity), eight (Time)
Fifth lumbar: point 9 - Soul
Fourth lumbar: point 11 - Transmutation
Third lumbar: point 12 - Connection
Second lumbar: point 13 - Yin
First lumbar: point 14 - Yang
Twelfth thoracic: point 15 - Polarities
Eleventh thoracic: point 16 - Similarities
Tenth thoracic: point 17 - Harmony
Ninth thoracic: point 18 - Freedom
Eighth thoracic: point 19 - Kundalini

Seventh thoracic: point 20 - Mastery
Sixth thoracic: point 21 - Abundance
Fifth thoracic: point 22- Clarity
Fourth thoracic: point 23 - Knowledge
Third thoracic: point 24 - Creation
Second thoracic: point 25 - Manifestation
First thoracic: point 26 - Alignment
Seventh cervical: point 27 - Peace
Sixth cervical: point 28 - Wisdom
Fifth cervical: point 29 - Enjoyment
Fourth cervical: point 30 - Forgiveness
Third cervical: point 31 - Faith
Second cervical: point 32 - Grace
First cervical: point 33 - The Principal of the 33rd

The axis serves as a pivot for which the atlas holds the head and allows the head to swivel. The atlas makes the connection with the higher spiritual centers through the thirty-second energy point (sixth cervical), the Grace and Divine Source consciousness center. This is the connection point to the golden kundalini energy.

Dale says this of the axis:

> It has neither a physical nor a spinal process. It is ring-like in shape with a front and back arch. Metaphysically, the axis pertains to the Principle of the Thirty-third, which is a protective energy that must be used to safely work with any of the higher energy points. This principle is that of Love. Not just love, the feeling we feel when infatuated, but the energy of Love, the feeling the Divine Source has for itself and for us.[223]

In mystical traditions the twelve thoracic or dorsal vertebrae reflect the twelve signs of the zodiac and the twelve houses of the astrology chart. They define the heart of our superior and mundane life experience. Because they are located in the same area as the ribs, they are also in connection with the third chakra and the heart chakra. It is notable, too, that they are heart-shaped. Esoteric teachings indicate that the major function of these vertebrae is to integrate the higher spiritual energies that support the desires of the heart and help us realize our dreams. These represent our individual journeys through the Land of Egypt, meaning the world of the material and beyond to the higher aspect of ourselves, connecting through that journey with the One.

The five lumbar vertebrae bear witness to Leonardo da Vinci's *Canon of Man*, the number of the pentagram, or, as Fisher says, "The archetype of the physical body of man and the connecting link between the infernal and mundane worlds in man."[224]

These five vertebrae are some of the largest vertebrae in the spine, which means they are good energy conductors and add stability to the whole of the body's energy system. They are connected to the second chakra, which relates to issues of sex, money, personal power, relationships, and creativity. Each of the five vertebrae has connections to the chakra system and other spiritual energy points located outside the physical body. The fifth lumbar is associated with the ninth chakra, the soul chakra, located just above the head. This chakra holds the blueprint for this incarnation and all other incarnations. Dale suggests that for healing to be permanent, the blueprint must be re-imprinted. The fourth lumbar vertebra is associated with the eleventh chakra, the chakras of the hands and feet, through which we can transform negative energy into the energy of love. The third lumbar vertebra is associated with spiritual points within and without the physical body. Refer to the twelfth secondary chakra system in this work to identify these points. The second lumbar vertebra is associated with the yin point, and the first lumbar vertebra is associated with the yang point.

The nine sacral and coccygeal vertebrae are symbolized, according to Fisher, "in the 666, the 'number of man;' the 'Land of Egypt;' the *infernal world of man*, the nine lesser initiations[,] and the nine occult strata of the Earth."[225] The "Land of Egypt" refers to the time Moses spent in Egypt being raised as a prince, with all the privileges that accompanied the title. It was when he became aware of the struggles of the people around him, especially the Hebrews, that he faced the internal world that we all have the opportunity to face in our own life experience. We may get so invested in the material world of things that we lose sight of *living*. Metaphorically, Moses leading the Hebrews out of bondage and into the Light is the journey we all must make. Whether we do or not is an individual choice.

According to Cyndi Dale, "The coccyx, commonly called the tailbone, performs critical physical and metaphysical functions. . . . Metaphysically, I believe it relates to our most basic self and is associated with our reproductive capacities."[226] She also says that the first coccygeal vertebra is our connection to the tenth chakra, which grounds us in the reality of the third dimension and is the access point to red kundalini energy. Kundalini has been described as "sleeping coiled energy" at the base of the spine. It is a higher spiritual energy that, when made active, moves up the spinal column like two snakes coiled around a column, their heads meeting at the top. The Hindus speak of these two snakes as the Ida and the Pingala, and when they meet at the top, they activate the pineal gland, which allows for a greater ability to "see" intuitively and psychically. There are many schools of thought both ancient and modern concerning the activation of the kundalini. Nevertheless, the general consensus seems to be that kundalini is undiluted raw life energy and is necessary for all developmental stages of life. It is said to activate our sexuality and stimulate us in the drive to achieve our purpose. Inherent in red kundalini is the energy of fire, which lends itself to violence and abusive behaviors when stagnant. When kundalini energy is connected with golden kundalini of the seventh chakra, the raw energy of fire kundalini can be tempered with higher spiritual energy of love, elevating fire kundalini into a higher mode of expression.

Dale says that activation of kundalini energy is different in men than in women, and some consider female kundalini energy inherent in a woman's natural biological processes, such as the menstrual cycle and the birthing process. This indicates that kundalini activation of women must make its way through the second chakra, which is where women find their strength, courage, and creative expression. Men, on the other hand, must move kundalini through the solar plexus chakra, where they connect with their emotional nature.

My own deep dive into the spinal column, paired with the spinal nerves associated with each, led me to connect associated feelings and core negative beliefs to each of the vertebrae, as listed below. When Matrix XI makes the indicator change during a defusion process, these connections can be an invaluable way to help the patient recognize the patterns of limitation in their life.

Spinal Area	Vertebra	
Coccygeal	Fourth (lowest)	1 pair spinal nerves
	Third	
	Second	
	First	
Sacral	Fifth	5 pair of spinal nerves
	Fourth	
	Third	
	Second	
	First	
Lumbar	Fifth	5 pair of spinal nerves
	Fourth	
	Third	
	Second	
	First	
Thoracic	Twelfth	12 pair of spinal nerves
	Eleventh	
	Tenth	
	Ninth	
	Eighth	
	Seventh	
	Sixth	
	Fifth	
	Fourth	
	Third	
	Second	
	First	
Cervical	Seventh	7 pair of spinal nerves

Sixth
Fifth
Fourth
Third
Second
First[227]

When spinal column/nerve conditions make the indicator change in the EMCS process, it is the emotional connection that tells the story. Through many years of working with clients accessing information from their systems via muscle testing led to the universalization of beliefs associated with the spinal column and associated nerve conditions. The work of these authors only echoes my own conclusions: *Messages from the Body: Their Psychological Meaning* by Narayan Singh Khalsa, Ph.D.; *You Can Heal Your Life* by Louise Hay; and *The Joy of Feeling* by Marshaa Iona Teeguarten. Use all your tools as an energician to clear any blockages that come up during the defusion process. This includes all Matrix systems and Living in Choice Gem and Mineral Essences.

First Cervical - *Principle of the 33rd*

Possible associated feelings: fear, confusion, self-destruction, rejection, unappreciation

Possible core negative beliefs: "I am not good enough." "The only way I can get love is if I am perfect."

Second Cervical - *Holds the meaning of life*

Possible associated feelings: resentment, blame, worthlessness, defeat, desertion

Possible core negative beliefs: "If I know the truth, it will only cause me pain." "God is my enemy." "It is dangerous to tell the truth or be accountable."

Third Cervical - *The self's ability to be itself.*

Possible associated feelings: shame, blame, guilt, fear, anxiety, belligerence

Possible core negative beliefs: "I always get exploited." "It is always my fault." "I can never get it right."

Fourth Cervical - *The right to decide who we want to become or not*

Possible associated feelings: guilt, bitterness, disconnection, rage, resignation, joylessness

Possible core negative beliefs: "I feel guilty for everything." "It is always my fault." "I have to magically have all the answers." "I have to magically know how to fix it."

Fifth Cervical - *The knowledge that we deserve joy*

Possible associated feelings: fear of making mistakes, fear of ridicule, nothing good can ever happen for me, control is everything

Possible core negative beliefs: "I just can't figure it out." "I am responsible for everything that goes wrong." "My intuition only gets me in trouble." "They just think I am a psychic freak."

Sixth Cervical - *Sacred Wisdom - collected wisdom from the ages*

Possible associated feelings: burdened, overloaded, inflexible, rigid, legalistic

Possible core negative beliefs: "I cannot be out of control." "The only way to be safe is to be rational and logical." "It is my job to fix everyone."

Seventh Cervical - *Self-acceptance mirrored by the acceptance of Divine Source*

Possible associated feelings: abandonment, rejection, confusion, anger, helplessness, deprivation, blame

Possible negative core beliefs: "I can never be rich and beautiful." "I have no right to be me." "I can't trust anyone or anything, least of all myself." "I must have done something awful for God to hate me so."

First Thoracic - *Respect for the process of alignment and the energy to flow with it*

Possible associated feelings: hopelessness, despair, apathy, grief, anger toward self

Possible core negative beliefs: "There is nothing more to do; there is no hope." "Life is just too hard; I can't cope with its difficulties." "I have no options left but to withdraw."

Second Thoracic - *The energy necessary to defend our right to self-actualize*

Possible associated feelings: fear, hurt, distrust, indifference, pride

Possible core negative beliefs: "I can't trust God." "The pain is so great that I can't let myself feel or I will be destroyed." "Love can only destroy me." "I am not lovable and will never have any peace."

Third Thoracic - *Holds the gem of our innocence*

Possible associated feelings: desire to return to innocence, connection to self-love, issues of good/bad self

Possible core negative beliefs: "I am bad," "I don't have a right to exist," and "I am not deserving of love."

Fourth Thoracic - *Alignment and flow*

Possible associated feelings: shame, guilt, grief, blame, separation, inadequacy

Possible core negative beliefs: "I can never be good enough." "The world is an evil place." "I don't deserve happiness."

Fifth Thoracic - *Search for innocence*

Possible associated feelings: confusion, dissatisfaction, disappointment, feeling lost

Possible core negative beliefs: "I just don't know what to think." "I can never get better." "This pain will never end."

Sixth Thoracic - *Getting needs met*

Possible associated feelings: envy, greed, sorrow, jealousy, fear of loss

Possible core negative beliefs: "I am inherently evil." "I can never have enough." "I don't deserve good in my life."

Seventh Thoracic - *Our connection to the greater universe and the belief it holds about us*

Possible associated feelings: low self-esteem, lack of worth and value, depression, apathy

Possible core negative beliefs: "I don't deserve success." "Life is not worth living." "I can never master life itself." "I am doomed to mediocrity."

Eighth Thoracic - *Natural energy needed to create and maintain life or Kundalini*

Possible associated feelings: When started, Kundalini energy fuels the entire physical system as it travels up the spine, making active each of the chakra centers. It connects the material to the spiritual. It is raw life force energy.

Possible core negative beliefs: Sexual inhibitions, low-iron blood, lack of money (first chakra issues), as well as work addictions and violent behavior

Ninth Thoracic - *Aligns us with our abilities and right to choose that which unites us with our higher purpose and essential needs*

Possible feelings: loss, abandonment, confusion, fear, anxiety, betrayal, victimhood

Possible core negative beliefs: "I can never be me." "I feel like an alien." "I don't know how to choose for myself."

Tenth Thoracic - *Necessary perceptions required to express authentically*

Possible feelings: a lack of harmony, struggle between good and evil, a lack of attunement with others

Possible core negative beliefs: "I can never be in harmony with the world around me." "I am a freak—I just don't fit in."

Eleventh Thoracic - *Understanding similarities*

Possible feelings: disgust, arrogance, indifference, hostility, rage, judgmental attitudes

Possible core negative beliefs: "They are all fools." "They need to be done away with." "They are the cause of all ills in the world." "Everyone should live as I do."

Twelfth Thoracic - *Understanding oppositional qualities*

Possible feelings: apathy, insecurity, worry, inadequacy, internal struggle, indecision·

Possible core negative beliefs: "I can never be safe." "What is the use? Nothing works," "I

am so confused; I just can't figure it out." "I just don't know what my purpose is." "I give up."

First Lumbar - *Perceptions of male universal energies*

Possible feelings: empowerment, courage, anger, rage, helplessness

Possible core negative beliefs: "I must achieve no matter what." "I am worthless unless I can achieve and defend those I love." "I must stand up for what I believe or else."

Second Lumbar - *Perceptions regarding universal feminine energy*

Possible feelings: grief, sorrow, loss, fear, powerlessness, lack, insecurity.

Possible core negative beliefs: "I will never be enough." "I must be in control of everything to be safe." "I must find the answer."

Third Lumbar - *the twelfth chakra - connection between natural forces and the physical body*

Possible feelings: anger, control, depression, fear, lack, limitation

Possible core negative beliefs: "It is my heredity that is the problem." "I just can't stomach the world." "I have to work very hard to get ahead." "There is no joy in Bloodville."

Fourth Lumbar - *connected to the eleventh chakra, transmutation of energy*

Possible feelings: capable, strong, perceptive, transformational, expressive, frustrated

Possible core negative beliefs: "Opportunities never come my way." "I never get the help I need."

Fifth Lumbar - *connected to the soul chakra or ninth chakra, programming the soul*

Possible feelings: déjà vu, archetypal symbols and myths may bring insight and clarity.

Possible core negative beliefs: "This has happened to me before, and I can't change it." "I don't know what's wrong, but it is my destiny."

First Sacral - *connected to the Eighth Chakra - seat of the Akashic Records*

Possible feelings: unbalanced, procrastination, rebellious, antagonistic, frustrated

Possible core negative beliefs: "I can never get anywhere on time." "I always seem to be off-balance, out of sync." "I seem to keep having the same problems repeatedly."

Second Sacral - *connected to the seventh chakra - the crown chakra - reception of higher levels of information*

Possible feelings: depression, lack of direction, ungrounded, inability to self-reflect

Possible core negative beliefs: "I must not have a purpose for being here."

Third Sacral - *connected to the sixth chakra - the third-eye chakra – self-image and the means of shaping ones's worldview*

Possible feelings: intuition, insight, "seeing" the bigger picture emotionally

Possible core negative beliefs: "It is evil to be psychic." "I don't dare share my intuitive insights for fear of retaliation."

Fourth Sacral - *related to the fifth chakra - throat chakra - ability to defend ourselves in the world*

Possible feelings: fear, insecurity, inadequacy, lack, limitation

Possible core negative beliefs: "I have no responsibility for my life." "I don't know how to say no." "I don't have any power over what happens to me."

Fifth Sacral - *related to the fourth chakra - the heart chakra - ability to relate*

Possible feelings: compassion, love, hate, resentment, betrayal, acceptance, forgiveness, joy, misery

Possible core negative beliefs: "I am not lovable." "No one cares about me." "I will never be able to achieve my dreams."

First Coccygeal - *related to the third chakra - solar plexus chakra - opinions and beliefs*

Possible feelings: low self-esteem, self-denigration, apathy, shame, resentment, hostility

Possible core negative beliefs: "I have no power in the world." "I don't measure up." "I need someone to take care of me."

Second Coccygeal - *related to the second chakra - reproductive chakra - feeling concerned for self and others*

Possible feelings: rage, anger, hurt, disappointment, fear, resentment, worry, guilt, inadequacy, victimhood

Possible core negative beliefs: "If I get angry, that makes me a bad person." "I must take care of others to be important."

Third Coccygeal - *related to the first chakra - the base chakra - where we store our roots and our heritage, our right to be here and to occupy space, to be loved and to love, to get our needs met.*

Possible feelings: passion, rage, terror, joy, entitlement, excitement, enthusiasm

Possible core negative beliefs: "I don't belong here." "I don't deserve happiness." "I don't have the right to have more than enough."

Fourth Coccygeal - *related to the tenth chakra - the grounding chakra at the feet*

Possible feelings: confusion, paranoia, fear, anxiety

Possible core negative beliefs: "I can never be safe in this world." "They are all out to get me." "The only way I can survive is to dissociate from the world."

CHAPTER EIGHTEEN

MATRIX XII

SEVEN RAYS

Ray energy is the focus of Matrix XII of the Energy Matrix Clearing System. I chose it as the final matrix because of its complexity. Ray energy holds the final key to the patterns inherent in the human psyche and, ultimately, the manifestations of human endeavor. Let me say at the outset of this chapter that in no way is it possible for me to cover the extensive material regarding ray energy. Therefore, for further education and understanding of the impact of ray energy on the human species, I suggest the student read the work of Alice Bailey, who wrote five volumes on the rays, and David Tansley, who brought the language of the rays to radionics work; and Arthur E. Powell's compilation of Theosophical thinking on the subject.

"Each aspect of the esoteric constitution of man is qualified by a ray energy," Tansley suggests. "So there is the ray of the monad or spirit, the ray of the soul, the ray of the mental body, the ray of the emotional body[,] and those of the etheric body and personality."[228]

It is common knowledge in energy work that humans are pulsating, vibrating beings of light and sound. Human-emitted frequencies can be translated into color using the Resonant Field Imaging system developed by the Institute of Technical Energy Medicine. The RFI, perhaps best described as a type of external MRI, gives information regarding physical health, mental/emotional health, and the chakra system. This energetic diagnostic system is significant in educating the client regarding the health and wellbeing of each system. The energy we generate through our thoughts, feelings, and emotions plays an important role not only in our personal physical, mental, emotional, and spiritual health but also in how we interact with the external world. It is a truth that "what you think you create."

I utilized the RFI technology for fifteen years or more in my practice because it was the best diagnostic technology available for energy work at the time. The Institute of Technical Energy Medicine closed its doors in 2019 as technology advanced and RFI became outdated. In 2020, I shifted to a system developed by Solex called AO Scan™, a comprehensive tool for measuring and optimizing frequencies.

Previous chapters and matrices have focused on the energy of the chakras, meridian system, and subtle energy bodies. Each of these systems vibrates with its own frequencies and, therefore, colors. The question then arises: "Are these systems generating specific colors based on each individual system's base of operation, or are each of these systems driven by an energy/vibration downloaded from beyond the individual human energy system?"

Tansley states, "These rays then form the life-pattern of the individual and confer upon him his strengths and weaknesses, his potential and limitations. In times of inner crisis, an understanding of these ray energies and their effects can serve as a focal point from which a new awareness and orientation can be achieved."[229]

Many questions may arise from Tansley's observation: From whence do the rays originate? What is their purpose? What is their effect on humanity? Are they divinely created? Can they be human-directed or changed? What part do they play in health and wellbeing? Answering these questions would take a lifetime of study involving astrology, energy systems, star systems, planetary systems, solar systems, and more.

My aim is to answer, at least in part, the questions that are pertinent to EMCS. In chapter thirteen I explain the connection between the twelve cranial nerves and the twelve houses of the astrology chart. Here, you will learn that the astrological signs are included in the system of ray energy.

Before beginning a more in-depth study of the rays, it is necessary to have knowledge of the fundamental propositions upon which this information is founded. Alice Bailey suggests, "They are for me, a humble worker in the Hierarchy, as they are for the Great White Lodge as a whole, a statement of fact and of truth, for students and seekers they must be accepted as an hypothesis."[230]

As Bailey outlines, these propositions are as follows and are reprinted here with permission from the publisher:

PROPOSITION #1: There is one Life, which expresses Itself primarily through seven basic qualities or aspects, and secondarily through the myriad diversity of forms.

PROPOSITION #2: These seven radiant qualities are the seven Rays, the seven Lives, Who give Their Life to the forms and give the form world its meaning, its laws, and its urge to evolution.

PROPOSITION #3: Life, quality and appearance, or spirit, soul and body constitute all that exists. They are existence itself, with its capacity for growth, for activity, for manifestation of beauty, and for full conformity to the Plan. This Plan is rooted in the consciousness of the seven ray Lives.

PROPOSITION #4: These seven Lives, Whose nature is consciousness and Whose expression is sentiency and specific quality, produce cyclically the manifested world; They work together in the closest union and harmony, and co-operate intelligently with the Plan of which They are the custodians. They are the seven Builders, Who produce the radiant temple of the Lord, under the guidance of the Mind of the Great Architect of the Universe.

PROPOSITION #5: Each ray Life is predominantly expressing Itself through one of the seven sacred planets, but the Life of all the seven flows through every planet, including the Earth, and thus qualifies every form. On each planet is a small replica of the general scheme, and every planet conforms to the intent and purpose of the whole.

PROPOSITION #6: Humanity, with which this treatise deals, is an expression of the Life of God, and every human being has come forth along one line or other of these seven ray forces. The nature of his soul is qualified or determined by the ray Life which breathed him forth, and his form nature is colored by the ray Life which—in its cyclic appearance on the physical plane at any particular time—sets the quality of the race life and of the forms in the kingdoms of nature. The sour nature or quality remains the same throughout a world period; its form life and nature change form life to life, according to its cyclic need and the environing group condition. This latter is determined by the ray or rays in incarnation at the time.

PROPOSITION #7: The Monad is the Life, lived in unison with the seven ray Lives. One Monad, seven rays and myriad of forms— this is the structure behind the manifested worlds.

PROPOSITION #8: The Laws which govern the emergence of the quality or soul, through the medium of forms, are simply the mental purpose and life direction of the ray Lords, Whose purpose is immutable, Whose vision is perfect, and Whose justice is supreme.

PROPOSITION #9: The mode or method of development for humanity is self-expression and self-realization. When this process is consummated the self expressed in the One Self or the ray Life, and the realization achieved is the revelation of God as the quality of the manifested world and as the Life behind appearance and quality. The seven ray Lives, or the seven soul types, are seen as the expression of one Life, and diversity is lost in the vision of the One and in identification with the One.

PROPOSITION #10: The method employed to bring about this realization is experience, beginning with individualization and ending with initiation, this producing the perfect blending and expression of life-quality-appearance.[231]

As Bailey writes, "This is a brief statement of the Plan. Of this the Hierarchy of Masters in Its seven divisions (the correspondences of the seven rays) is the custodian, and with Them lies the responsibility in any century of carrying out the next state of that Plan."[232]

As defined, a ray is a particular force or type of energy, with the emphasis upon the quality of the force and not its form-aspect.

Each ray has a color attribute and has a relationship with a particular chakra. There are seven rays or "builders," according to Tansley, but having said that, the ray we are interested in here is the second ray of love/wisdom because that is the ray being developed on planet Earth. Christ and Buddha introduced the second ray of love/wisdom to humanity. From this point on I will speak to the subset seven rays of the second ray. Let's look first at an overview of the rays.

The Rays of Aspect expressing from the Father Nature:

- First Ray   Power, will, and purpose
- Second Ray   Love/wisdom
- Third Ray   Active intelligence

The Rays of Attribute expressing from the Mother Nature:

- Fourth Ray   Harmony through conflict
- Fifth Ray   Science and knowledge
- Sixth Ray   Idealism and devotion
- Seventh Ray   Order and ceremonial magic

- First Ray   Red   Crown chakra

- Second Ray   Blue   Heart chakra
- Third Ray   Yellow   Throat chakra
- Fourth Ray   Orange   Brow chakra
- Fifth Ray   Green   Sacral chakra
- Sixth Ray   Violet   Solar plexus chakra
- Seventh Ray   Indigo   Base chakra

The Energy Matrix Clearing System incorporates the seven rays in the tradition of Alice Bailey and David Tansley. Tansley determined the method for identifying ray energy in his patients using the dowsing method over seven symbols which he determined represented the seven rays. They are as follows:

- First Ray: circle and dot
- Second Ray: Christian cross
- Third Ray: equilateral triangle
- Fourth Ray: wave
- Fifty Ray: Pentagram
- Sixth Ray: four petals
- Seventh Ray: swastika

The First Ray: Power, Will, and Purpose

The First Ray of Will and Power can through destruction lead to liberation, which is similar to the Chinese philosophical belief that creation precedes destruction and destruction precedes creation, always leading to choice.

Some esoteric titles given the first ray are:

- The Lord of Death
- The Liberator from Form
- The Most High
- The Will that Breaks into the Garden
- The Lord of the Burning Ground

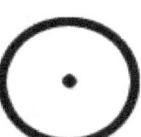

Its qualities include a purposeful attitude, natural leadership, positive drive, directness in personal relationships, and the ability to initiate activities and govern men. First Ray people tend to be ambitious and arrogant, with a love of power. They may lack compassion and tend to be impatient, irritable, and inflexible. Some examples of First Ray people from the past are: Roosevelt, Napoleon, Genghis Khan, Alexander the Great, Hitler, and Mussolini. We could add from the present Donald Trump and Hillary Clinton.

Bailey and Tansley both tell us that each ray has four distinct qualities: special virtues, vices, glamours, and virtues to be acquired.

SPECIAL VIRTUES: Strength, courage, steadfastness, truthfulness arising from absolute fearlessness, power to rule, capacity to grasp great questions and concepts in a large-minded way, and ability to handle men and their actions.

VICES: Pride, ambition, willfulness, hardness, arrogance, desire to control others, anger, and obstinacy.

GLAMORS: Love of power and authority, pride, selfish ambition, impatience, irritation, coldness, aloofness, and selfishness.

VIRTUES TO BE ACQUIRED: Tenderness, sympathy, humility, tolerance, patience, and compassion.

The Second Ray: Love and Wisdom

Characteristics of this ray include universal love, intuition, insight, cooperation, philanthropy, and wisdom. From this ray emerges the healers, teachers, sages, and reformers of humanity. Their mission is to save their fellow man by healing, serving, and elevating their consciousness to ever higher levels of vibration. The higher octaves of teaching from this ray produce the initiatory processes of the Illumined Ones, and the lower octaves express through religion.

Second Ray people tend to be naturally sympathetic, concerned for others, and well liked. As such, they mix easily with others. They are the peacemakers but can tend toward pessimistic attitudes and can be easily deflected from their purpose. Their weaknesses lie in sentimentality, sensuality, and impracticality. Mother Teresa of Calcutta and Pope John Paul II are examples of Second Ray people.

SPECIAL VIRTUES: Calm, strength, patience, endurance, love of truth, faithfulness, intuition, serene temper, and clear intelligence.

VICES: Coldness (if the wisdom aspect is overemphasized), indifference to others, contempt for mental limitations in others, and over absorption in studies.

GLAMORS: Fear, negativity, poor self-image, feelings of inferiority and inadequacy, depression, anxiety, and self-pity.

VIRTUES TO BE ACQUIRED: Love, compassion, and unselfishness.

Second Ray energy has been referred to as:
- The Displayer of Glory
- The Radiance in the Form
- The Great Geometrician
- The Cosmic Christ
- The Lord of Eternal Love

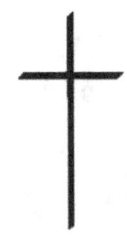

For the healer, these names are potential states to move toward through meditation and internal focus.

The Third Ray: Active Intelligence

Qualities of this ray are creative ideation, adaptability, impartiality, dignity, comprehension, and understanding. It is the ray of industry, business, technology, communications, and transport. This ray has the power to evoke form. Third Ray people are the true builders; they enjoy success in business and have great money sense and physical coordination. They are the astrologer, scholar, diplomat, philosopher, judge, bander, economist, chess player, strategist, and director, according to Tansley.

SPECIAL VIRTUES: Ability to see the bigger picture, sincerity of purpose, clear intellect, capacity for concentration on philosophic studies, patience, caution, and an absence of worry over trivial matters.

VICES: Intellectual pride, coldness, isolation, inaccuracy in details, absent-mindedness, obstinacy, selfishness, and overly critical of others.

GLAMORS: Business, materialism, preoccupation with detail to the point of causing paralysis of action, efficiency, feelings of self-importance and intellectual superiority, manipulative, and devious.

VIRTUES TO BE ACQUIRED: Tolerance, devotion, common sense, accuracy, and sympathy. Healers on this ray work best using herbs and minerals belonging to the Third Ray.

Third Ray energy names:
- The Builder of the Foundation
- The Great Architect of the Universe
- The Dispenser of Time
- The Lord of Memory
- The Illuminator of the Lotus

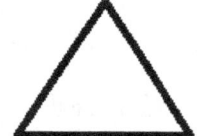

The Fourth Ray: Harmony through Conflict

This is the ray of the artist, the mediator, and the interpreter. Inherent in this ray is the sensitivity to color and form in the right proportion, but there is also an inertia aspect of this ray that may prevent Fourth Ray people from fully expressing their. Fourth ray people may be depressed, despondent, and discontent. They may tend to be ambivalent, vacillate between options, and can be emotionally unstable. They may overreact to situations and be hyperactive one moment and indolent the next. Since conflict is a major component of this ray, harmony is the ultimate aim.

SPECIAL VIRTUES: Strong affection, sympathy, physical courage, generosity, devotion, and quickness of intellect and perception.

VICES: Self-centeredness, worrying, inaccuracy, lack of moral courage, strong passions, indolence, and extravagance.

GLAMORS: Diffusion of interests and energy, impracticality and the and the glamour of imagination, grandiose schemes, vagueness, lack of objectivity, inner and outer conflict causing argument and acrimony, and dissatisfaction because of overly sensitive response to that which is better, and more beautiful.

VIRTUES TO BE ACQUIRED: Serenity, confidence, self-control, accuracy, mental and moral balance, and unselfishness.

Fourth Ray energy names:

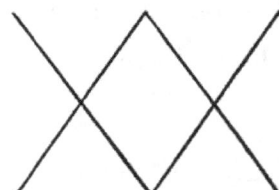

- The Perceiver on the Way
- The Divine Intermediary
- The Corrector of the Form
- The Dweller in the Holy Place

Bailey suggests the path of the fourth ray leads to the "Birth of Horus" or the Christ within.

The Fifth Ray: Concrete Knowledge and Science

The influence of this ray is on the lower mind, giving rise to science and the meaning of colors. The lawyer, scientist, mathematician, physicist, and astronomer are found on this ray. People on this ray analyze and quantify; they are intolerant of cloudy thinking and need everything measured and proven according to the scientific standards of the time. They have narrow convictions, intellectual pride and prejudice, and are intensely materialistic. Healers of this ray are locked into the use of crude and destructive drugs. It has proven to be, however, the quantum physicist who has led the way into the esoteric realms, as predicted by Alice Bailey in the 1930s.

SPECIAL VIRTUES: Perseverance, common sense, justice without mercy, strictly accurate statements, uprightness, independence, keen intellect, and perceptive mental penetration and application.

VICES: Narrowness, lack of sympathy, an unforgiving temper, harsh criticism, prejudice, and little reverence.

GLAMORS: Constant analysis and splitting of hairs, criticism, overemphasis of form while neglecting the life aspect, cold mental assessment and disparagement of feeling, intellectual pride, reason, holding proof and intellectuality as sacrosanct.

VIRTUES TO BE ACQUIRED: devotion, sympathy, love, and open-mindedness.

Fifth Ray names:

- The Revealer of Truth
- The Dispenser of Knowledge
- The Dividing Sword

- The Guardian of the Door

The Sixth Ray: Devotion

This ray fuels idealism and nationalistic attitudes. It is also the ray of the archetypal expressions of the saint, martyr, mystic, and evangelist. Sixth Ray energy dominated during the Crusades and subsequent religious wars. Tansley states, "The Inquisition was a manifestation of [Sixth Ray] energy, and those carrying it out felt it quite in order to burn people at the stake in order to 'save' their souls."[233] This ray is about blind devotion to those they perceive as gurus. Sixth Ray people can be bigoted and fanatical, such as those we find with the militant Sunni-Salafi-jihadist organization ISIL today. They are loyal to a cause, no matter if it is good or bad.

SPECIAL VIRTUES: Devotion, single-mindedness, love, tenderness, intuition, loyalty, and reverence.

VICES: Partiality, over-dependence on others, selfish and jealous love, self-deception, prejudice, sectarianism, fiery anger, and over-rapid conclusions.

GLAMORS: Fanaticism, narrow-mindedness, love of the past and existing forms, possessiveness, exaggerated devotion, reluctance to change, rigidity, too much intensity of feeling, and hero worship.

VIRTUES TO BE ACQUIRED: Strength, purity, self-sacrifice, truth, tolerance, serenity, balance, common sense, and flexibility.

Sixth Ray names:

- The Divine Robber
- The Crucifier and the Crucified
- The Devotee of Life
- The Hater of Forms
- The Warrior on the March

Prayer, faith, and inspiration are the tools of the healer on the sixth ray path. Christianity and spin-off religions are the higher expressions of the Sixth Ray. King Arthur and his Knights of the Round Table, with their high ideals and altruistic deeds, are expressions of the sixth ray.

The Seventh Ray: Ceremonial Magic or Order

The rules for law and order flow from this ray. Seventh Ray people are the ceremonialist, ritualist, magician, producer, and pageant-master. Shamans, high priests, and court chamberlains are a product of this ray path. Seventh Ray people are also born organizers and synthesizers, governing the areas of ceremony, sex, money, and government. Ordered daily functions, such as the routines involved in getting up—showering, dressing, eating breakfast, going to work—are a reflection of the Seventh Ray. Tansley says of the method of using subtle force fields and energies in the diagnosis and treatment of disease, "Radionics is certainly a [Seventh Ray] healing technique very much allied to ceremonial and ritual white magic, and to life-force which sustains man through the chakras, most notably the base chakra which it governs."[234]

Seventh Ray people have a distaste for the loss of outer power, humiliation, discourtesy, rudeness, frustration, and adverse criticism coming from one of lesser standing. Grace, precision, and ordered beauty is their forte.

SPECIAL VIRTUES: Strength, perseverance, courage, courtesy, extreme care in details, and self-reliance.

VICES: Formalism, bigotry, pride, narrowness, superficial judgement, fussiness, over-indulgence of one's self-opinion, fastidiousness, excessive organization.

GLAMORS: Rigid adherence to law and order, over-emphasis on organization and form, love of the secret and the mysterious, psychism, the glamour of ritual and ceremony, and a deep interest in omens and superstition.

VIRTUES TO BE ACQUIRED: Realization of unity, open-mindedness, tolerance, humility, gentleness, and love.

Seventh ray names:
- The Unveiled Magician
- The Worker in the Magical Art
- The Keeper of the Magical Word
- The Divine Alchemical Worker
- The Orienting Force
- The Key to the Mystery
- The One Who Lifts to Life

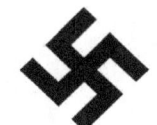

This brief overview of the rays only touches the tip of the iceberg, but it gives a starting point for understanding ray energy and how it shows up in the lives of humans. Tansley says that, "As a rule this type of information is of use to those patients who are consciously following the spiritual path, to those who are passing through a crisis point in their lives, or who really need the insight to re-orient themselves or alter their lifestyle to include the call of the inner way."[235]

Muscle checking for current ray influence

When testing a client for their ray energy in EMCS, test the symbols by the number, beginning with the symbol for the transpersonal self. Use this language when testing:

"Give me an indicator change for the monad ray, one through seven," followed by:

"Give me an indicator change for the symbol indicating which ray the soul of the client is utilizing in this incarnation by the number one through seven."

Next, repeat the process for each of the subtle energy bodies—astral, mental, and causal—and then test for the personality ray.

After testing for the personality ray, muscle check for which body the soul ray is predominantly working through.

Finally, muscle check for which ray the personality is working through.

This information will help identify for the client which characteristics, capacities, and limitations will be reduced or enhanced. This will clarify issues for defusion work toward continued spiritual growth.

The seven rays are also divided into the rays of love and the rays of will. Rays two, four, and six are rays of love. Rays one, three, five, and seven are rays of will. This knowledge will help in understanding certain subtleties, like why Tansley says, "A person with a [fifth] ray mental body and a [third] ray physical will have the capacity to bring ideas through from the mind to the brain with ease[;] on the other hand if the physical body is on the [second] ray then there might be some resistance."[236]

Once you have identified the rays as discussed above, identify the qualities of each and determine how each of the rays helps or challenges the client's quest for soul growth. The challenges become issues for EMCS defusion work.

CHAPTER NINETEEN

CONCLUSION

PUTTING IT ALL TOGETHER

I began the main body of this book with this quote from the fifteenth-century vitalist physician Paracelsus: "External nature moulds the shape of internal nature, and if nature vanishes, the inner nature is also lost; for the outer is the mother of the inner."

There is another axiom that forms the fundamental principle of all spiritual science as well: "As above, so below," which has become known as the Hermetic Axiom. This is the basis upon which the Energy Matrix Clearing System is founded.

Within this simple statement lies the understanding, illuminated through spiritual science, that the world we humans access through our five senses, the world "below," is not all there is. There is a deeper world that is hidden behind that which we comprehend with our five senses and our intellect. That is the spiritual world, which the Hermetic Axiom calls "above."

Paracelsus and Hermes, as well as many other master teachers throughout history, clearly understood that the world of the five senses was not all there was. They knew that what they were seeing was a reflection, or, as Fisher explains:

> Rather, a kind of physiognomy which he recognizes as the expression of a world of soul and spirit, just as when you gaze upon a human countenance, you must not stop at the form of the face and the gestures, paying attention only to them, but must pass, as a matter of course, from the physiognomy and the gestures to the spiritual element which is expressed in them.[237]

The process of EMCS takes the world of "below" and, step by step, interprets that world, enabling the world of "above" to emerge little by little until, at last, the greater truth is seen.

It begins with the energician connecting with the client in a sacred way and in a sacred space, listening with the heart and mind to the story of the client. This story, or the "below," becomes the access point to the world of the "above." It is a sacred journey, and it unfolds in an elegant and graceful manner, making it possible for the client to see the journey through the eyes of the higher self. There is no judgment in the process, only compassion and forgiveness for the unknowing. Each component of EMCS is designed to open the gates of the "above" in which the "below" is revealed, illuminating the darkness and flooding it with the light of wisdom and truth. Thus, the Energy Matrix Clearing System effects a vibrational shift from "within" that naturally flows into "without" in an elegant flow of light, illuminating life from a whole new perspective.

I conclude this work with a quote from Bruce Fisher's *Man, Grand Reflection of the Greater Cosmos: Studies in Occult Anatomy*:

What actually constitutes wisdom? Spiritual science has always maintained that human wisdom has something to do with experience and *that* painful experience. He who is actually in the throes of suffering manifests in this suffering something that is an inward lack of harmony. He, however, who has overcome the pain and suffering and bears their fruits within him, will always tell you that through suffering, he has gained some measure of wisdom. The joys and pleasures of life, all that life can offer me in the way of satisfaction, all these things do I receive gratefully; yet were I far more loath to part with my pain and suffering than with those pleasant gifts of life, for it is to my pain and suffering that I owe my wisdom. And so it is that in wisdom, occult science has ever recognized what may be called crystallized pain - pain that has been conquered *and thus changed into its opposite.* Occult investigation shows decisively that all things which surround us in this world - the mineral foundation, the vegetable covering, and the animal world - should be regarded as the physiognomical expression, or the "below," of an "above" or spirit life lying behind them.[238]

AFTERWORD

I began this journey into the world of human bioenergy with a single thought: "I think the cause of relapse is cellular shame." I was the clinical director of an outpatient chemical dependency program at a local hospital at the time, and I saw many clients who had been through treatment return at a later date after relapsing. I wondered what we were missing. Looking for answers to the cause of relapse, I explored a myriad of therapies, from psychodrama to inner child work, Ericksonian hypnosis to Transcendental Meditation. It wasn't until I was introduced to Transformational Kinesiology in 1991 that I was sure I had the answer—cellular shame—and the method that would access and release that shame. Those realizations led to the creation of the Energy Matrix Clearing System that I use today.

What started as a way to help me treat addiction and prevent relapse eventually became my treatment modality for a host of ailments. As a result, the system has morphed since its inception to include more systems and options for clearing not only cellular shame but also limiting beliefs, trauma, and other energy blockages that create distortions of life energy.

There are many stories of success that have come out of my thirty-plus years of working with clients from all walks of life, but none more poignant than that of an infant who was born premature and with a prognosis of a short life lived in a vegetated state. This was in 1992, the first year I was in private practice. The infant's grandmother, with home I had worked clearing her fear of flying, brought her to me with the hope that my method would help her granddaughter.

The newborn was almost lifeless, her eyes blank and her arms and legs tiny and motionless. I held my hand palm down over the top of her head, seeking a connection to her energy field. After a minute or two, I began to feel an electrical pulse in my palm. In order to gain permission to work with her in this specific way, I began to ask a series of questions intended to communicate with her higher self. Permission was granted to begin the work. While her grandmother held her, I explored her energy systems to determine if there were blockages in those systems. First, the meridian system, then the chakras, and finally, the subtle energy systems and their chakras. I found blockages in the kidney and lung meridians and the lower three chakras. I cleared the blockages using homeopathic gem and mineral essences. Her grandmother helped me administer the drops. With that done, the session was over. The report from the medical community was bleak at best. They did not expect the infant to live more than five years, and with that, no quality of life. Given these assessments, neither I nor the grandmother had any expectations of a positive outcome. Still, we were willing to try. We agreed on another session for the following week.

The grandmother reported that shortly after the last session, her granddaughter's bowels had begun to work naturally. She also noticed that the infant was able to track movement with her eyes. She said it was like she had woken up. We were both excited at the change and hopeful that other changes could be made as well, even though the doctors did not think that she would have any cognitive ability or be able to walk or communicate in any meaningful way.

I began our second session in the same way, with my palm over the baby's head, waiting until I received a connection with her energy field. The connection came much more quickly this time, and I continued to search for blockages in her energy system. At the time, I was wearing an antique Edwardian-style ring set with a faceted aquamarine stone. The ring had rotated so that the stone was on the underside of my finger rather than on the top. It was that hand that I was holding over the infant's body to access her information from her energy field. She reached up to touch the stone of the ring. Her grandmother and I were amazed—not only had she noticed the stone, but she had reached up to touch it.

That was the beginning of the infant's healing. I continued to work with her throughout the years. She was never able to walk, but her mind and verbal skills were phenomenal. She is in her twenties today and has completed both a bachelor's and master's degree in counseling and is employed doing virtual therapy. She is also a prolific writer.

If I ever questioned the efficacy of the Energy Matrix Clearing System, working with that tiny baby and watching her progress allayed all those doubts.

APPENDIX I

ENERGY MATRIX CLEARING SYSTEM

SCRIPT

1. Show me a yes.
    Show me a no.

2. What's a yes?
    What's a no?

3. You are here and present and communicating energetically on every level: body, mind, emotional, essential, etheric, astral, mental, causal.

    You are somewhere else.

4. I have permission to work with you in this way.

    I do not have permission to work with you in this way.

5. You commit to taking 100 percent responsibility for: noticing, acting on, and benefiting from the positive change without self-punishment for that change.

    You are not willing to commit.

6. I have permission to focus this process on diffusing _____that would support that belief that _____.

    I do not have permission.

    This is the highest priority.

    It is not the highest priority.

I need to add something to the statement.

I need to take something away from the statement.

7. Our command is that any miasm, universal subconscious negative prompters, belief systems, life experiences, past life experiences, genetic imprinting, karmic ties, or any other kind of distorted

energy that would in any way cause or support these effects, be extirpated from your holographic human energy system, cancelled on a compass of time, re-patterned on all soul levels, all dimensions, known and unknown, and transformed into the universal law of light, love, balance, and rhythmic interchange.

You understand and accept the command.

You do not understand and/or accept the command.

8.   You are willing to act on that command.

You are not willing.

9.   Give me an indicator change for all that apply: Core negative belief: 1–5, 5–10, etc., through 190.

There are others under that category to identify.

10.   Shadow belief: 1–119.

Historical_____. (Past Lives) 1–5, 5–10, etc.

Past lives questions:
- Where lived: This planet? If so, what location on the planet? Other planets? If so, which one?
- Age of death in that lifetime?
- Cause of death?
- Marital status: single or married?
- Social status?
- Genetic: Which genetic line, mother's or father's? How far back (one genetic age is approximately forty years)?
- Ancestral age (this is epigenetic influence): Which line? Time period? Actual

- Grandparent?
- Lost Will: 1–19
- Dimensional Level: 1–10

11.   Give me an indicator change for the subtle bodies that hold blockages: physical, etheric, astral, mental, causal.

12.   Give me an indicator change for the level of responsibility from the EMCS Chart for this issue: emotion, feeling, thought . . .

13.   Give me an indicator change for the negative emotional energy (NEE).

Less than infinity. Less than a million. More than a million.

If less than a million, 900 thousand, 800, 700, etc., until indicator changes.

If more than a million, 50 million, 100, 200, etc., until the indicator changes.

14.   The positive emotional energy (PEE).

More than a million. Less than a million.

15.   Give me an indicator change for all that apply: Pleiadian Glyph (16).

16. The Avoidant Behavior: 1-5, 6-10, 11-15, 16-20, 21-26 . . .

17. The Universal Fear: 1-5, 6-10, 11-15, 16-20, 21-24 . . .

18. The Reflective Mirror: 1-5, 6-10, 11-15, 16-20, 21-23 . . .

19. The priority of the ten elements: earth, fire, wood, water, metal, star, aether, stone, air, light (dark/light/Rose Gold).

20. The archetypes: Major category I-XIII
    I. Traditional Archetypes. Subs: 1-12
    II. EMCS Pantheon of Gods: 1-6
    III. Archangels: 1-15
    IV. Angels 1: 1-75
    V. Major Arcana/Angels: 1-21
    VI. Ascended Masters: 1-15
    VII. Buddha Fire: 1-5
    VIII. Earth Essences: 1-13
    IX. Egyptian Magic: 1-23
    X. Angels #2: 1-40
    XI. Archangels: 1-18
    XII. Goddesses: 1-45
    XIII. Power Animals: 1-21
    XIV. Sacred Geometry: 1-21

21. The level of consciousness: 1-17

22. Gene Keys/I Ching: 1-64

23. The priority of the 72 Names: 1-72

24. Give me an indicator change for the matrix system effected: 1-13

25. Give me an indicator change for subcategory.

26. There are others to identify.

27. Drainers: how many and where are they located in the holographic human energy?

28. Entities: how many and where?

29. Curse: where is it attached?

30. A miasm, or a symptom of a miasm.

TALK ABOUT INFORMATION GATHERED IN PRESENT TIME then proceed.

31. Show me a yes.
    Show me a no.

32. I am putting the information that we have gathered, read, and discussed in the circuit.

    It is loaded.

    It is not loaded.

33. I have permission to age recess at this time.

    I do not have permission to age recess at this time.

34. Give me an indicator change for the ages on line, age of cause, age of best understanding, and best age to correct for this issue. (Example: 50 to 45, etc.)

35. Give me an indicator change for the negative emotional energy on this issue at this age.

    Less than infinity

More than infinity

36. The level of responsibility: emotion, feeling, thought

37. FlorAlive—Level I: 1-42; Level II 1-22

38. The Avoidant Behavior: 1-26

39. The Universal Fear: 1-24

40. The Reflective Mirror: 1-23

41. The priority of the ten elements: earth, fire, wood, water, metal, star, aether, stone, air, light (dark/light).

42. The archetype: 1-13, Subcategory

43. The subtle energy bodies: physical, etheric, astral, mental, causal.

44. The matrix system for correction for the systems holding blockage: 1-13

    Subcategory under each.

45. There are others to identify.

46. Drainers involved.

47. Entities involved.

48. A miasm or a symptom of a miasm.

49. Negative energetic cord: ritual, belief, trauma, hex, vow

    If vow, identify what kind of vow: poverty, chastity, religious, retribution, etc.

50. Give me an indicator change for the method of clearing the vow.

51. Category of Essences: 1-55

52. Subcategory

53. Number of drops

54. Method of use: on the tongue, under the tongue, in water

55. Repeat 51 through 53 for each identified matrix outage.

TALK ABOUT INFORMATION GATHERED IN PAST TIME

56. Show me a yes.
    Show me a no.

57. What's a yes.
    What's a no.

58. One hundred percent of all blockages have absolutely, totally, and completely been extirpated from your holographic human energy system and have been transformed into the Universal Law of Light, Love of Balance Rhythmic Interchange?

    This is true on all levels, all dimensions known and unknown, and on all points on the compass of time, from beginning of time to the end of time and all points in between.

    Any reason that is not absolutely true?

59. The negative energy is 0, and the positive 100.

It is not.

60.   We are infusing the energy of the _____.
We are infusing anything else.

Instruct the testee to imagine the energy of the infusion symbol.

Bring that energy of _____ forward in time from the age of recession in increments of five years, gently pumping their arms at each increment until reaching the present time.

Verifying: You are right here, right now, in the present time.

You are not.

The negative energy is 0 on this issue in present time.

It is not.

There will be withdrawal or residual from this process.

There will not be withdrawal or residual from this process.

The blockages holding this/these negative patterns in place have absolutely, totally, and completely been cleared from your holographic human energy.

They have not.

61.   There is some aspect remaining.

There is not.

Verify in all arm positions: Extension, contraction, and active circuit right and left.

Cleared in this position.

Not cleared in this position.

Repeat for each position.

62.   There is homework.

There is not homework. (Identify homework from the Elements or the Archetype.)

Length of focus: Number of days and number of times a day.

APPENDIX II

HUMAN BODY MERIDIANS

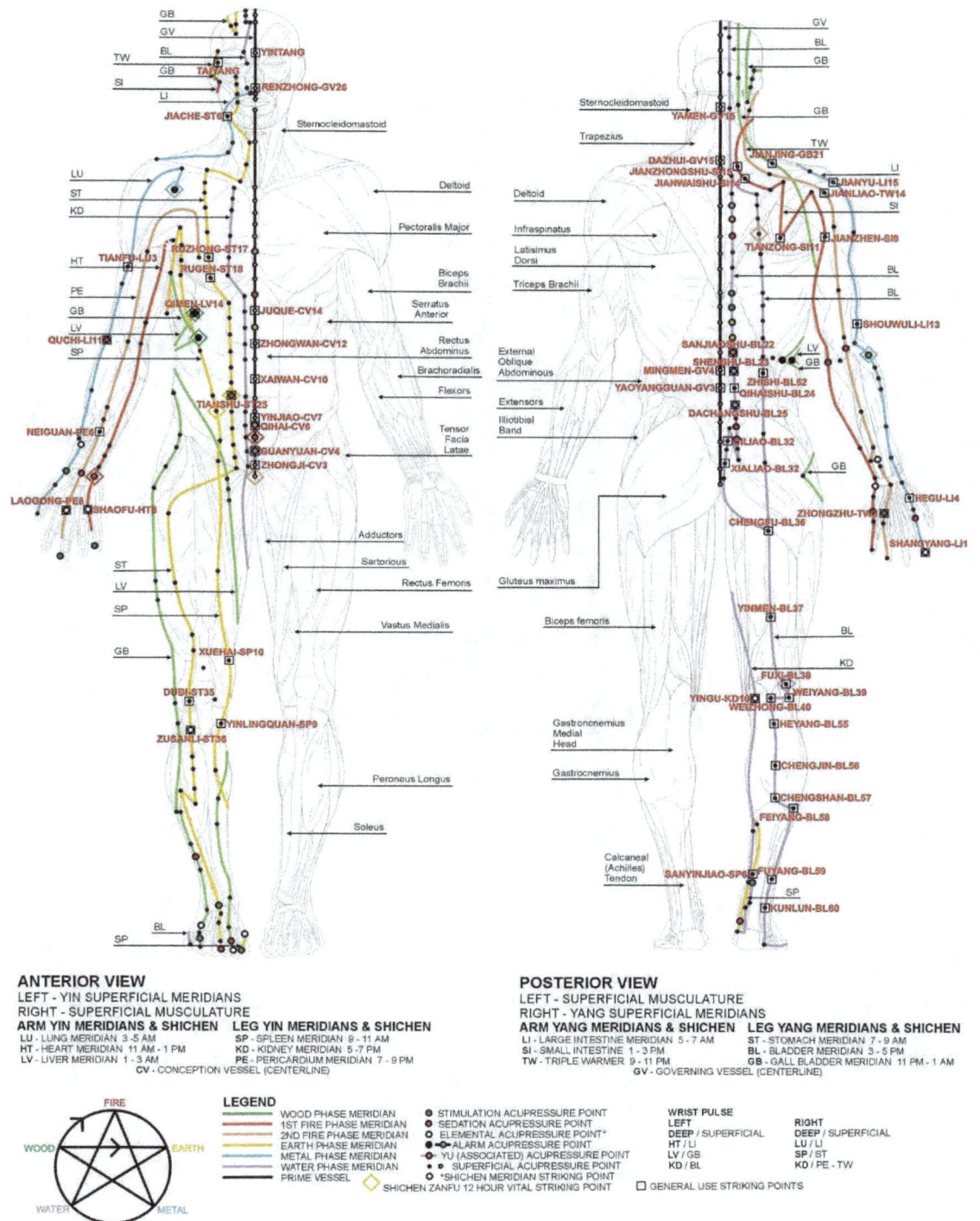

ANTERIOR VIEW
LEFT - YIN SUPERFICIAL MERIDIANS
RIGHT - SUPERFICIAL MUSCULATURE

ARM YIN MERIDIANS & SHICHEN
LU - LUNG MERIDIAN 3-5 AM
HT - HEART MERIDIAN 11 AM - 1 PM
LV - LIVER MERIDIAN 1 - 3 AM

LEG YIN MERIDIANS & SHICHEN
SP - SPLEEN MERIDIAN 9 - 11 AM
KD - KIDNEY MERIDIAN 5-7 PM
PE - PERICARDIUM MERIDIAN 7 - 9 PM
CV - CONCEPTION VESSEL (CENTERLINE)

POSTERIOR VIEW
LEFT - SUPERFICIAL MUSCULATURE
RIGHT - YANG SUPERFICIAL MERIDIANS

ARM YANG MERIDIANS & SHICHEN
LI - LARGE INTESTINE MERIDIAN 5 - 7 AM
SI - SMALL INTESTINE 1 - 3 PM
TW - TRIPLE WARMER 9 - 11 PM

LEG YANG MERIDIANS & SHICHEN
ST - STOMACH MERIDIAN 7 - 9 AM
BL - BLADDER MERIDIAN 3 - 5 PM
GB - GALL BLADDER MERIDIAN 11 PM - 1 AM
GV - GOVERNING VESSEL (CENTERLINE)

LEGEND

— WOOD PHASE MERIDIAN
— 1ST FIRE PHASE MERIDIAN
— 2ND FIRE PHASE MERIDIAN
— EARTH PHASE MERIDIAN
— METAL PHASE MERIDIAN
— WATER PHASE MERIDIAN
— PRIME VESSEL
◇ SHICHEN ZANFU 12 HOUR VITAL STRIKING POINT

● STIMULATION ACUPRESSURE POINT
● SEDATION ACUPRESSURE POINT
◎ ELEMENTAL ACUPRESSURE POINT*
●─● ALARM ACUPRESSURE POINT
◆─● YU (ASSOCIATED) ACUPRESSURE POINT
● SUPERFICIAL ACUPRESSURE POINT
● *SHICHEN MERIDIAN STRIKING POINT

□ GENERAL USE STRIKING POINTS

WRIST PULSE

LEFT	RIGHT
DEEP / SUPERFICIAL	DEEP / SUPERFICIAL
HT / LI	LU / LI
LV / GB	SP / ST
KD / BL	KD / PE - TW

FIRE
WOOD — EARTH
WATER — METAL

APPENDIX III

NEUROLYMPHATIC MASSAGE POINTS

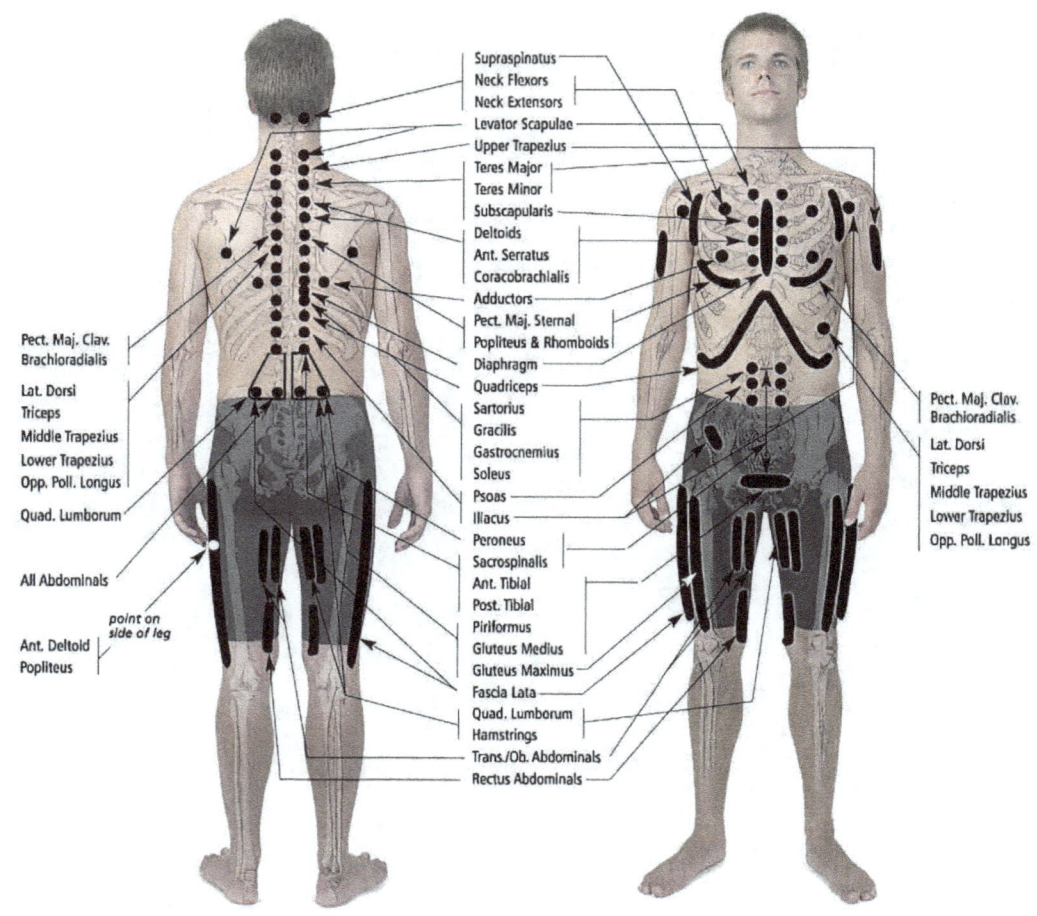

Supraspinatus
Neck Flexors
Neck Extensors
Levator Scapulae
Upper Trapezius
Teres Major
Teres Minor
Subscapularis
Deltoids
Ant. Serratus
Coracobrachialis
Adductors
Pect. Maj. Sternal
Popliteus & Rhomboids
Diaphragm
Quadriceps
Sartorius
Gracilis
Gastrocnemius
Soleus
Psoas
Iliacus
Peroneus
Sacrospinalis
Ant. Tibial
Post. Tibial
Piriformus
Gluteus Medius
Gluteus Maximus
Fascia Lata
Quad. Lumborum
Hamstrings
Trans./Ob. Abdominals
Rectus Abdominals

Pect. Maj. Clav.
Brachioradialis

Lat. Dorsi
Triceps
Middle Trapezius
Lower Trapezius
Opp. Poll. Longus

Quad. Lumborum

All Abdominals

point on
side of leg

Ant. Deltoid
Popliteus

Pect. Maj. Clav.
Brachioradialis

Lat. Dorsi
Triceps
Middle Trapezius
Lower Trapezius
Opp. Poll. Longus

APPENDIX IV

EMCS SHADOW BELIEFS

This is by no means an exhaustive list of shadow beliefs. As you do the defusion work of EMCS, you will discover others. Please add them to the list as they arise.

1. God is punishing me.
2. I was conceived in original sin.
3. I should never have been born.
4. I am not the man I want to be.
5. I am not the woman I want to be.
6. I will suffer even more than I do.
7. I am bad, no good.
8. I am helpless, powerless.
9. I am insane.
10. I am scary.
11. I am ugly.
12. I am dirty.
13. It is my fault.
14. I am hopelessly flawed.
15. It is all or nothing.
16. I owe my parents.
17. I don't deserve love.
18. I don't deserve to live.
19. I am alone.
20. Nobody loves me.
21. Nobody cares about me.
22. There is never enough love to go around.
23. I need someone special to make me happy.
24. Nobody takes care of me.
25. Nobody listens to me.
26. I have to scream, rant, rage, or have a tantrum to get you to listen to me.
27. When I am abusive or violent, I'm strong.
28. I do not matter.
29. Who I am and what I want doesn't matter.
30. I don't count.
31. I am not appreciated.
32. I am not wanted.
33. I wasn't wanted.
34. I am not worthy of friends.
35. I am not ready yet.
36. I am not creative.
37. I never had any luck.
38. I will never change.
39. I will never be enough.
40. I can never get ahead.
41. I am not good enough. I'm not worthy of love.
42. I am not worthy of health.
43. I am not worthy of friends.
44. There is something wrong with me.
45. I am wrong for being a boy.
46. I am wrong for being a girl.
47. I am wrong for not being a boy.
48. I am wrong for not being a girl.
49. Men have all the breaks in life.
50. Women have all the breaks in life.
51. There is no help for people like me, people with my problems.
52. No one can save me.
53. This will never stop.
54. It makes no sense.
55. It is not safe to be me.
56. I must be making all this up.
57. I have to be strong.
58. I have to be perfect.
59. I have to prove myself.
60. I have nothing of value to offer.
61. I never have enough time.
62. I never have enough money.
63. I am not worthy of money.
64. Even if I get or make money, I will just lose it.
65. If I get money, I'll abuse it.
66. I can't get what I want.

67. I can't do anything right.
68. I don't deserve to live.
69. I don't deserve to be alive.
70. I don't deserve happiness.
71. I don't deserve success.
72. I can't trust women.
73. I can't trust men.
74. I can't trust anyone.
75. I can trust no one but myself.
76. People hurt me.
77. People "use" me.
78. Men hurt me.
79. Women hurt me.
80. All men are insensitive.
81. All women are insensitive.
82. Life is hostile.
83. Life is hell.
84. Everyone is out to get me.
85. People are out to get me.
86. People don't like me.
87. People always abandon me.
88. I always get taken advantage of.
89. It is safer not to confront anyone because then you can't get hurt.
90. It is not safe for me to express my distrust.
91. It is not safe for me to express my emotions.
92. It is not safe for me to speak out.
93. People don't like to see my emotions.
94. Others are more important than me.
95. I am afraid of my emotions.
96. I am always last or left out.
97. I have to fight to get what I need or want.
98. Somebody it trying to kill me.
99. I don't now what to think.
100. I don't know what I trust.
101. I don't know what to trust.
102. I don't know who I trust.
103. I don't know what to do.
104. Nothing is worth doing.

105. It is difficult to be successful no matter how intelligent I am.
106. I should be able to do it all myself.
107. I should have known.
108. I should have known better.
109. You have to work very hard to get ahead.
110. I am the only one who can get the job done.
111. I can't let people down; they depend on me.
112. I am better than everybody else.
113. Life is not fair.
114. Life is hostile.
115. I hate God for putting me here.
116. I don't want to be here if this is all there is.
117. I have to fight to survive.
118. I have to fight to get what I need or want.
119. I will get even for this pain.
120. I cause people pain.
121. I need pain to survive.
122. I am queer.
123. I am disgusting.
124. I must be in control.
125. I must be right or else.
126. I must "get even" to have value and worth so that you will respect me.

APPENDIX V

Universal Fears are a form of archetypal energy addressed in the EMCS process. They are covered in depth in chapter fourteen but listed again here for quick reference:

1. Fear of abandonment and separation
2. Fear of self-worth
3. Fear of surrendering and trusting
4. Fear of our own divinity
5. Fear there is no God
6. Fear of death
7. Fear of not understanding what God is trying to teach us
8. Fear there is no recourse, so we only have ourselves to blame
9. Fear of being unsafe and unprotected
10. Fear of love
11. Fear of the Light
12. Fear of splendor
13. Fear of the death of the ego
14. Fear of being punished
15. Fear of prophecy
16. Fear of the consequences of speaking the truth
17. Fear of sexual power
18. Fear of change
19. Fear of the judgement of right versus wrong
20. Fear of being incapacitated
21. Fear of oneness
22. Fear of perfect faith
23. Fear of justice
24. Fear that we are not ready
25. Fear that we will never have a place in this world
26. Fear of present technology

APPENDIX VI

EMCS REFLECTIVE MIRRORS

Reflective Mirrors are a form of archetypal energy addressed in the EMCS process. They are covered in depth in chapter fourteen but listed again here for quick reference:

1. Reflective mirror of the moment
2. Reflective mirror of judgment
3. Reflective mirror of loss
4. Reflective mirror of self-love
5. Reflective mirror of mother/father/creator
6. Reflective mirror of the dark night of the soul
7. Reflective mirror of compassion for oneself
8. Reflective mirror of illusion
9. Reflective mirror of the illuminator of darkness
10. Reflective mirror of the power of the Light
11. Reflective mirror our journey's purpose
12. Reflective mirror of guilt
13. Reflective mirror of God/fear of splendor
14. Reflective mirror of creative work
15. Reflective mirror of free will
16. Reflective mirror of recognizing that which is hidden
17. Reflective mirror of the subconscious
18. Reflective mirror of the opened stargate
19. Reflective mirror of transformation
20. Reflective mirror of the illusion of time
21. Reflective mirror of ethics
22. Reflective mirror of the illusion that humanity can malfunction
23. Reflective mirror of being

APPENDIX VII

EMCS LEVELS OF AVOIDANCE

The EMCS levels of avoidance are drawn from the world of chiropractic medicine and are specifically associated with the ways in which we avoid taking responsibility for our recovery from illness and pain. Research has shown these levels of avoidance to be progressive, beginning with the first level of avoidance (that one's life revolves around pain), and increasing in intensity to the final (twenty-sixth) level (avoiding geopathic stress).[239]

These levels of avoidance are life limiting and eventually life threatening. I present them here as a method for determining the level of denial or fear supporting dysfunction, whether physical, mental, emotional, or spiritual (emotional and spiritual pain can be as debilitating as physical pain), and what taking responsibility looks like.

Life Revolves Around Pain

Nothing but pain matters. The pain excuses self-destructive behavior in every aspect of life: relationships, jobs, finances, negative behaviors. Doctor appointments and monitoring of pain symptoms are all I care about.

Taking responsibility: I own the responsibility for my own recovery. My life flows naturally because I live in the moment.

Dependence on Medication

I am so unhappy with my life that the only way I can get through it is by numbing the pain with medication, be it prescription drugs, illegal substances, food, relationships, exercise, or some other form of numbing agent. Whatever it is, I cannot function without it.

Taking Responsibility: I choose to take time for myself. Meditation, centering, and grounding are helping me find my life again.

Anxiety and Depression

I am anxious because I feel like I can no longer handle life's problems. I feel totally immobilized, which causes me to feel depressed. I have no self-esteem. When others point out my inability to handle life, I just get more depressed.

Taking Responsibility: I know that I have all I need within me to create the kind of life I desire. I have the courage to create a joy-filled life.

Looking to Someone Else

I just want someone to fix the symptoms. I don't want to have to do any work myself. After all, that's why they make the big bucks, right? If this one can't fix it, I will find someone else who can. (This pattern works the same in relationships, i.e., "If this relationship doesn't work, I'll find another one that will.")

Taking Responsibility: I am the source of my own happiness.

Withdrawal From Social Activities

I am in too much pain to be around people. It takes too much effort to get ready, and I don't feel like small talk. I feel more comfortable staying at home except when I have a doctor's appointment.

Taking Responsibility: I am willing to share my life with others. I am a valuable person, and I feel better when I give of myself.

Sex: "Who needs it?"

Sex is uncomfortable and painful. Besides, it is just too much trouble. I just fake it anyway. The only reason I have sex is to please someone else, so what is the use?

Taking Responsibility: I choose to sexually express myself in a loving and enjoyable way.

Hysteria

The pain is so intense that I get hysterical. I am so sick of this pain; even my closest family members don't seem to understand. I scream and yell at them because I feel so pitiful and desperately want help. I know they understand how badly I feel, but I realize my outbursts cause a wall to go up between us.

Taking Responsibility: I choose to see my suffering with empathy. I accept responsibility for getting better.

Codependency

I take on everyone else's pain and ignore my own. My thought is, "If I can help them get better, somehow I will feel more important." I am a rescuer; that is just how I am.

Taking Responsibility: I choose to take responsibility for my own health and wellbeing.

Pain as Permanent

My pain is so severe that it is likely to be permanent. There is no way I can do anything new, and doing so might make the pain even worse. I can manage this, but that is all. Besides, if the pain increases, no one will want to be around me anyway. They hardly come around now.

Taking Responsibility: I trust the bigger picture; I know this pain is not greater than I am. I *can* get better.

Giving Up

I'll never get better. I have tried everything and nothing has helped. I feel so hopeless; there is nothing more to do.

Taking Responsibility: I have the courage to succeed. There is a bigger picture, and I am willing to see it.

Guilt

I must have done something horrible, in this lifetime or some other, to deserve this pain. Otherwise, it wouldn't be happening to me. Nothing I try works. I don't see how anyone could love me; I am so "bad!"

Taking Responsibility: I am lovable. I accept the love of the Divine.

I Have No Other Problems

It doesn't matter that everyone has left me. Or that I have lost my job, and I am about to lose my house. So what? The pain consumes me, and I can't do anything about that.

Taking Responsibility: I realize "pain" is a part of life, but it is not greater than I am. I take full responsibility for getting on with my life. I own the right to enjoy living.

It's Not My Fault

"They" tell me the choices I have made in my life contribute to this pain. "They" tell me that if I watched what I ate, if I exercised, if I stopped smoking, drinking, and abusing my medications, I would heal faster. I just think I am a victim of my genes and other life circumstances. I couldn't possibly be at fault.

Taking Responsibility: I choose to take responsibility for my own actions. Having fun is my priority.

Using Suffering to Get What I Want

The only attention I get is when I have a crisis. Otherwise, without this suffering, no one would care about me.

Taking Responsibility: I choose to openly ask for what I need.

Addiction to the Pain

I have had this pain for so long that I don't know how to live any other way. I am afraid to get well. What will happen to me if I do get better? Even if I do get better, I know there will be some other pain to replace it.

Taking Responsibility: I willingly accept the responsibility for reclaiming my life.

Judging to Avoid Responsibility

When we judge that which we have created, all growth stops. Judgment is a projection of that which we do not want to feel onto the other or the situation, therefore missing the opportunity to grow from the experience.

Taking Responsibility: I willingly accept the responsibility for that which I have created.

Avoiding Balance and the "Now"

Yin and yang only come together as they flow one into the other in a moment of "balance." "Ultimate balance can only be achieved through transcendence beyond the intellect or personality. The only way to achieve this is by accessing the primordial spiritual quality of energy."[240]

Taking responsibility: I joyfully live in the flow of every moment!

Avoiding Mastermind and Developing Psychic Powers/Avoiding the Divine Nature of Man:

Living through the "what is." We have expectations of how life "should" be and when it isn't what we expect we go into survival mode, causing pain and suffering.

Taking Responsibility: I use all my faculties to make appropriate decisions.

Avoiding Justice:

Not liking what we see, blaming others for our pain.

Taking Responsibility: I know I am a co-creator of my world. I am always making choices.

Avoiding Achievement (Enneagram #3)[241]

I have no value other than what I have achieved.

Taking Responsibility: I love knowing that I am valuable simply because I exist.

Avoiding the "Shadow"

My life is driven by my insecurities, fears, doubts, and limiting beliefs. I do all I can to avoid others seeing how "faulty" I really am.

Taking Responsibility: I realize I can heal the past by being present to my upsets and living through them.

Avoiding Loyalty (Enneagram #6)

I have no support and/or security. I follow the rules to get others to be loyal.

Taking Responsibility: I know that the universe is benevolent and supports me completely.

I Am Not Loved by God

I am so "bad" that God does not love me.

Taking Responsibility: I absolutely know that God and I are One.

Avoiding the Moment

I have learned to survive by focusing on the past and fearing the future.

Taking Responsibility: I am fully responsible for what I create. There is no past or future; there is only now.

Avoiding Freeing the Soul from the Body

I am afraid of death. I am only my body; nothing else exists.

Taking Responsibility: We are spiritual beings having a human experience. We are not our physical body. As spiritual beings, we are eternal.

Avoiding Geopathic Stress:

It doesn't matter what I do to the Earth, it doesn't affect me.

Taking Responsibility: We could not be without the Earth. The Earth is our home. It is a living entity and how I treat my home is a reflection of how I treat myself and others.

APPENDIX VIII

EMCS ARCHETYPAL ENERGIES

Category I
Traditional Archetypes

Anima/Feminity
1. Goddess
2. Queen
3. Mother
4. Gaia
5. Princess
6. Damsel
7. Lover

Child/Innocence
1. Innocent
2. Orphan
3. Wounded
4. Divine
5. Puck
6. Puer/Puella

Animus/Masculinity
1. God
2. King
3. Father
4. Knight
5. Prince
6. Lover

Spirituality/Divinity
1. Mystic
2. Priest/Priestess
3. Nun
4. Monk
5. Shaman
6. Pantheist
7. Alchemist
8. Exorcist

9. Rabbi
10. Celibate
11. Disciple

Security/Protection
1. Warrior
2. Mercenary
3. Hero
4. Detective
5. Soldier
6. Firefighter
7. Police
8. Rescuer
9. Midas
10. Aggressor
11. Bully
12. Destroyer
13. Thief
14. Murderer
15. Moneymaker
16. Banker

Oracle/Wisdom
1. Visionary
2. Prophet
3. Crone
4. Actor
5. Sage
6. Storyteller
7. Philosopher

Artistic/Aesthetics
1. Author

2. Artist
3. Poet
4. Musician
5. Chef

Entertainer/Humorist
1. Clown
2. Fool
3. Magician
4. Trickster

Mercurial/Reality
1. Scientist
2. Wizard
3. Teacher
4. Scholar
5. Inventor
6. Scribe
7. Engineer

Lawmaker/Arbiter of Justice
1. Judge
2. Politician
3. Statesperson
4. Attorney
5. Legislator
6. Rebel

Healer/Self-esteem Builder
1. Therapist
2. Physician
3. Nurse
4. Psychologist
5. Counselor

6. Victim
7. Prostitute
8. Saboteur
9. Coward
10. Slave

Category II
EMCS Pantheon of Gods

Egyptian
1. Nut - female
2. Geb - male
3. Sho - love
4. Re - creative
5. Osiris - resurrection
6. Isis - divine mother
7. Horus - divine Son
8. Hathor - joy of life
9. Thoth - wisdom
10. Set - death
11. Sekmet - war
12. Imhotep - healing

Greco-Roman
1. Uranus - Father
2. Gaia - Mother
3. Kronos - time
4. Rhea - Earth
5. Aphrodite/Venus - love
6. Hermes/Mercury - communication/healing
7. Zeus/Jupiter - final judge
8. Hera/Juno - motherhood

11. Olympian
12. Martyr
13. Perfectionist

Explorer
1. Wanderer

9. Poseidon - ocean
10. Demeter - Earth
11. Apollo - Sun
12. Artemis/Diana - moon/chastity
13. Ares/Mars - war
14. Athena/Minerva - wisdom
15. Hephaestus - metal/fire
16. Hestia - home/hearth
17. Hades - underworld
18. Persephone - spring
19. Atropos - fate that determines the length of life
20. Aesculapius - healer

Hindu
1. Brahma - The All
2. Vishnu - creative aspect
3. Shiva - destructive aspect
4. Shakti/Kali – Shiva's female aspect

2. Hermit
3. Pioneer
4. Missionary
5. Astronaut

5. Krishna - later manifestation of The All

Other Deities
Scandinavian
1. Woton - Father
2. Frigga - Mother
3. Thor - thunder/war
4. Freya - youth/beauty
5. Norn - fate
6. Loki - mischief

Eastern
1. Mohammed
2. Buddha
3. Lao Tze (Zen)
4. Confucius

Western
1. The Great Spirit - Native American
2. Quetzacoatl - Aztec Christ
3. Jesus - The Son/Savior

Category III
Archangels

1. Ariel: Helps us to display courage and stand up for our beliefs as wells as realize that our material needs are provided for as we follow our intuition and manifest our dreams into reality. Ariel reminds us not to hold back. Spread your wings and fly. You are ready to soar.

2. Azrael: Comes in time of need to bring comfort and healing to our hearts. Azrael lets us know that our loved ones who have passed on are fine and helps us to feel their love and support from beyond.

3. Chamuel: Known as the "beloved one," Chamuel helps with spiritual soulmate relationships and with career transitions, letting you know your life purpose is triggering a blessed career change. He reminds us to remember that peace comes from the truth that only love is real.

4. Gabriel: As the archangel of creative writing, it helps us to express ourselves through the written word. Gabriel also helps us assume our leadership power to lovingly guide others, showing us that nurturing others helps us to nurture ourselves.

5. Haniel: Helps us to use the cycles of the moon to release anything we are done with and helps us to focus on manifesting desires and intentions. Haniel also helps us to trust and follow our passion in our love lives and careers and to realize that it is safe to be sensitive to our emotions.

6. Jeremial: Lets us know that all is well, that everything is happening exactly as it's supposed to and with hidden blessings that we will soon understand. Jermial also helps us assess and take inventory of our lives and to resolve, change, or heal any imbalances.

Jeremial also helps us overcome difficulties, showing us when the worst is behind us and that we are stronger for our efforts in overcoming those obstacles.

7. Jophiel: Urges us to get rid of clutter and clear both the space and energy of our physical environments (feng shui is one useful tool in this endeavor). He also helps us connect to nature, which improves our own timing and rhythms, leading us to cultivate patience in the process of life.

8. Metatron: Clears chakras using sacred geometry and helps us to recognize Indigo and Crystal Children, which in turn allos us to strengthen our bond with those who are sensitive to spirit.

9. Michael: Governs crystal-clear intentions and helps us to be clear about that which we desire and focus upon with unwavering faith. Michaels also reminds us of who we are as powerful, loving, and creative children of God and that we are much loved. Michael lets us know we are safe and that he is protecting and guarding us, our loved ones, and our homes.

10. Raguel: As the archangel of clairsentience (the psychic ability to pick up other people's emotional energy), Raguel helps us communicate through physical and emotional feelings that are divinely guided. Raguel also reminds us that everything is in divine right order.

11. Raphael: Think of Raphael as angel therapy, to whom we can give our cares and worries. Raphael also teaches us to breathe deeply to release old destructive patterns and advises us to live a healthy lifestyle by eating

nutritious foods, rising early, and getting plenty of exercise.

12. Raziel: As the archangel of clairvoyance (the psychic ability to perceive future events or occurrences beyond normal sensory input), Raziel helps us communicates through mental images, dreams, recurring sights in the physical world, auras, and apparition experience. Raziel brings spiritual understanding to esoteric information and clarity to spiritual truths, thus enabling God-given power and intention to manifest blessing in our lives.

13. Sandalphon: Urges us to be gentle with ourselves and to surround ourselves with gentle people, situations, and environments. Sandalphon also encourages us to be open to receiving gifts from our Creator, knowing that our prayers have been answered—have faith.

14. Uriel: The archangel of brilliant, divinely guided ideas, Uriel sends the message, "Take action; you know what to do." Trust your inner knowledge and act upon it without fear or delay.

15. Zadkiel: As the archangel of clairaudience (the psychic ability to "hear" that which is inaudible), Zadkiel helps us communicate by hearing divine guidance. Zadkiel also helps us to forgive ourselves and others and to compassionately see other points of view. Zadkiel teaches us to keep an open mind, learn new ideas, and pass them on to others.

Category IV
Angels

1. Adriana: leads us toward the answers to our prayers; communicates through intuition, thoughts, and dreams.

2. Akasha: bestows the ability of spiritual counseling

3. Amitiel: attunes us to a high level of truth

4. Ananchel: opens our hearts to unimaginable love and grace from God

5. Angel Vibration: emanations from the source of divine love

6. Arielle: helps create change and expand consciousness via psychic and spiritual experiences, including study, prayer, and meditation

7. Astara: helps us to raise our standards and believe we deserve the best

8. Athena: helps us to reveal our power to ourselves; enhances relationships, self-esteem, and life purpose

9. Aurora: encourages patience and faith and prevents negativity about desired outcomes

10. Bethany: helps us to learn to relax and treat ourselves as we treat others; pampers the self-energy

11. Azure: helps one to have patience and faith and not to slip into negativity about desired outcomes.

12. Bridgette: helps us to trust our gut feelings and look before continuing

13. Caressa: eases the end of a life cycle and urges self-care during the transition

14. Celest: ushers in positive energy when it's time to make a move; helps us stay positive during the transition

15. Cerviel: brings courage

16. Chantall: as the angel of romance, encourages new romance and is open to giving and receiving love

17. Chamuel: grounds the feelings of adoration.

18. Charmiene: heals by balancing all negative feelings with great appreciation and love for the self.

19. Crystal: represents the seeds we have sown coming to fruition

20. Daniel: the angel of marriage, heals past wounds that relate to marriage and the pain of our parent's marriage

21. Desiree: tells us when conditions are not favorable for action, wait, look, and think before acting

22. Fiona: helps us remain open to receiving help when we ask for it

23. Fortunata: creates a balance between the abundance of energy, spiritual growth, and the enjoyment of material prosperity

24. Francesca: helping you to make your own decisions concerning what you truly want. Helps one not to be afraid of making a wrong decision.

25. Gabriel: brings renewal on every level, reminds us of our life purpose

26. Grace and Antoinette: helps us to heal the situation by seeing the other person's point of view with compassion

27. Gratitude Angel: encourages us on our path; our watchful and helpful protector

28. Hadraniel: awakens our knowledge of God's eternal, unconditional love for us

29. Hamied: creates miracles

30. Iofiel: honors the vibration of exquisite beauty in all things

31. Indriel: helps light workers clear away cords or toxins that may result from helping others

32. Isabella: reveals when the timing is right for a new venture

33. Isaiah: helps us move forward on new ideas and situations in life

34. Israfel: transports us with ecstatic, soothing music from angelic realms

35. Jamaerah: elevates our vibration to a place where our vision and desires attract the energy to manifest, and they move on lightbeams to the material plane, ready to manifest

36. Jophiel: empowers our imagination with creativity and the energy to manifest on the material plane

37. Kaeylarae: brings the peaceful state of the heavens to our soul

38. Leila: urges us to spend time alone in nature to get clear on our desires and intentions

39. Maya: helps us with schooling, study, and education in pursuit of our life's purpose

40. Metatron: prepares us to receive the truth of our divine self through the release of negative thought patterns and judgments that can lead to unhappiness

41. Merlina: helps us to overcome confusion and indecisiveness by gathering more information

42. Micah: guides us in our choices, working through lifetimes of patterning, to become our authentic selves, free to experience our destiny

43. Michael: protects by transmuting negativity and self-imposed limitations

44. Mihr: blesses relationships of all kinds, maximizing their potential

45. Mystique: urges us to keep charging ahead and not take "no" for an answer

46. Nathaniel: responds to the commitment to move more fully into our divinity by burning away our illusions and limitations

47. Nisroc: encourages us to break free of our limitations

48. Oceana: urges us to take action, for we are in touch with our truth in the situation—we need to trust and assert ourselves

49. Omega: victory! Our desires are coming to fruition

50. Ongkanon: connects soul-level communication with our conscious self
51. Opal: guardian angel of children
52. Patience: now is the time to learn, study, and gather information
53. Paschar: sees through God's eyes and through God's heart, helps us manifest our beauty
54. Phanuel: brings hope
55. Ramaela: heals our bodies, hearts, and minds; guides healers in their work
56. Raye: governs yoga and physical exercise or movement
57. Raziel: enhances our ability to access understanding of universal knowledge
58. Remliel: wakes us from illusions and brings us to the truth
59. Rochelle: helps heal negative beliefs, emotions, and associations with money
60. Rosetta: brings us opportunities to help children
61. Sandalphon: empowers our hearts and strengthens the belief that we deserve to be loved.
62. Serena: angel of abundance in all forms
63. Seraphina: angel of families
64. Shanti: angel of peace, brings tranquility to our souls so we can mirror the peace of mind that is our true divine nature.

65. Shekinah: helps to immerse us in the vibration of God's light and love
66. Sushienae: purifies internal space as well as that of the entire planet
67. Sonya: guardian angel of deceased loved ones
68. Soqed Hozi: supports nurturing, true partnerships
69. Stamera: encourages honesty with our feelings, release of hurt, and forgiveness.
70. Teresa: alerts us to the necessity of stopping and taking a break
71. Uriel: arrives with love when the name of God is spoken
72. Uzziel: helps us transcend the everyday realm, aspiring to find the trust in God called faith
73. Vanessa: helps us make decisions by revealing the path that brings us closer to our divine purpose
74. Yvonne: guards our relationships with animals and helps us learn from them
75. Zanna: helps heal our hearts from past upsets and trauma, worry, or fear; helps to release self-sabotaging thoughts or behavior; renews feelings of safety and peace

Category V
Arcana Archetypes

1. Aeon: a non-judgmental perspective developed over lifetimes, which creates an understanding that can transform all aspects of our lives
2. Magician: the skilled and cunning master of all he/she surveys; represents an individual in control of life's tools and techniques, as well as the power to communicate and manifest on many levels of consciousness, to receive messages from the subtle realms, and to create in the ethers
3. Art/Temperance: creative, alchemical genius; demonstrates that moderation can serve as a bridge to wholeness

4. Chariot: the vehicle for accomplishing things effortlessly and well
5. Death/Rebirth: allows for new life, growth, and new patterns through detachment and respect for impermanence
6. Devil: a light, Pan-like approach to ourselves and the world, humor and laughter with insight
7. Emperor: powerful ability to create and construct new worlds and ideals for the planet
8. Empress: spiritual feminine, guidance with love and wisdom
9. Fool: the trusting soul, moving through the journey of our life without fear
10. Hanged Man: breaking patterns in a state of conscious surrender to our highest self
11. Hermit: an inner place of contemplation where clarity and truth can guide us
12. Hierophant: structures faith and resolves the family hierarchy within, taking what is valuable and letting go of the rest

13. High Priestess: powerful intuition and wisdom
14. Justice: aligned, balanced, inspired energy from which right action flows
15. Lovers: enlightened co-creation and cultivation of relationships, the highest vibration of the relationship
16. Lust/Strength: fiery strength to overcome fear of our shadow and live in our fullest life expression
17. Moon: the deep feminine aspect guiding our life's course on our journey to express our authentic self
18. Star: a state of radiant confidence resulting from a strong connection to one's own value and inner wisdom
19. Sun: unlimited life force, the master of energy
20. Tower: healing through dissolving limiting structures
21. Universe: conscious mastery of self and the entirety of which we are a part

Category VI
Ascended Masters

1. Buddha: silence and all its enlightenment chakras
2. Divine Mother: emanates compassion and conditional love
3. Djwal Khul: brings messages in absolute clarity
4. El Morya: aligns personal will with divine will
5. Kuthumi: understands universal truths
6. Lady Nada: aligns the power of love and spiritual growth with the earthly plan
7. Lady Portia: brings the quality of confidence in our connection to the divine.

8. Maha Chohan: helps us expand our awareness to the galactic consciousness
9. Orion and Angelica: connect us with the essence of pure love
10. Quan Yin: nurtures spiritual knowledge and cultivates dignity
11. Saint Germain: transmutes with the high vibrational flame
12. Sananda: light and divine love and compassion integrated into the physical world
13. Sanat Kumara: spiritual consciousness of the Earth

14. Serapis Bey: infuses us with the power of light and expanded awareness

15. Source: white light imbued with vast power and all knowledge

Category VII
Buddha Fire Archetypes

1. Ascension: facilitates traveling, on a golden ray, to our highest expression of self
2. Dorje: brings powerful alignment with spiritual knowledge
3. Golden Aura: infuses the auric field with the vibration of gold
4. Homecoming: connects the body and soul in a state of acceptance of the limitations of the Earth's plane
5. Soul/Cell Renewal: regenerates the body with an infusion of soul perfection and light

Category VIII
Earth Essences Archetypes

1. Collective Rain: used to bring about a gentle release of pent-up energy
2. Mars Fire Storm: used to push through a tight place in the heart or mind
3. Mother Earth: used to connect with the "mother" energy of the earth, accepting self unconditionally
4. Mountain Seeds: stimulates a "reframing" or new picture of an old topic
5. Night Air Storm: pushes through old, deeply held beliefs that no longer serve
6. On the Edge: gives an added sense of strength to "hang on" when it is appropriate to do so
7. Rain (creative): releases creativity
8. Rain (jewel of joy): releases and opens joy
9. Rain (joy and healing): releases the fear of healing and opens up the joy
10. Rain (safe to cry): releases fear of crying due to feeling unsafe
11. Raindrops: gentle, general releasing of energy
12. River Calm Free: reminds us of flowing in freedom and peace
13. Santa Fe Mountain Flowers: a general soothing and joyful energy for feeling alive

Category IX
Egyptian Magic Archetypes
These open pathways to our own ancient wisdom

1. Air: keep things moving, wind
2. Ankh: life force, spiritually enlightening, key to understanding ourselves as God
3. Anubis: watchful protector, can assist us in finding what we need
4. Bast: joy and happiness, psychic protection
5. Buckle of Isis: fertility, sacred manifesting of all things

6. Crook and Flail: manifests through alignment of self-discipline and confidence
7. Earth: grounding wealth, brings etheric energy into tangible reality for all things growing
8. Fire: creative spark, personal fire, being in touch with your own ideas
9. Hathor: goddess of beauty and love, strengthens and protects women
10. Horus: appreciation of beauty and awakening creativity
11. Isis: nurturing, caring, maternal love, stillness, contentment
12. Nephthys: spiritual use of intuition
13. Osiris: discernment through alignment with spiritual truth
14. Ptah: best aspects of the masculine, especially when applied to problem-solving

15. Pyramid: acceptance of life's events as directed by our soul's evolution
16. Scarab: aligns us with a more fulfilling path; may involve great change
17. Sirius: unlimited possibilities
18. Sphinx: develops wisdom as the observer in the cosmic scheme of things
19. Thoth: understands the complexity of universal laws, communicator of knowledge
20. Twins: attracts a partner with harmonious energy
21. Uraeus: ability to see with powerful capacity
22. Water: flowing feelings and energy, cleansing
23. Winged Disk: connects with inspiration and communicates with higher realms.

Category X
Goddesses

1. Abundantia: Prosperity. Roman and Norse goddess of prosperity, success, good fortune, and abundance.
2. Aeracura: Blossoming. As a Celtic and Germanic Mother
3. Earth deity: she is a fairy queen that bridges earthly life and the hereafter. Also helps us put goals and challenges into perspective.
4. Aine: Leap of faith. Celtic goddess and fairy queen who gave birth to incarnated fairies from her romances with moral men. Helps us to have faith and take action.
5. Aphrodite: Inner Goddess. Greek goddess of passion and love associated with the planet Venus. She represents unabashed female sexual energy.

6. Artemis: Guardian. Greek goddess who is the twin sister of Apollo, the sun god. Exuding tomboy energy, she prefers the woods, her bow and arrow, and the company of wild animals. As a guardian goddess, she helps us focus, take aim, and reach our mark.
7. Athena: Guardian. Greek goddess who is both powerful and wise, overseeing and protecting those who call upon her.
8. Bast: Independence. Egyptian goddess represented by a cat. She is our protector throughout the night. She is graceful, independent, playful, and intuitive Both a moon and a sun goddess.
9. Brigit: "Don't back down." Celtic triple goddess represents three aspects of woman:

the young virgin, the nurturing mother, and the crone/sage/wise woman. She is a female archangel Michael, a warrior energy who tirelessly protects those who call upon her.

10. Butterfly Maiden: Transformation. Hopi kachina spirit who ensures healthy and bountiful harvests. Helps us escape from any cocoon that's trapping us or impeding our growth or joy. Guided us through the transition.

11. Cordelia: Nature. Celtic goddess who watches over flowers that bloom in spring and summer.

12. Coventina: Purification. Celtic goddess of waters. She protects bodies of water and their inhabitants. Helps us purify our bodies, as they are primarily water.

13. Damara: Guides children. Celtic fertility goddess whose name means "gentle." She helps bring peace and harmony to families and households and helps maintain the youthful innocence of children.

14. Dana: High priestess. Celtic goddess who was worshipped as the Creator Mother Goddess. She is extremely powerful and helps us with manifestation, alchemy, and divine magic.

15. Diana: Focused Intention. Roman moon goddess who carries a silver sword. She is associated with healthy childbirth, helping to ensure a painless process. She loves to spend time in nature and is very fond of oak trees. She helps animals and facilitates the connection between humans and the natural world.

16. Eireen: Peace. Greek goddess who brings peace to all who call upon her. The Romans referred to her as Pax, and she helped replace worry with faith.

17. Freyja: Bold. Nordic earth goddess of fertility, celebration, and passion. She teaches us to appreciate our attractiveness and enjoy ourselves. Friday is named after her.

18. Green Tara: Delegates. Hindu and Buddhist goddess whose name means "star." She is known as a speedy helper who offers emergency aid and provides a rapid understanding of situations and relationships. She rescues us by empowering us to save ourselves.

19. Guinevere: True Love. Celtic triple goddess whose name means "white one." She was invoked for both fertility and as a bridge to take the dead to the afterlife. She helps ensure that we partner with our true love and assists us in keeping that love alive.

20. Hathor: Receptivity. Egyptian goddess represented by the head of a cow to symbolize the sacred animal's life-giving milk and mothering. She is a goddess of the sky and sun who helps with all aspects of child conception, birthing, and raising. She is called upon to guide us in nurturing ourselves and our loved ones.

21. Ishtar: Boundaries. An ancient Mesopotamian goddess worshiped as the embodiment of womanly energy. She represents the divine feminine in all her aspects, including nurturing, mothering, sensuality, fertility, healing, protection, and wisdom.

22. Isis: Past Life. Egyptian high-priestess moon goddess. She is simultaneously motherly and businesslike, feminine and ultra-strong. She is also known as the goddess of divine magic and alchemy and can be called upon for help with past-life memories.

23. Isolt: Undying Love. Celtic goddess who was caught in a tragic love triangle between her betrothed, King Mark of Cornwall, and his nephew, Sir Tristan. She dealt with this

situation with courage and thus can help us with our relationships, including familial, romantic, parental, and friendship. She reminds us that regardless of the situation, our love is real, powerful, and undying.

24. Ixchel: Medicine Woman. Mayan moon goddess who gave birth to all other Mayan gods. She is connected with the tides of the water and is believed to control rain flow and all aspects of water. The goddess of fertility and childbirth, she is a powerful healer who remembers the origin of human life on the planet. She can connect us with our own roots as spiritual healers.

25. Kali: Endings and beginnings. This Hindu goddess is feared by those who do not understand the cycles of birth, death, and rebirth. She embodies Mother Nature and cleanses away the old with natural storms and fires to make the ground fertile for new crops and life. She is a get-things-done goddess who is a wise mother, pushing us beyond our comfort zone to reach our highest potential.

26. Kuan Yin: Compassion. Buddhist goddess who hears all prayers and is the essence of purity, nurturing love, and gentle power. She has vowed to stay on the Earth until all of us reach enlightenment.

27. Lakshmi: Bright future. Hindu goddess who brings abundance to those who call upon her. She has a connection to the lotus flower and elephants. Water represents her absolute faith, fertility, and abundance.

28. Maat: Fairness. Egyptian goddess of integrity, fairness, and justice. At the time of one's death, she holds the scales that weigh the soul against a feather to detect one's measure of guilt.

29. Maeve: Cycles and rhythms. Celtic goddess who celebrates her femininity. She has a

legendary sexual appetite and can be called upon to relieve pain associated with feminine cycles, labor, delivery, and menopause.

30. Mary Magdalene: Unconditional love. Christian representation of unconditional love and forgiveness and overlooking false judgments. She helps us to keep our hearts open to love.

31. Mawu: Mother Earth. West African moon goddess who, along with her husband, the sun god Liza, is believed to have created all life. She helps us to learn to live in harmony with nature and respect its resources.

32. Mother Mary: Expect a miracle. Mother of Christ, who is known as the queen of angels because of her healing work. She works closely with child advocates, teachers, and healers.

33. Nemetona: Sacred space. Celtic goddess who protected ancient ceremonial sites, especially those connected to nature. She helps us to build our own sacred space.

34. Oonagh: Rest and relaxation. Celtic goddess who helps with transitions and guides us in creative and magical ways.

35. Ostara: Fertility. Teutonic goddess of fertility is celebrated during the spring equinox as the bringer of increased light. She is the balance between nighttime and daytime hours. She is invoked to increase fruitfulness and fertility or to help us embark on new ventures.

36. Pele: Divine Passion. Hawaiian goddess of volcanoes. She shows us that fire can purify, release us from the old to make way for the new, and ignite our passions. Without fire, nothing would change. She helps us get in touch with our true passions.

37. Rhiannon: Sorceress. Welsh lunar goddess whose name means "great queen." She is the inspiration or muse for poets, artists, and

royalty. She carries souls from Earth to the afterlife, helping them to adjust to the transition of life after death.

38. Sarasvati: The Arts. Hindu goddess of the arts who helps us with all creative expressions.

39. Sedna: Infinite supply. Inuit Eskimo and Alaskan sea goddess who provides sustenance for the body and soul.

40. Sekhmet: Strength. Egyptian sun goddess whose name means "strong and mighty." She is connected with lions, symbolizing her fiercely protective nature, and sometimes appears with a lion's head and a human woman's body. Call upon her for strength and power.

41. Sige: Quiet time. Gnostic goddess considered to be the "great silence" or "void" from which all creation springs. She reminds us that words create duality and that in silence, we find our true origin.

42. Sulis: Bodies of water. Celtic sun goddess who oversees bodies of water associated with healing.

43. Vesta: Home. Roman goddess of home and hearth. She is a fire goddess who brings warmth to households.

44. White Tara: Sensitivity. Buddhist and Hindu goddess Mother Creator. She represents purity, maturity, and compassion and helps us live long and peaceful lives.

45. Yemanya: Golden Opportunity. Brazilian goddess who is credited for creating the sea. She is a protector, supplier, and one who grants wishes.

Category XI
Power Animal Archetypes

1. Ant: patience, focus, discipline, determination, hard work
2. Bear: wisdom, strength, quiet inner space, introspection
3. Bee: majesty, wealth
4. Coyote: the trickster, opportunity, cleverness, strategic thinking
5. Deer: gentleness, grace
6. Dog: loyalty, playfulness, unconditional love
7. Dragon: firepower with wisdom
8. Eagle: the big picture, the unification of inner and outer sight
9. Hawk: precise vision wherever focused
10. Horse: power, strength of heart, individuality
11. Jaguar: the ability to stalk the underworld, to reveal what is hidden
12. Lion: worry-free, fearless, impulsive
13. Lizard: the message of the dreamer and a reminder to pay attention to their dreams and symbols.
14. Rabbit: speed, heightened awareness, timidity
15. Raven: magic, challenges us to go to powerful, mysterious places
16. Red-tail hawk: a messenger that leads us to our life purpose
17. Snake: awakens energy, initiates transformation, moves us through death to new life
18. Snowy owl: magic, ancient wisdom
19. Spider: dreaming, creativity, channels ideas and designs
20. Wolf: community, reliability, teaching
21. Wren: confidence, resourcefulness

For information on all fifty-two animals, refer to a set of animal medicine cards.[242]

Category XII
Sacred Geometry as Archetype
The elegant and abstract language of form

1. Circle: has a point as its center and a point revolving around it, thus representing unity, continuity, containment
2. Cross: intersection of two realities, meeting of the end and the beginning
3. Cube: stable, solid base, earth element
4. Dodecahedron: made of pentagons, a spirit element, a structure in which the vastness of spiritual energy moves powerfully
5. Ellipse: has two centers, graceful evolution
6. Equilateral triangle: simple structure, all lines and angles equal, stable, ordered
7. Hexagram: two equilateral triangles pointing in opposite directions, six-pointed star, harmonious resolution of conflict
8. Human canon: unifies our personal self with the cosmos; the geometric hologram which makes up the human body is the same as that which makes up the universe
9. Icosahedron: this pattern creates receptivity, water element
10. Line: connects two points through infinity
11. Octagram: eight-pointed star, interlaces two squares, coming together of two stable forces
12. Octahedron: eight equilateral triangles joined, air element, mediator
13. Pentagram: five-pointed star, power directed and focused
14. Point: beginning, moment of conception
15. Right triangle: has one right angle, rearranging priorities to move into unity
16. Sphere: three-dimensional circle, energetically represents limitlessness
17. Spiral: unfolding what is hidden
18. Square: solid construction, stable
19. Squaring the circle: complete, success, achievement
20. Tetrahedron: made up of four equilateral triangles, fire element, draws power into center, energy
21. Vesica Piscis: overlapping circles, unity resulting in creation

CELESTIAL BLENDS

The celestial spirit infused into the gem and mineral essences enhances and strengthens the inherent gem/mineral qualities. Each of these blends was created with the intention of promoting positive health and optimum functioning at all levels: physical, etheric, astral, mental, and causal. The energetic harmonics of each blend combine uniquely with the spirit it meets with to work for the highest good of all concerned.

Shamanic Spirit (Navajo Turquoise and Silver): Healer of the spirit, drawing out all forms of negativity. Awakens the visionary aspect of the self at all levels and brings peace of mind.

Brilliant Radiance (Diamond, Pearl, Gold): Strengthens all aspects of the higher self. Promotes charity, faith, truth, courage, integrity, and spiritual knowledge. Activates the internal purity of the universal spirit and the development of consciousness.

Luminous Creation (Rubellite Tourmaline, Gold): Releases blockages so energy can be free-flowing and physical vitality activated. Illuminates the higher self for inspired creativity.

Harmonic Light (Sapphire, Gold): Stimulates and strengthens the desire for inner peace through prayer, devotion, and spiritual enlightenment. Releases self-judgement to allow a healing space within.

Perfect Manifestation (Amber, Silver): Focuses and clarifies the energy for each chakra. Creates a spiritual intellect for manifestation of what is desired. Balances mental processes to improve memory and decisiveness.

Heavenly Abundance (Azurite, Clear Quartz, Emerald): Allows eloquent expression of the positive emotions of the heart and the communication of gratitude for the experience of universal abundance.

Sacred Clarity (Turquoise, Azurite, Lapis Lazuli): Releases emotional bondage, expands awareness, and encourages connection to celestial realms. Creates serenity through recognition and manifestation of the good within.

Inner Beauty (Rose Quartz, Emerald, Tiger Eye): Heightens awareness of the beauty around us. Allows spiritual attunement to the energy of love and enhances personal power through self-reliance on the dynamic beauty within.

Transcendent Purity (Pearl, Emerald, Clear Quartz): Creates a stable, positive energy flow for spiritual expansion through faith, charity, and truth. Promotes gratitude for the abundance of love in the universe.

Master Release (Lapis Lazuli, Malachite, Gold, Pyrite): Strengthens the desire for spiritual truth and allows the release of fear, guilt, self-doubt, limiting patterns of thought or behavior, and all physical toxins in the body. Activates all the regenerative energies of the body.

Freedom (Fire Opal, Pearl, Tiger Eye): Creates emotional stability and mental clarity, allowing us to seek higher inspiration. Clears beliefs that may interfere with our unlimited freedom, independence, and productivity.

Vision Quest (Pipestone, Turquoise, Silver): Awakens visionary communication; calls forth positive guidance from the universe. Moves us to the place of no time and all time and oneness with the Creator. Promotes detachment from and integration of the lessons of the great mystery.

Revelations (Diamond, Herkimer Diamond, Fire Opal): Radiates the energy of acceptance for the gifts of the universe. Creates receptivity to divine creation and manifestation within and without. Cleanses the physical temple and all the surrounding energetic fields to allow disbursement of light and love.

Ascendance (Dark Pearl, Moonstone, Gold): Makes active, elevates, and empowers the feminine energy of the spirit. Attunes body fluids to lunar tides and magnetism. Balancing, introspective, and intuitive. Related to acceptance of life changes at all levels. Balances and develops the heart chakra, opens and makes active the third eye and crown chakras, rebuilds the nervous system, and rejuvenates the endocrine system.

Transformation (Kinoite, Green Calcite, Magnetite [POS], Green Tourmaline): Enhances our spirituality during the initial stages of growth. Provides a reflection of the self. Clears and makes active all the chakras. Dispels fear, grief, anger, and attachment.

APPENDIX X

ETHERIC BODY CHAKRA ESSENCES

These essences were created to assist and strengthen the chakras of the etheric body. They cleanse the body and etheric template of toxins. They call into consciousness the cellular memories that promote positive change and acceptance of the individual life path. They provoke the physical manifestation of this process as bodily symptoms, dreams, heightened awareness, clarity of thoughts, increased or decreased energy, etc.

Base Chakra (Clear Quartz, Moldavite): Connects the physical dimension to the mental dimension for harmonious transformation. Clears and makes active the physical energy centers of the body. Expands our understanding of who we are in relation to the universe, moves us out of limited thinking about ourselves and our lives, reconnects us with spirituality.

Reproductive Chakra___(Citrine, Yellow Carnelian): Synthesizes our creative forces, strengthens intuition, and provides a sense of clarity in all forms of communication with self and others. Inspires optimism, but with moderation and tolerance toward self and others. Increases sensitivity to the environment by opening awareness to the vibrant life force of all things.

Solar Plexus Chakra (Emerald, Black Tourmaline Quartz): Allows the experience of unconditional love and gratitude. Symbolizes love, prosperity, kindness, and goodness. Provides a sense of emotional safety and protection as we let go of expectations and have a sense of being surrounded by the light.

Heart Chakra (Fire Opal, Chalcedony): Clears beliefs that limit freedom and independence. Helps initiate new ways of thinking and a more spontaneous approach to life. Unblocks creative channels. Releases anger and reclaims self-worth. Brings calm and peace by helping us express our emotional needs. Provides an opening for honesty and for asking for support.

Throat Chakra (Blue Tourmaline, Peacock Ore): Strengthens understanding and the ability to value our intuition, especially when it conflicts with the expectations of others. Helps us find our rhythm with the harmonies of the universe that guide our spiritual service. Makes active personal will and helps us release that which is no longer useful. Protects from negativity and transforms negative forces into beneficial energy.

Third Eye Chakra (Lapis Lazuli, Peridot): Allows clear sight to what is truth and strengthens the desire for it. Clears what is stored in the subconscious mind to a space where action can be initiated and changes made. Helps us look at things we have been avoiding. Revitalizes our sense of inner joy, opens us to balanced giving and receiving, and helps us recognize our true beauty.

Crown Chakra (Amethyst, Fluorite): Heightens spiritual awareness so that we recognize the divinity within us. Prepares us for spiritual work and transformation. Provides a state of fulfilment and attunement to the present time. Helps release addictive tendencies at all levels.

APPENDIX XI

ASTRAL BODY CHAKRA ESSENCES

Base Chakra (Kinoite and Aragonite): Enhances one's spirituality during the initial stages of growth. Provides a reflection of the self and the inner workings of the body, allowing one to see into its emotional, mental, and physical structures. Helps us center ourselves and provides insight into the basis of our problems. Enhances patience and helps us to "maintain" in the face of a myriad of responsibilities.

Reproductive Chakra (Cut Green Tourmaline, Rhodonite): Creates a clear path to balance the yin-yang energy, synthesizing the qualities of attainment with the spiritual universe and balancing the energies of the earth plane. Helps us reach our greatest potential. Transforms negative energy to a positive state without releasing it into the atmosphere, inspires creativity, and attracts success, prosperity, and abundance.

Solar Plexus Chakra (Purple Fluorite, Green Calcite, Marble): These essences, in combination, balance the positive and negative relationships of the mind, revealing the reality and truth behind illusion. Produces polarizing prismatic energy, which engenders a spectrum of energy to clear and activate all chakras. Provides both clarity and suspension during states of meditation. Activates the normally unused portions of the mind, providing for the strength of self-control, mastery of thought, and the power of serenity.

Heart Chakra (Citrine and Kinoite): This combination balances the yin-yang energy and aligns the chakras with the ethereal plane. Stabilizes the emotions and dispels anger. Encourages us to "look at the sunrise," the freshness of beginnings, and the reality of excellence. Helps us to refrain from delusional thinking and to recognize and extinguish self-limiting ideas.

Throat Chakra (Herkimer Diamond and Tanzanite): This combination provides a delicate harmony, enhancing distinct awareness and unbridled spontaneity. Helps us to "be." Also helps clear the body-mind systems of unconscious fears and repressions, allowing for total relaxation and expansion of the life energy. Tanzanite, specifically, produces the perfect symmetry of personal power and actualization.

Third Eye Chakra (Azurite/Malachite and Blue Goldstone): This combination helps to create a deep meditative state in order to be reborn into the light. Allows us to reach into the inner depths without fear so that we are sustained, absolved, and aware of the genesis of all time. Goldstone (a manmade sparkling opaque glass dating to the 1100s) is believed to transmit healing energy, increase self-acceptance, aid in learning, and is an ideal stone for empaths.

Crown Chakra (Amazonite, Galena, and Unakite): This combination aligns the physical, etheric, and astral bodies, producing a balancing and preventive energy. It balances the male/female energies, bringing the qualities of clarity and a clear spirit. Provides grounding, enhances energy, and helps to open the pathway between the physical and ethereal bodies to stimulate the nervous system. Can bring the emotional body into alignment with the higher forces of spirituality.

APPENDIX XII

MENTAL BODY CHAKRA ESSENCES

The mental body is the energy field in which concrete thought forms occur. Coming in from the higher consciousness, the thoughts are translated into forms that can make sense at the astral, etheric, and physical levels. These essences provide for clear reception and transmission of these important message energies so that they can manifest for us without distortion or blockages.

Base Chakra (Botswana Agate, Red Coral, and Wonderstone): This combination facilitates and reinforces the state of tranquility, eliminating worries, distress, and depression. Helps maintain a forthright character and sustain an attentiveness to detail, which further facilitates the sensitivity to, and the recognition and understanding of, the complete picture. Helps us to achieve harmony with the natural forces of the universe, opens and activates the base chakra, and stimulates the energetic pursuit of pre-determined goals.

Reproductive Chakra (Limonite and Vanadinite): This combination helps us alter our lives in order to achieve stability and comfort, to leave the "marsh of existence" and to further gain the "aspirations of the mountain," reaching toward the infinite powers of the mind. Promotes order, helps us define our goals, and shows us how to pursue those goals in an orderly manner.

Solar Plexus Chakra (Jade [Red] and Fire Opal): Jade is known as a "dream stone" and as a "stone of fidelity," bringing realization to our potential and devotion to our purpose. It is used to release suppressed emotions via the dream process. It was known in the Mayan culture as the "Sovereign of Harmony," facilitating peace within the physical, emotional, and intellectual structures, as well as within the materialistic world. Fire Opal assists in "maintaining" during stressful situations and provides added energy to ameliorate feelings of "burn-out."

Heart Chakra (Peacock Ore, Red Calcite): Allows the release of that which is no longer useful. Transforms negative energy into positive benefits. Encourages optimism and faith about life changes and transformations.

Throat Chakra (Yellow Carnelian, Copper): Encourages tolerance and optimism toward the self. Fine-tunes decision making and allows a broader perspective on things. Frees any life force energy constricted by restrictive thinking and allows its expression.

Third Eye Chakra (Harmonic Light, Peridot): Stimulates a desire for prayer, devotion, and spiritual enlightenment. Amplifies thoughts and balances the right and left brain functioning. Revitalizes our sense of inner joy and helps us recognize our true inner beauty.

Crown Chakra (Botswana Agate, Clear Quartz): Stimulates the desire to explore the unknown and seek further states of enlightenment. Harmonizes and aligns energy of all areas. Connects the physical and mental dimensions. Facilitates the giving and receiving of information.

APPENDIX XIII

CAUSAL BODY CHAKRA ESSENCES

The causal body is our primary contact with the spiritual essence of the universe. It is relatively immortal in that it is constant throughout human evolution in the physical form. The causal body holds the information of all the soul's incarnations (what theosophists call the Akashic records). These records hold the history of positive accomplishment or that which is in alignment with "the law," as defined by theosophists. The thought-process powers it holds are intention, memory, inductive and deductive reasoning, intuition, imagination, and internal will.

The causal body is where abstract thoughts and ideas exist in the symbolic form of a triangle. It acts as the vehicle for the ego and stores the germs of the qualities to be carried over into the next incarnation. It is the only true register of a person's growth. The possession of a causal body is what constitutes individuality; it develops until it becomes fit for the divine spirit to dwell in humanity. The causal body is literally our spiritual connection, and these gem essence combinations were created to allow that energy to flow freely and lovingly.

Base Chakra (Citrine and Spessartine Garnet): This combination recognizes that our consciousness is ready to both absorb and assimilate the higher levels of inner dynamics of growth and structural balance. Signals the balance of the yin-yang energy and the activation of the chakras with the ethereal plane. The combination illuminates the energy of the base chakra, delivering both comfort and optimism.

Reproductive Chakra (Green Calcite, Corundum, and Kinoite: This combination stimulates ambition and confidence. It dispels harsh and irritating attitudes, subdues emotions, and helps one to release anger in a positive manner. It reminds us of the state of perfection so that we can return to the natural state of flawlessness.

Solar Plexus Chakra (Amber and Sweatlodge Cobblestone): Amber, specifically, is a stone dedicated to the connection of the conscious self to universal perfection. Together with Sweatlodge Cobblestone, it assists in the art of manifestation, bringing that which is desired to the state of reality. It also transmutes the energy of physical vitality so that it can activate unconditional love. Amber specifically kindles the realization and subsequent response of choice, helping one to choose and to be chosen.

Heart Chakra (Gold and Wulfenite): This combination symbolizes the purity of the spiritual aspect of "all that is." Gold, specifically, is known as the "master healer." It can clear negativity from the chakras and the energy fields of the physical, emotional, intellectual, and spiritual bodies. This combination promotes the acceptance of the existence of the negative aspects that exist in the world, allowing us to recognize our issues and refuse to let "roadblocks" impede or limit our progress.

Throat Chakra (Diamond and Pearl): This combination brings similar qualities of innocence, fidelity, and love, thus grounding purity, constancy, and the loving and open nature with which we came into the physical world.

Third Eye Chakra (Red Jade, Black Coral, and Azurite/Malachite): This magical combination absorbs and transforms negativity, elevates the aspects of significant creative forces, and imparts tranquility to action. It dispels the fear of darkness and can bring hidden matters to the forefront. Helps us cherish our desires and make our dreams a physical reality. It bestows the cleansing of the immutable forces and freshens our outlook to be the "wind in the willow."

Crown Chakra (Amethyst Magnetite [positive] and Obsidian): This combination helps balance emotions with intellect, encourages trust in intuition, and produces the mental clarity needed to determine which minerals would also benefit our lives. Facilitates transmutation of lower energies into higher frequencies of both the spiritual and ethereal levels. Represents the principles of complete metamorphosis. Creates protective energy, shields against negativity, disperses unloving thoughts, and connects one to the center of the earth, thus aligning the above and the below in perfect harmony.

End Notes

[1] John Randolph Price, *The Superbeings* (Austin: Quartus Foundation for Spiritual Research, Inc., 1981), xiii.

[2] Price, *The Superbeings*, 49.

[3] Bruce Fisher, *Man, Grand Reflection of the Greater Cosmos: Studies in Occult Anatomy* (Prescott, AZ: Subru Publications, 1996), 1:4.

[4] Fisher, *Man, Grand Reflection of the Greater Cosmos*, 1:4.

[5] Fisher, 32–33.

[6] Arthur E. Powell, *The Mental Body* (London: Theosophical Publishing House, 1967), 16.

[7] Fisher, 33.

[8] Fisher, 33.

[9] Fisher, 15.

[10] Fisher, 34.

[11] Richard Gerber, *Vibrational Medicine for the 21st Century* (New York: Harper Collins, 2000), 39.

[12] William Tiller, *Science and Human Transformation* (Walnut Creek, CA: Pavior, 1997), 145.

[13] Julia Melges Jablonski, "Psychophysics: A Wholistic Approach to Energy Healing," *Psychic Journal* (1996): accessed April 13, 2002, http://www.spiritofra.com/psychophysics.htm.

[14] Claude Swanson, *Life Force, The Scientific Basis: Breakthrough Physics of Energy Medicine, Healing, Chi and Quantum Consciousness* (Tucson: Poseidia, 2010), 1.

[15] Arthur E. Powell, *Etheric Double: The Health Aura* (Wheaton, IL: Quest Books, 1996), 8.

[16] Powell, *The Etheric Body*, 9.

[17] Powell, 10.

[18] Barbara Starfield, "Is US Health Care Really the Best in the World?" *Journal of American Medical Association*, vol. 284(4) (2000): 483–485.

[19] Swanson, *Life Force*, 8.

[20] Carl Johan Calleman, *The Purposeful Universe: How Quantum Theory and Mayan Cosmology Explain the Origin and Evolution of Life* (Rochester, VT: Bear & Company, 2009), 14.

[21] Calleman, *The Purposeful Universe*, 14.

[22] Calleman, 15.

[23] W. Edward Mann, *Organ, Reich & Eros: Wilhelm Reich's Theory of Life Energy* (New York: Simon & Schuster 1973), 195.

[24] Candice Pert, *Molecules of Emotion* (New York: Simon & Schuster, 1997), 39.

[25] David Hawkins, *Power vs Force* (Sedona: Veritas, 2004), 8.

[26] Gordon Stokes and Daniel Whiteside, *Tools of the Trade: For Understanding and Trusting Our Self,* (Carson City, NV: Thoth Publishing, 2004), 38.

[27] Hawkins, *Power vs Force*, 44.

[15] Maggie la Tourelle with Anthea Courtenay, *Thorsons Introductory Guide to Kinesiology* (London: Harper Collins, 1992), 13.

[29] Association for Comprehensive Energy Psychology (ACEP), *Training Module 3*.

[30] Association for Comprehensive Energy Psychology (ACEP), *Training Module 3*.

[31] Association for Comprehensive Energy Psychology (ACEP), *Training Module 3*.

[32] Stokes and Whiteside, *Tools of the Trade*, 30.

[33] Stokes and Whiteside, 32.

[34] Torkom Saraydarian, *The Ageless Wisdom*, (Cave Creek, AZ: TSG Publishing Foundation, 1990), 40.

[35] Ceanne DeRohan, *The Unseen Role of Denial Series: The Right Use of Will* (Santa Fe: Four Winds, 1986).

[36] Bruce Fisher, *Man, Grand Reflection of the Great Cosmos,* 1:14–15.

[37] Fisher, *Man, Grand Reflection*, 14–15.

[38] Barbara Hand Clow, *Alchemy of Nine Dimensions: Decoding the Vertical Axis, Crop Circles, and the Mayan Calendar* (Charlottesville: Hampton Roads, 2004), 49.

[39] Clow, *Alchemy*, 49.

[40] Rudolph Ballentine, *Radical Healing* (New York: Harmony, 1999), 100.

[41] Byron Gentry, *Miracles of the Mind: How to Use the Power of Your Mind for Healing and Prosperity* (Highland City, FL: Rainbow Books, 1998), 169.

[42] Gentry, *Miracles*, 169.

[43] Gentry, 169.

[44] Barbara Stone, *Invisible Roots* (Santa Rosa, CA: Energy Psychology Press, 2008), 176.

[45] Stone, *Invisible* Roots, 176.

[46] Gentry, 180.

[47] Myles Seabrook, *I Ching for Everyone* (New York: Barnes & Noble, 1994).

[48] Yehuda Berg, *The 72 Names of God: Technology for the Soul* (New York: The Kabbalah Center, 2004).

[49] Gordon Stokes and Daniel Whiteside, *Body Circuits, Pain and Understanding* (Carson City, NV: Thoth, 1990), 17.

[50] Jeff Harris, "Relationship of the 5 Elements and Polar Meridians," *Institute of Energy Medicine*, www.edenenergymedicine.com/relationship-of-the-5-elements-and-polar-meridians/ (accessed February 25, 2013).

[51] Tiller, *Science and Human Transformation*, 117.

[52] Richard Gerber, *Vibrational Medicine for the 21st Century* (New York: HarperCollins, 2001), 176.

[53] Iona Marsaa Teeguarden, *The Joy of Feeling: Bodymind Acupressure* (Tokyo/New York: Japan Publications, 1984), 158.

[54] Teeguarden, *The Joy of Feeling*, 106.

[55] Cyndi Dale, *New Chakra Healing: The Revolutionary 32-Center Energy System* (St. Paul, MN: Llewellyn, 1997), 117.

[56] Michio Kushi, *Oriental Diagnosis: What Your Face Reveals* (London: Sunwheel Publications, 1978), ix.

[57] Kushi, *Oriental Diagnosis*, ix.

[58] Kushi, x.

[59] Kushi, xi.

[60] Stokes and Whiteside, *Body Circuits,* 80-84.

[61] Tiller, *Science and Human Transformation*, 117.

[62] George Goodheart, "Overview and Update of the Bennett Neurovascular Reflexes," International College of Applied Kinesiology, 1999, https://www.icakusa.com/sites/default/files/Overview%20and%20Update%20of%20the%20Bennett%20Neurovascualr%20Reflexes.pdf (accessed January 18, 2022).

[63] Megan Bath, Amanda Nguyen, and Bruno Bordoni, "Physiology, Chapman's Points," *National Library of Medicine*, May 8, 2022, https://www.ncbi.nlm.nih.gov/books/NBK558953/ (accessed January 18, 2023).

[64] Calleman, *The Purposeful Universe*, 14–15.

[65] Walter Wink, *Engaging the Powers* (Philadelphia: Fortress Press, 1992), 13.

[66] Ester and Jerry Hicks, *The Astonishing Power of Emotions* (Carlsbad, CA: Hay House, Inc. Publishing, 2007), 34.

[67] Pert, *Molecules of Emotion*, 307.

[68] Pert, *Molecules of Emotion,* 441.

[69] Pert, 141.

[70] Melody, *Love is in the Earth* (Wheat Ridge, CO: Love Publishing, 1998), 32.

[71] Gurudas, channeled through Kevin Ryerson, *Gem Elixirs and Vibrational Healing* (San Rafael, CA: Casandra Press, 1989), 1:3.

[72] Gurudas, *Gem Elixirs and Vibrational Healing*, 1:18.

[73] Gary Cone, *The Cone Center for Living in Choice Celestial Blends* (Oklahoma City: Cone Center, 2003), 5–15.

[74] See Appendix IX for the complete list of Celestial Blends.

[75] Julio Rocha do Amaral and Jorge Martins de Oliveira, "The Limbic System: The Center of Emotions," The Healing Center On-Line, www.healing-arts.org/n-r-limbic.htm (accessed May 28, 2002).

[76] *Rand McNally Atlas of the Body and Mind* (Chicago: Rand McNally Publisher, 1976), 119.

[77] Rocha do Amaral and Martins de Oliveira, "The Limbic System: The Center of Emotions."

[78] *Rand McNally Atlas of the Body and Mind*, 119.

[79] Tim Dalgleish, "The Emotional Brain," *Nature Reviews Neuroscience,* no. 5 (2004): 582–585.

[80] Rocha do Amaral and Martins de Oliveira, "The Limbic System: The Center of Emotions."

[81] David Bohm, *Wholeness and the Implicate Order* (Oxfordshire, England: Routledge, 1988).

[82] Edmond Bordeaux Szekely, *The Teachings of the Essenes from Enoch to the Dead Sea Scrolls* (San Diego: International Biogenic Society, 1999), 53.

[83] Gregg Braden, *Walking Between the Worlds: The Science of Compassion*, (Bellevue, WA: Radio Book Press, 1997), xiv.

[84] While not a part of the endocrine system, the liver plays an important role in that system's health and well-being.

[85] Bruce Fisher, *Man, Grand Reflection of the Great Cosmos,* 1:31.

[86] Teeguarden, *The Joy of Feeling*, 154.

[87] Teeguarden, 263.

[88] Teeguarden, 118.

[89] The Sal Goldman Pancreatic Research Center, http://pathology.jhu.edu/pc/BasicOverview3.php?area=ba (accessed February 20, 2013).

[90] Teeguarden, 199.

[91] Trebbe Johnson, "The Joy of the Maze," *Parabola Magazine* Vol. 17.2 (1994): 66–67.

[92] Drunvalo Melchizedek, *The Ancient Secret of the Flower of Life* (Flagstaff: Light Technology Publishing, 2000), 2:320.

[93] Shahriar Afshar, "Sharp complementary wave and wave particle behaviors in the same welcher weg experiment," July 2005, https://irims.org/quant-ph/030503/index.htm (accessed January 26, 2023).

[94] Jose Arguelles, *The Mayan Factor: Path Beyond Technology* (Santa Fe: Bear & Company, 1987), 120.

[95] Arguelles, *The Mayan Factor*, 122.

[96] Charles Breaux, *Journey into Consciousness: The Chakras, Tantra and Jungian Psychology* (York Beach, ME: Nicholas-Hays, Inc., 1989), 33.

[97] Barbara Brennan, *Hands of Light: A Guide to Healing Through the Human Energy Field* (New York: Bantam Books, 1987), 45–46.

[98] Brennan, *Hands of Light*, 72.

[99] Anodea Judith, *Wheels of Light* (St. Paul, MN: Llewellyn, 1998), 66.

[100] Caroline Myss, *Anatomy of the Spirit* (New York: Harmony Books, 1996), 80.

[101] Breaux, *Journey into Consciousness*, 80.

[102] Arthur E. Powell, *The Astral Body* (Wheaton, IL: Theosophical Publishing House, 1972), 32.

[103] Judith, *The Wheels of Light*, 120.

[104] Anodea Judith, *The Truth about Chakras* (St. Paul, MN: Llewellyn, 1998), 21.

[105] Carol Pearson, *The Hero Within* (San Francisco: Harper Collins, 1986), 3.

[106] Hawkins, *Power vs Force*, 126.

[107] Breaux, *Journey into Consciousness,* 84.

[108] Myss, *Anatomy of the Spirit, 192.*

[109] Breaux, *Journey into Consciousness*, 101.

[110] Judith, *Wheels of Life*, 193.

[111] Myss, *Anatomy of the Spirit*, 199.

[112] Judith, *Wheels of Life*, 205.

[113] Breaux, *Journey into Consciousness*, 106.

[114] Myss, *Anatomy of the Spirit*, 219.

[115] DeRohan, *The Right Use of Will*, 116.

[116] Judith, *Wheels of Life*, 243.

[117] Dale, *New Chakra Healing*, 121.

[118] Myss, *Anatomy of the Spirit*, 234.

[119] Hawkins, *Power vs Force*, 53.

[120] Myss, *Anatomy of the Spirit*, 234, 239.

[121] Judith, *Wheels of Life*, 304.

[122] Breaux, *Journey into Consciousness*, 197.

[123] Judith, *Wheels of Life*, 320.

[124] Breaux, *Journey into Consciousness*, 200.

[125] The ancient Maya had developed a complex writing system using over eight hundred hieroglyphs. Efforts to decipher this "code" have been going on for centuries, and scholars have made progress on about 90 percent of the symbols. They were used in the Maya's elaborate calendar system, which served a host of purposes, from marking civic and religious cycles to making astronomical calculations to tracking the passage of days, months, and years.

[126] Cyndi Dale, *The Subtle Body: An Encyclopedia of Your Energetic Anatomy* (Boulder: Sounds True, Inc., 2009), 298.

[127] Dale, *New Chakra Healing*, 21, 28.

[128] Jude Currivan, *The 8th Chakra* (Carlsbad, CA: Hay House Publishing, 2007), 108.

[129] Currivan, *The 8th Chakra*, 108.

[130] The ancient Greek philosopher Plato believed that the elements that make up our natural world fall into one of five shapes, each representing one of the five basic elements of earth, fire, water, air, and the universe.

[131] Currivan, *The 8th Chakra*, 109.

[132] Melchizedek, *The Flower of Life*, 2:361.

[133] *Wisdom's Door,* http://wisdomsdoor.com.

[134] Enochian is a language constructed by sixteenth-century English mathematician John Dee and his colleague Edward Kelly for the purposes of their investigations into otherworldly phenomenon.

[135] Dale, *New Chakra Healing*, 58–59.

[136] The Center of the Universal World Tree, according to esoteric traditions, is called the Central Sun.

[137] Carl Johan Calleman, *The Mayan Calendar and the Transformation of Consciousness* (Rochester, VT: Bear & Company, 2004), 104.

[138] *Ascension Glossary,* https://ascensionglossary.com/index.php/Main_Page.

[139] Franz Hartmann, *Paracelsus: Life and Prophecies* (Blauvelt, New York: Rudolph Steiner Publications, 1973), 30.

[140] Powell, *The Etheric Double,* 3.

[141] Michael Green, *Resonant Field Imaging: Technician's Manual for Scientific and Clinical Application* (Moscow: Institute of Technical Energy Medicine, Inc.,1999), xi.

[142] Walter Russell, *A Course in Cosmic Consciousness* (Vancouver: Contact Printing, 2001), 75.

[143] Powell, *The Etheric Double,* 75.

[144] Hartmann, *Paracelsus: Life and Prophecies*, 33.

[145] Powell, *The Astral Body*, 46.

[146] Powell, 47.

[147] Powell, 47.

[148] Dr. David Hawkins presents his findings in a video available on the Veritas Publishing website, https://veritaspub.com/product/drug-addiction-and-alcoholism/.

[149] Hartmann, *Paracelsus: Life and Prophecies*, 107.

[150] Carl Jung, *Analytical Psychology: Its Theory and Practice* (New York: Vintage Printing, 1968), 10.

[151] Lyall Watson, *Lifetide* (New York: Simon & Schuster, 1979), 147–148. Watson, who holds degrees in anthropology, biology, and zoology, among others, coined this phrase to describe a phenomenon he observed in his work with a group of monkeys in Japan. He theorized that it is possible for a behavior adopted by members in one group to rapidly spread by unexplained means to other groups, even those that are physically separated and have no apparent means of communicating with each other.

[110] Yasuhiko Genku Kimura, *The Twilight Manifesto* (Vancouver: The University of Science and Philosophy Press, 2000), 24.

[153] https://VXM.com/1.CompTheory.html.

[154] Powell, *The Mental Body*, 13.

[155] Powell, 7.

[156] Fisher, *Studies in Occult Anatomy*, 33.

[157] Russell, *A Course in Cosmic Consciousness*, 4.

[158] Russell, *A Course in Cosmic Consciousness*, 219.

[159] Powell, 139.

[160] Russell, *A Course in Cosmic Consciousness*, 16.

[161] A. E. Powell, *The Causal Body and the Ego* (London: Theosophical Publishing House, 1967), 1.

[162] Powell, *The Causal Body and the Ego*, 2.

[163] Sacred Wisdom Chart #12, Helion Publishing.

[164] Powell, *The Causal Body and the Ego*, 89.

[165] Powell, *The Causal Body and the Ego*, 108.

[166] Powell, *The Causal Body and the Ego*, 101.

[167] Calleman, *The Purposeful Universe*, 239.

[168] Calleman, 288.

[169] Calleman, 12.

[170] 250.

[171] 250.

[172] 261.

[173] Calleman, 262.

[174] 263.

[175] Calleman, 27.

[176] Gurudas, *Gem Elixirs and Vibrational Healing*, 1:3.

[177] Gurudas, 1:53.

[178] Aubrey Westlake, "Miasms," *Psionic Medicine* (Winter, 1969), 71-72.

[179] David V. Tansley, *Chakras: Rays and Radionics (Saffron Walden, Essex: C.W. Daniel Co. Ltd., 1972), 102.*

[180] Gurudas, 1:82.

[181] Gurudas, 1:83.

[182] Gurudas, 1:83.

[183] Gurudas, 1:83.

[184] Machaelle Small Wright, "Flower Essences: Reordering Our Understanding and Approach to Illness and Health," https://www.perelandra-ltd.com/Perelandra-Papers-C831.aspx (accessed February 6, 2023).

[185] Tansley, *Chakras: Rays and Radionics,* 103.

[186] David Little, "Miasms in Classical Homeopathy," 1996, http://simillimum.com/education/little-library/constitution-temperaments-and-miasms/mch/article.php.

[187] Tansley, *Chakras: Rays and Radionics*, 107.

[188] *Essential Oils Desk Reference,* (USA: Essential Science Publishing, 2000), 3.

[189] A subclass of terpenes (the chemical compounds found in plants that are responsible for aroma and flavor) that seem to have antimicrobial and anti-tumor properties.

[190] *Essential Oils Desk Reference,* 2.

[191] *Essential Oils Desk Reference,* 2.

[192] The Burton Goldberg Group, *Alternative Medicine: The Definitive Guide* (USA: Future Medicine Publishing, Inc. 1997), 54.

[193] Stokes and Whiteside, *Body Circuits,* 81.

[194] Karol Kuhn Truman, *Feelings Buried Alive Never Die* (USA: Olympus Publishing Company, 1991).

[195] Michael Lincoln, *Messages from the Body*: *Their Psychological Meaning.* USA: Talking Hearts, 2019).

[196] Stokes and Whiteside, *Body Circuits*, 81.

[197] Robert and Kerri Broe, *Advanced Medical Awareness* (Aripeka, FL: Tuberose Publishing, 1997), 151.

[198] Fisher, *Man, Grand Reflection of the Great Cosmos*, 1:123.

[199] Carl Jung, *The Archetypes and the Collective Unconscious* (Princeton: Princeton University Press, 1968), 2.

[200] Jung, *The Archetypes and The Collective* Unconscious, 4.

[201] Jung, 1.

[202] Jung, 5.

[203] Jung, 30.

[204] Jung, 39.

[205] Gary Cone, "Living in Choice: A Workshop," (self-published, 2002).

[206] James M. Robinson, editor, *The Nag Hammadi Library: The Definitive Translation of the Gnostic Scriptures Complete in One Volume* (San Francisco: HarperOne, 1990), 277.

[207] Ernest Holmes, *The Science of Mind* (New York: G.P. Putnam's Sons, 1998), 151.

[208] Braden, *Walking Between the Worlds*, 128.

[209] Helen Schucman and William Thetford, *A Course in Miracles*, (New York: Viking: The Foundation for Inner Peace, 1976).

[210] Gary Renard, *Disappearance of the Universe: Straight Talk about Illusions, Past Lives, Religion, Sex, Politics, and the Miracles of Forgiveness* (Napa, CA: Fearless Books, 2003), 171.

[211] Renard, *The Disappearance of the Universe,* 199.

[212] Caroline Myss, *Vision, Creativity & Intuition: Part II Sacred Contracts* (St. Louis: self-published, 1998), 1.

[213] Seabrook, *I Ching for Everyone*, 32.

[214] Richard Rudd, *The Gene Keys* (London: Watkins Publishing, 2015), xiii.

[215] Siddhi is the name ancient Hindus gave to the spiritual gifts that come with enlightenment.

[216] DeRohan, *Right Use of Will*, vi.

[217] Gentry, *Miracles of the Mind*, 169.

[218] Fisher, *Man, Grand Reflection of the Great Cosmos*, 1:10.

[219] Charles Ponce, *Kabbalah: An Introduction and Illumination for the World Today* (Wheaton, IL: Quest Books, 1973), 101.

[220] Fisher, *Man, Grand Reflection of the Greater Cosmos*, 2:45.

[221] Fisher, 2:45.

[222] Dale, *New Chakra Healing,* 227.

[223] Dale, 229.

[224] Fisher, 2:45.

[225] Fisher, 2:45.

[226] Dale, 217.

[227] http://www.spineuniverse.com.

[228] Tansley, 20.

[229] Tansley, 20.

[230] Alice Bailey, *The Seven Rays of Life* (New York: Lucis Publishing Company, 2003), 1.

[231] Alice Bailey, *Esoteric Psychology Volume I: A Treatise on the Seven Rays* (New York: Lucis Publishing Company, 2002), 141–143.

[232] Bailey, *The Seven Rays of Life*, 3.

[233] Tansley, 32.

[234] Tansley, 33.

[235] Tansley, 37.

[236] Tansley, 42.

[237] Fisher, *Man, Grand Reflection of the Great Cosmos*, 2:21.

[238] Fisher, *Man, Grand Reflection of the Great Cosmos*, 2:22.

[239] Gordon Stokes and Daniel Whiteside, *Structural Neurology* (Burbank: Three In One Concepts, Inc., revised edition 1999), 30.

[240] Ibrahim Karim, *Back to a Future for Mankind: BioGeometry* (Amazon Publishing: CreateSpace, 2010) p. 112.

[241] Don Riso and Russ Hudson, *The Wisdom of the Enneagram* (New York: Bantam Books, 1999), 151. The Enneagram is a geometric figure that maps out the nine fundamental personality types of human nature.

[242] Jamie Sams and David Carson, *Medicine Cards*: *The Discovery of Power Through the Ways of Animals* (New York: St. Martin's Press, 1999).